Ringworm and Irradiation

Ringworm and Irradiation

The Historical, Medical, and Legal Implications of the Forgotten Epidemic

EDITED BY SHIFRA SHVARTS, PHD

PROFESSOR (EMERITA)
MOSHE PRYWES CENTER FOR MEDICAL EDUCATION,
FACULTY OF HEALTH SCIENCES, BEN-GURION
UNIVERSITY OF THE NEGEV, ISRAEL

SIEGAL SADETZKI-JACKOBSON, MD-MPH

MINISTRY OF HEALTH; THE GERTNER INSTITUTE FOR
EPIDEMIOLOGY & HEALTH POLICY RESEARCH; SACKLER
FACULTY OF MEDICINE, TEL AVIV UNIVERSITY, ISRAEL

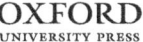

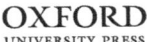

Oxford University Press is a department of the University of Oxford. It furthers
the University's objective of excellence in research, scholarship, and education
by publishing worldwide. Oxford is a registered trade mark of Oxford University
Press in the UK and certain other countries.

Published in the United States of America by Oxford University Press
198 Madison Avenue, New York, NY 10016, United States of America.

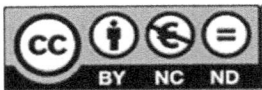

© Oxford University Press 2022

Some rights reserved. This is an open access publication, available online and distributed under the
terms of the Creative Commons Attribution-Non Commercial-No Derivatives 4.0 International
licence (CC BY-NC-ND 4.0), a copy of which is available at http://creativecommons.org/licenses/
by-nc-nd/4.0/. Enquiries concerning use outside the scope of the licence terms should be sent to the
Rights Department, Oxford University Press.

Library of Congress Cataloging-in-Publication Data
Names: Shvarts, Shifra, editor. | Sadetzki-Jackobson, Siegal, editor.
Title: Ringworm and irradiation : the historical, medical, and
legal implications of the forgotten epidemic /
[edited by] Shifra Shvarts, Siegal Sadetzki-Jackobson.
Description: New York, NY : Oxford University Press, 2022. |
Includes bibliographical references and index.
Identifiers: LCCN 2021046182 (print) | LCCN 2021046183 (ebook) |
ISBN 9780197568965 (paperback) | ISBN 9780197568989 (epub) |
ISBN 9780197568996 (online)
Subjects: MESH: Tinea Capitis—history | Tinea Capitis—radiotherapy |
Radiation Effects | History, 20th Century
Classification: LCC RL780 (print) | LCC RL780 (ebook) | NLM WR 11.1 |
DDC 616.5/79—dc23
LC record available at https://lccn.loc.gov/2021046182
LC ebook record available at https://lccn.loc.gov/2021046183

DOI: 10.1093/med/9780197568965.001.0001

This material is not intended to be, and should not be considered, a substitute for medical or other
professional advice. Treatment for the conditions described in this material is highly dependent on
the individual circumstances. And, while this material is designed to offer accurate information with
respect to the subject matter covered and to be current as of the time it was written, research and
knowledge about medical and health issues is constantly evolving and dose schedules for medications
are being revised continually, with new side effects recognized and accounted for regularly. Readers
must therefore always check the product information and clinical procedures with the most up-to-date
published product information and data sheets provided by the manufacturers and the most recent
codes of conduct and safety regulation. The publisher and the authors make no representations or
warranties to readers, express or implied, as to the accuracy or completeness of this material. Without
limiting the foregoing, the publisher and the authors make no representations or warranties as to the
accuracy or efficacy of the drug dosages mentioned in the material. The authors and the publisher do
not accept, and expressly disclaim, any responsibility for any liability, loss, or risk that may be claimed
or incurred as a consequence of the use and/or application of any of the contents of this material.

The manufacturer's authorised representative in the EU for product safety is Oxford University Press
España S.A. of El Parque Empresarial San Fernando de Henares, Avenida de Castilla, 2 – 28830
Madrid (www.oup.es/en or product.safety@oup.com). OUP España S.A. also acts as importer into
Spain of products made by the manufacturer.

CONTENTS

Acknowledgement vii
Contributors ix
Introduction xi

1. Ringworm of the scalp: the history of an ancient disease 1
   Ciro Bursztein

2. Radiation epilation for tinea capitis: scientific and historical aspects 11
   M. Raphael Pfeffer

3. The ringworm children at the Hôpital Saint-Louis, Paris: from medical neglect to biosocial obsession 31
   Gérard Tilles

4. Ringworm: a disease of schools and mass schooling in the United Kingdom 77
   Aya Homei and Michael Worboys

5. The JDC-Joint and OSE campaign for eradication of ringworm in the Jewish communities in Eastern Europe and North Africa 115
   Shifra Shvarts, Pnina Romem, Itzhak Romem, and Mordechai Shani

6. The ringworm campaign in Serbia (former Yugoslavia) in the 1950s 163
   Shifra Shvarts, Goran Sevo, Marija Tasic, Mordechai Shani, and Siegal Sadetzki-Jackobson

7. The ringworm campaign in Portugal, 1940–1970: historical review and present evaluation of x-ray–epilated individuals 181
   Paula Boaventura, Dina Pereira, Paula Soares, and José Teixeira-Gomes

8. "Deadly Medicine": Michael Reese Hospital's Pandora's box and the campaign to warn the public of the late health effects of ionizing radiation in the United States 215
   Itai Bavli and Shifra Shvarts

9. Healing the children and the nation: the campaign to eradicate ringworm in Israel, 1925–1960 245
   Shifra Shvarts, Aya Bar Oz, Eli Shachar, Sari Levi, Sigal Samchi, and Itai Bavli

10. "Think before you act": ringworm research in Israel, 1965–1995 293
    Siegal Sadetzki-Jackobson

11. The muted voices of the ringworm patients and their families worldwide 331
    Liat Hoffer

Index 353

ACKNOWLEDGEMENT

We would like to thank the Gertner Institute—the Sheba Medical Center and the Ben Gurion University, Israel for supporting the publication of this book.

CONTRIBUTORS

Itai Bavli, PhD
Department of the History of Science
Harvard University
Cambridge, Massachusetts, USA
and
The University of British Columbia
Vancouver, BC, Canada

Paula Boaventura, PhD
IPATIMUP-Institute of Molecular Pathology and Immunology of the University of Porto, Porto, Portugal
i3S—Instituto de Investigação e Inovação em Saúde
Porto, Portugal

Ciro Bursztein, MSc, MA
Biovac Pharmacueticals LTD
Or-Akiva, Israel

José Teixeira-Gomes, MD-PhD
IPATIMUP-Institute of Molecular Pathology and Immunology of the University of Porto
i3S—Instituto de Investigação e Inovação em Saúde
Porto, Portugal

Liat Hoffer, PhD
Faculty of Health Sciences, Ben-Gurion University of the Negev
Beer-Sheva, Israel

Aya Homei, PhD
Japanese Studies, Modern Languages and Cultures
University of Manchester
Manchester, GB, UK

Sari Levi, MA
Ministry of Health, Sheba Medical Center
Ramat Gan, Israel

Aya Bar-Oz, MA
University of Toronto
Toronto, ON, Canada

Dina Pereira, PhD
Center for Neuroscience and Cell Biology
Coimbra, Portugal

Raphael Pfeffer, MBBS
Assuta Medical Center
Tel Aviv, Israel

Itzhak Romem, MD
Soroka Medical Center
Beer Sheva, Israel

Pnina Romem, PhD
Faculty of Health Sciences, Ben Gurion University
Beer Sheva, Israel

Siegal Sadetzki-Jackobson, MD-MPH
Ministry of Health; The Gertner Institute for Epidemiology & Health Policy Research; Sackler Faculty of Medicine, Tel Aviv University
Tel Aviv, Israel

Sigal Samchi, MA
Ministry of Health
Ramat Gan, Israel

Goran Sevo, MD, PhD, Epidemiologist
Institute for Geriatrics and Palliative Care
Belgrade, Serbia

Eli Shachar
Ministry of Health
Ramat Gan, Israel

Mordechai Shani, MD
The Sheba Medical Center and the Sackler Faculty of Medicine, Tel Aviv University
Tel Aviv, Israel

Shifra Shvarts, PhD
Moshe Prywes Center for Medical Education, Faculty of Health Sciences, Ben Gurion University of the Negev
Beer Sheva, Israel

Paula Soares, PhD
IPATIMUP-Institute of Molecular Pathology and Immunology of the University of Porto
i3S—Instituto de Investigação e Inovação em Saúde
Porto, Portugal

Marija Tasic, Prim. Mr Sc, MD
Institute for Geriatrics and Palliative Care
Belgrade, Serbia

Gérard Tilles, MD, PhD
Hôpital Saint Louis
Paris, France

Michael Worboys, DPhil
Centre for the History of Science, Technology and Medicine (CHSTM)
University of Manchester
Manchester, GB, UK

INTRODUCTION

In July 1973, a study at the University of Chicago linked radiation treatment in childhood to a variety of diseases, including thyroid cancer. A few months later, a worker at Michael Reese Hospital in Chicago found a registry of 5,266 former patients treated with radiation during the 1950s and 1960s. Hospital officials decided to contact these patients and arrange for follow-up medical examinations. Media coverage of Reese's campaign had a snowball effect, prompting more medical institutions to follow suit and the National Cancer Institute (NCI) to launch a nationwide campaign warning the medical community and public about the late effects of ionizing radiation.

The practice of using x-rays for the medical treatment of benign diseases began in the 1920s and peaked in the 1940s and 1950s. Radiation therapy was considered good medical practice and was very effective at eliminating ringworm, often with immediate results. X-ray treatment gradually came to an end in the 1960s when other effective treatments were developed (e.g., griseofulvin for ringworm) and studies started to suggest that benign and malignant tumors of the thyroid gland, as well as leukemia, were detected in individuals who had been exposed to radiation treatment during childhood.

In the United States, tens of thousands of children were treated with radiation therapy for ringworm of the scalp. In Yugoslavia, a UNICEF-assisted campaign to eliminate ringworm resulted in the treatment of approximately 50,000 children with radiation. In Portugal, health authorities treated approximately 30,000 children with scalp ringworm using radiation, and tens of thousands in France, the United Kingdom, Canada, Australia, North Africa (mainly Morocco), and the Middle East underwent similar treatments. In Israel, approximately 31,000 children with ringworm were treated with radiation.

This volume on ringworm, the use of irradiation in its treatment, and the latent health risks discovered decades later is not simply a medical history. Rather, it offers a learning experience still relevant to the practice of medicine today concerning the introduction of *any* new medical technology that provides immediate relief but carries potential long-term risks to the patient and the public. From a public policy standpoint, irradiation of ringworm constitutes a case study yielding insights into both the possible consequences of a well-intended practice that was hastily adopted and poorly executed, and how these consequences have been addressed—country by country—after discovery of the latent health risks patients face.

1

Ringworm of the scalp

The history of an ancient disease

CIRO BURSZTEIN

INTRODUCTION

This chapter will describe different aspects of the classification, categorization, and treatment of ringworm of the scalp from ancient times until the beginning of the use of x-rays for the cure of the disease in 1897. In addition, some of the key figures in different scientific fields who played an important role in the research of the disease over the centuries will be presented, along with some of their most important publications on the subject.

The history of tinea capitis can be divided into three eras:

1. From ancient times until the introduction of modern medical science in the 17th century (which in my opinion is characterized by the invention of the microscope)
2. From the 17th century until 1897 with the introduction of Roentgen rays (x-rays) for the cure of the disease
3. From 1897 until today.

The second era may also be divided into various sub-eras, according to the key figures who played a very important role in the research of the disease (e.g., David Gruby, Raymond Sabouraud). This chapter will describe the first and second eras, focusing on the second one, since most of the scientific progress in the research of tinea capitis was achieved during it.

Ringworm of the scalp (tinea capitis) is a fungal infectious disease that attacks the hair and scalp of humans. It produces localized alopecia, scaling, reddening, and crusting of the scalp. It can also lead to secondary microbial infections. The disease varies from a benign scaly, noninflamed, subclinical colonization to an inflammatory disease characterized by the production of scaly erythematous lesions and by alopecia that may become severely inflamed. It is very contagious and widespread in crowded and dirty places.[1]

THE FIRST ERA

The earliest mentions of tinea capitis and other mycoses go back many centuries and even millennia ago. The biblical disease of leprosy (*tzara'at*) may well have been confused with mycotic infection of the scalp and/or body.[2,3] Fungal diseases has been confirmed in Egyptian mummies by DNA analysis. According to the Ebers Papyrus, one of the most ancient medical documents (c. 1550 B.C.), skin, hair, and nail mycoses may have been treated by henna (known as *kupros* or *cyperus*).[4] Hippocrates first documented oral pseudomembranous candidosis with the name *aphthae albae*, a finding that was corroborated by Clarissimus Galen[5] (Galen [130–200 A.D] lived in the Roman Empire and was a well-known Greek physician[6]). Aulus Cornelius Celsus, in his encyclopedic *De medicina*, was the first to describe favus, which he did in the first century A.D. (Celsus [25 B.C.–50 A.D.] lived in Rome and was one of the greatest Roman medical writers[7]). He referred to cutaneous fungal disease as *porrigo* ("to spread" in Latin).[8]

Cassius Felix is thought to be the first to use the term *tinea*, which he did in about the year 400 A.D. in his summary of medicine[9] (Felix, a fifth-century physician from Cirta, Numidia, wrote a treatise called *De medicina*[10]). The word *tinea*, which was used to describe the tenacity of the disease, is found in the writings of Etienne of Antioch, who translated the work of Haly-Abbas[11] (Haly-Abbas [925–994] was a Persian physician and psychologist most famous for the *Kitab al-Maliki* ["Complete Book of the Medical Art"], his textbook on medicine and psychology[12]). Guy de Chauliac adopted this term and identified five types of tinea: tinea favosa, tinea ficosa, tinea amedosa, tinea uberosa, and tinea lupinosa (de Chauliac [1300–1368] lived in France and was the most eminent surgeon of the European Middle Ages. His *Chirurgia Magna* [1363] was a standard work on surgery until at least the 17th century[13]). This classification of the disease remained valid until the beginning of the 19th century and was even adopted by Jean-Louis Alibert, who represented the old tradition in French medicine[14] (Alibert [1768–1837] was the pioneer of French dermatology[15]). Physicians in the Renaissance era, like Hieronymus Mercurialis, used the term *tinea* or *teigne* to describe all diseases of the scalp[16] (Mercurialis [1530–1606] was an Italian philologist and physician, most famous for his work *De arte gymnastica*[17]).

Since Roman times, the literature has presented different kinds of remedies. Aulus Celsus anointed infected areas of the scalp with honey and *shumach*.[18] Gaius Plinius Secundus (23–79 A.D), a Roman author, naturalist, and natural philosopher, described in his publication *Historia naturalis* his treatment for tinea capitis, which included the use of goat's gall with Cimolian chalk and vinegar.[19] During the Middle Ages the treatment of choice for ringworm of the scalp was the use of a variety of ointments such as bell grease, celandine leaves, and soft creamy juice expressed from a houseleek, which were rubbed into the ringworm lesion.[20] Irritating ointment was also used in order to cause an artificial inflammation of the scalp, resulting in the falling out of the diseased hair in the inflamed area. These ointments were applied for months and even years with a low rate of success and in some cases led to serious sequelae.

Another method to treat the disease was the epilation of the scalp by using the *calotte* (skullcap) or *capellus piceus*. The calotte was a kind of helmet applied to the scalp with an adhesive ointment. It was left in place for 2 to 3 days and then forcibly removed. The logic of this treatment was to pluck out any diseased hair. It was followed by manual epilation of the remaining hair using tweezers or forceps. Needless to say, healthy hair was also removed, and this was a very painful and cruel method for treating the disease.

The use of forceps and tweezers for the epilation of the diseased hair was much more effective and much gentler than epilation with the calotte, and it replaced the latter in the beginning of the 19th century. This technique had been described by Mercurialis back in 1577.[21] The calotte was used much more commonly in France than in other parts of Europe.

Tinea capitis was not only described in the medical literature but was also presented in the arts. It is shown in some artworks by famous painters from the end of the Middle Ages (Figure 1.1).[22]

THE SECOND ERA

The greatest advances in the research of tinea capitis took place during the second era, especially in the 18th century, when we encounter many key figures who played a very important role in the research of the disease (e.g., David Gruby, Raymond Sabouraud, Johann Lukas Schöenlein, Samuel Plumbe, the Mahon brothers, Robert Remak, Daniel Turner, Robert Willan, Thomas Bateman). This section of the chapter will describe their work, their contributions to the research of the disease, some of their most important publications, and of course the advances made until the end of this era.

There is no exact date to the end of the first era and the beginning of the second one. It is possible to base this division on some processes and inventions that took place in Europe that greatly contributed to the development of science, such as the Renaissance, the Age of Enlightenment, the invention and subsequent refinement of the microscope, and many others. All this processes greatly contributed to the transition from the superstition-based "science" of the Middle Ages to a more

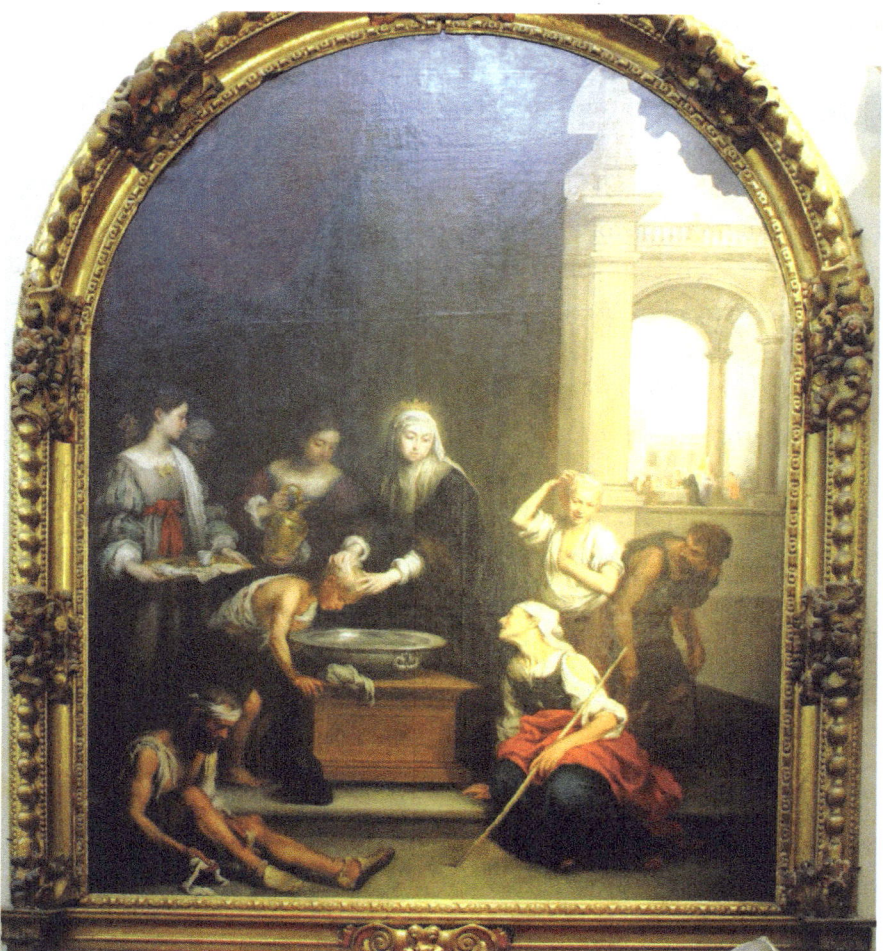

Figure 1.1 "Santa Isabela Reina de Hungria Curando a los Enfermos" by Bartolome Esteban Murillo (1617–1682), a Baroque painter from Seville. This 1672 painting illustrates Saint Elizabeth, daughter of Andrew II of Hungary, curing children infected with ringworm in the 13th century. The child near the pail has typical manifestations of ringworm.
Courtesy of the Hospital of Santa Caridad in Seville.

observation-based and rational science of the second era that greatly benefited the research of all fields of science.

In the second era, the research of tinea capitis, as well as other fields of cutaneous diseases and mycology, was mainly focused in England, France, and the German-speaking territories. The United States was somewhat of a latecomer to this field.

Skin diseases were not presented as a dedicated medical area until Mercurialis's *De morbis cutaneis* ("Diseases of the Skin") was published in 1572. Mercurialis classified skin disorders into two groups: ones involving the head and ones involving the rest of the body. The ninth chapter, on cephalic dermatoses, is called "Achores and Favus." *Achores* is a term close to tinea or to head ulcerations and was used to designate oozing cephalic dermatoses that were common in children.[23] The Englishman Daniel Turner's (1667–1741) *De Morbis Cutaneis: A Treatise of Disease Incident to the Skin*, published in 1714, was the first full book in English dedicated to the subject of skin diseases.[24] Later he described his treatment of the disease: "bleeding and general purgation . . . Pulling them [the hair] up by the roots with fine nippers, or drawing them up all at once by a Pitch or other plaster."[25] In *A Treatise of Disease Incident to the Skin*, he described the origin of the term *tinea*: It derived from Latin and describes the little holes visible in the scalp. It is also the name of a moth worm, and the damage the worm causes to fabrics resembles the damage seen on the scalp of the afflicted. Turner continued to describe the physiologic appearance of the disease on the scalp. Later on he proposed some remedies for the disease, including bleeding and repeat purgation. If there were dry scabs, he suggested, then it was possible to begin with local application of a different ointment. However, in order to do that, the hair must be removed (if it interferes with the use of the different remedies) by being pulled out with "fine nippers" or pitch (see the earlier discussion of the calotte). Turner warned of possible side effects of the epilation, such as fever and pain. Some of the ointments suggested by Turner are butter hog's lard covered with a cap made of hog's bladder, beeswax, oleum, calomel, and more.

Turner described an interesting incident in which he was asked to treat a 10-month-old baby suffering from ulcers upon the hairy scalp secreting some fluids (probably caused by some kind of tinea). Turner purged the baby with syrup of chicory twice a week. Between the treatments he rubbed the baby's head with 2 to 3 grains of calomel overnight. He clipped the baby's hair and attached leeches behind his ears. After that, the scalp was rubbed overnight with balfanum sulfur and a cap of hog's bladder was put over it. Turner reported that after a short time, the ulcers began to dry up and the baby's situation was improved; he did not reveal the exact time it took for the baby to recover.[26]

Alibert adopted de Chauliac's earlier classification of the different strains of tinea capitis. Later on, however, he made a serious mistake. Up to that time, tinea lupinosa represented the modern classification of favus, and the term *favus* indicated our modern classification of impetigo. Alibert abandoned (teigne) tinea lupinosa and called it *favus*. For this reason, our modern favus was given its name.[27] Alibert used the term *favus* to describe the honey-like exudate in some scalp infections.

In England, Robert Willan (1757–1812) and Thomas Bateman (the founder of modern British dermatology) renamed teignes as *porrigo* and classified them into six subcategories: porrigo lupinosa, porrigo scutulata (*teigne tondante* or scalp ringworm), porrigo larvalis (impetiginous eczema), porrigo furfurans (pityriasis capitis), porrigo decalvans (*la pelade* or alopecia areata), and porrigo favosa (impetigo contagiosa).[28] However, the mycologic origin of the disease remained unknown, and Bateman explained it as a spontaneous disease of the feeble-minded and malnourished: "to originate spontaneously in children of feeble and flabby habits, or in a state approaching marasmus, who are ill fed, uncleanly and not sufficiently exercised."[29] Bateman and Willan also described the features of tinea capitis: "appears in ... patches ... upon the scalp ... with clusters of small light yellow pustules ... which become thick and hard ... As the patches extend, the hair covering them becomes lighter in its color and sometimes breaks off short."[30,31]

It would take another 30 years for the parasitic origin of tinea capitis to be discovered by Gruby, Schönlein, and Remak (Figure 1.2). This turning point in the research of tinea capitis will be described extensively in this chapter.

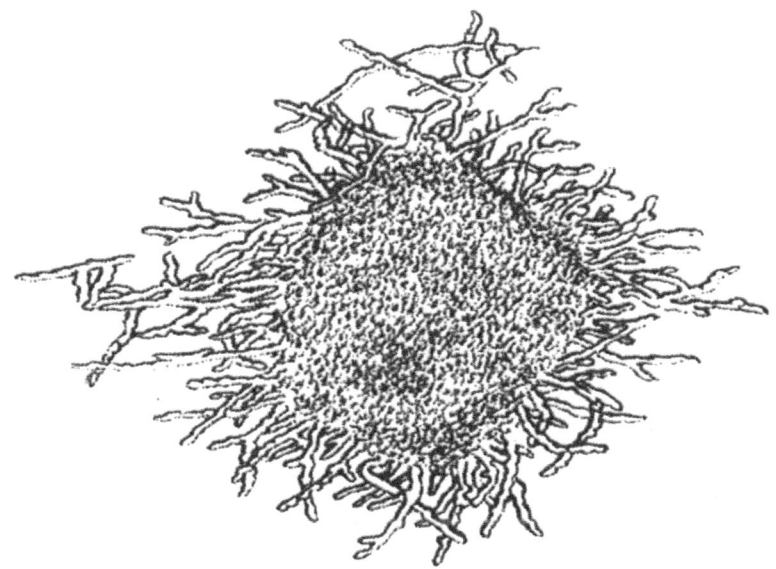

Figure 1.2 Schönlein's illustration depicting a ringworm infection as observed under a microscope lens
Archiu fiir Anatomie, Physiologie und wissenschaftliche Medicin@, 1839, p. 82.

NOTES

1. Rippon JW. *Medical Mycology: Pathogenic Fungi and the Pathogenic Actinomycetes* (2nd ed.). W.B.Saunders Co; 1982:169–177.
2. Marks RS. Dermatophytes in art. *J Med Vet Mycol.* 1991;29:1–8.
3. Ilkit M. Favus of the scalp: An overview and update. *Mycopathologia.* 2010;170:143–154.
4. Skellet AM, Levell N. Less work and good beer: An historical review of fungus of the skin. Norfolk University Hospital from the British Association of Dermatologists website, http://www.bad.org.uk/shared/get-ile.ashx?itemtype=document&id=1402
5. Negroni R. Historical aspects of dermatomycoses. *Clin Dermatol.* 2010;28:125–132.
6. Clarissimus Galen (130–200). *JAMA.* 1964;188:604–606. https://jamanetwork.com/journals/jama/article-abstract/1162991
7. *Encyclopedia Britannica*, web edition. https://www.britannica.com/biography/Aulus-Cornelius-Celsus.
8. Skellet and Levell.
9. Rosenthal T. Perspectives in ringworm of the scalp. *Arch Dermatol.* 1960;82:851–856.
10. Cameron ML. *Anglo-Saxon Medicine* (Cambridge Studies in Anglo-Saxon England). New York: Cambridge University Press; 1993:7.
11. Dochoa A. Consideraciones epidemiologicas y terapeuticas sobre las tinas. *Med Colonial.* 1947;9:431–448.
12. Browne EG. *Islamic Medicine.* New York: Goodword Books; 2001:53–54.

13. *Encyclopedia Britannica*, web edition. https://www.britannica.com/biography/Aulus-Cornelius-Celsus.
14. Rosenthal, 1960.
15. Everett MA. Jean-Louis Alibert: The father of French dermatology. *Int J Dermatol.* 1984;23:351–356.
16. Gupta AK, Summerbell RC. Tinea capitis. *Med Mycol.* 2000;38:255–287.
17. Ruhrah J. Hieronymus Mercurialis, 1530–1606. *Am J Dis Child.* 1928;36:819–821.
18. Skellet and Levell.
19. Pliny. *Historia naturalis*, Book XXVII, Chapter 47.
20. Marks, 1991.
21. Rosenthal, 1960.
22. Marks, 1991.
23. Bermann KC, Ring J. *History of Allergy.* Chem Immunol Allergy. Basel, Karger; 2014:83.
24. Royal College of Physicians of the United Kingdom. https://rcp.soutron.net/Portal/Default/en-GB/RecordView/Index/80775.
25. Turner D. *De morbis cutaneis: A Treatise of Diseases Incident to the Skin* (2nd ed.). J. Walthoe, R. Wilkin, J. and J. Bonwicke, S. Birt, T. Ward and E. Wicksteed, London; 1723:217.
26. Turner D. *De morbis cutaneis: A Treatise of Diseases Incident to the Skin* (4th ed.). J. Walthoe, R. Wilkin, J. and J. Bonwicke, S. Birt, T. Ward and E. Wicksteed; 1731, Part II, Chapter II.
27. Rosenthal, 1960.
28. Gupta & Summerbell, 2000.
29. Bateman T. *A Practical Synopsis of Cutaneous Diseases According to the Arrangement of Dr. Willan.* (2nd ed.). London: Longman; 1813:169.
30. Bateman, 1813.
31. Skellet & Levell.

2

Radiation epilation for tinea capitis

Scientific and historical aspects

M. RAPHAEL PFEFFER

INTRODUCTION

In November 1895 Conrad Roentgen experimented with a cathode-ray tube and covered the tube with a black shield. He noticed that despite the shield, some crystals nearby fluoresced. Roentgen realized that the tube produced invisible rays that were capable of passing through the black shield. He called them *x-rays*. The news of Roentgen's discovery rapidly spread around the world. The Crooke's cold cathode tube that Roentgen used to produce x-rays was widely available. Within months x-rays were being used to diagnose trauma and to locate foreign objects in the body. Several experimenters noted skin irritation and hair loss following the use of diagnostic x-rays and suggested the potential therapeutic use of x-rays.[1,2] Radiation was soon shown to be useful in the treatment of several benign skin disorders, including eczema, acne, and lupus. In March 1896 John Daniel at Vanderbilt University experimented on the dean of his university before attempting to use x-rays to locate a bullet in a child's skull. A 2-inch-diameter tube was held a half-inch from his hair for 1 hour; the outcome was a 2-inch circle of alopecia on the dean's head.[3] In October 1896 Freund in Vienna used radiation to successfully epilate a large hairy nevus covering the entire back of a 5-year-old girl.[4,5]

Radiation epilation became the recommended treatment of ringworm wherever the necessary equipment and expertise were available. Over the following 60 years hundreds of thousands of children with ringworm were successfully treated worldwide. I will review here some of the historical and scientific aspects of radiation epilation, together with the discovery of the long-term risk of such treatment and the development of radiation protection.

EARLY YEARS OF RADIATION

In the early years after Roentgen's discovery, the x-ray dose was measured by the degree of erythema on the operator's skin, later defined as erythema skin units (ESU). In 1907 Sabouraud and Noiré introduced x-ray–sensitive pastilles calibrated to the erythema dose. Placing the pastille on the patient's skin avoided the need to expose the operator's arm to the x-rays. The skin erythema dose remained in use until the 1930s, when ion chambers were adopted into regular use and consensus was reached on units of measurement of the quantity of x-rays. The quality of the x-rays (i.e., penetration into tissues) was defined by the half-value layer (HVL) concept, a crude but useful definition introduced in 1912. The HVL refers to the thickness of material placed in a beam that reduces the beam's intensity by 50%. Higher-energy (deeper-penetrating) x-rays have a thicker HVL. In 1913 Coolidge invented an x-ray tube with a tungsten filament in an absolute vacuum. This allowed the delivery of a steady stream of x-rays that could be calibrated to the depth of the hair follicles in order to produce epilation. Shanks summarized the development of the equipment and techniques used from 1922 to 1958. Over these years there were minor changes in technique and improvements in the stability of the machines, but the basic principles remained unchanged.[6]

It was noted early on that radiation of painful skin lesions and painful joints resulted in reduced swelling and pain relief in a wide range of benign skin conditions, including psoriasis, tuberculous ulcers, and lupus. X-rays were also used to treat to treat deeper-seated inflammations; for example, x-rays were used to treat tuberculous lymphadenitis until the successful development of appropriate antibiotics in the 1950s. In 1907 radiotherapy was reported to be effective to shrink enlarged thymus glands, which were thought to contribute to the risk of sudden infant death. Radiation for enlarged thymus glands in children was common practice in many countries, including the United States, until about 1950, around which time the increased risk of thyroid cancer in these irradiated children was first noted and this treatment was abandoned.[7]

The awareness of possible long-term sequelae of x-rays, especially in children, and the development of alternative medical treatments led to a reduction in the use of radiation therapy for benign diseases. Nevertheless, today radiation therapy is still sometimes recommended to treat benign diseases after judicious evaluation of the possible side effects and alternative treatments.[8] In several countries x-rays are prescribed to treat painful inflammatory conditions in adults.[9] Prospective randomized studies support the use of radiation to prevent painful heterotopic ossification after hip surgery.[10] High-dose radiotherapy may be recommended for some benign conditions in children, for example focal radiotherapy in children with low-grade or benign brain tumors situated at sites where surgery entails a high risk of neurologic deficit.[11] In the introduction to their textbook of radiation therapy in benign diseases, Order and Donaldson recommend:

> Consider radiation treatment if conventional methods of treatment have not succeeded in alleviating the condition, if the risk of other therapies is greater than the risk of radiation therapy, and if the potential consequences of no further treatment are unacceptable.[12]

RADIATION EPILATION

In the 19th century ringworm of the scalp reached epidemic proportions and was a major public health concern, resulting in thousands of children being removed and isolated from their homes for prolonged periods of time, at considerable expense to the health care system. In France several hospitals were dedicated to the inpatient treatment of tinea (see Chapter 3). There was no effective antiparasitic therapy, and treatment was based on removing the host site of the parasite in the base of the hair follicles. Mahon, in Paris, described the treatment of 39,719 patients with ringworm during a 20-year period from 1807 to 1828. Most were cured, but nevertheless he stated that epilation with forceps is almost as cruel as it is inefficient. Bulkley in New York in 1881[13] considered that epilation by forceps was impractical for the large numbers of patients seen in epidemics. Herbert Alder Smith, the resident physician of Christ's Hospital School in London, noted in 1897 that apart from epilation, "the treatment of extensive ringworm is still most unsatisfactory, the new remedies are no better than the old."[14] In 1896 Charles Allen in New York asked, regarding the spread of ringworm, "Should these cases be epilated?" He answered, "Yes, if it can be done with proper skill, care and intelligence, but to start to epilate several hundred children with ordinary hospital attendants is a task much worse than useless."[15] It is therefore clear that at the end of the 19th century tinea capitis was widespread in several countries, including France, England, and the United States, and there was a need for a more efficient and less painful method of epilation to treat ringworm and prevent its spread. As Sabouraud noted in his monograph on tinea in 1894, the only effective treatment for ringworm at this time was epilation achieved by manual removal of the hair of the entire scalp with tweezers combined with the application of wax or ointments. This was both time consuming and painful.[16]

Following his successful treatment of a girl with a hairy nevus, Freund together with Schiff in Vienna began using radiation to epilate children suffering from ringworm. Initially radiation epilation resulted in a high incidence of permanent alopecia, but within a few years the equipment and the technique of radiation required to produce epilation were refined. Sabouraud was appointed head of the ringworm school at Hôpital Saint-Louis in Paris in 1897. In 1904 he reported that 100 children with ringworm had been successfully treated with radiation epilation, with few cases of permanent alopecia. He noted that ringworm of the scalp was disappearing in France as a result of the new method of treatment, but in other countries, especially in England, the percentage of cases of permanent alopecia was too high.[17] The introduction of radiation epilation for ringworm had an important effect on health economics. Prior to the introduction of radiation epilation, around 300 children were hospitalized at Hôpital Saint-Louis at any one time; around 110 were cured each year, with an average stay of 27 months. Treatment involved prolonged hospitalization, and the cost to the city of each child treated was around 2,000 francs (around $400). After the introduction of radiation epilation, in 1 year 327 children were cured as outpatients at a cost of less than $1 each.[18] In 1906 a hospital building with 150 beds was returned to the Health Board, annually saving about 1.2 million francs. The provincial ringworm colonies in France were closed. Wherever the necessary equipment and expertise to deliver radiation epilation were available, children with ringworm could be treated with a high degree of success and minimal side effects, allowing them to return to school within weeks. Very few side effects were reported except for a small incidence of permanent alopecia. In England the introduction of radiation epilation allowed the health authorities to close one of two ringworm schools, and the remaining school was left with many vacancies.[19] By 1910 radiation epilation was offered at several of the major (private) hospitals in London. The authorities recommended establishing four public service ringworm centers, each with two treatment coils, in order to avoid a situation in which many children lost months or even years of schooling.[20] Initially children under 3 years of age were not offered radiation epilation, but by 1926 Macleod stated that there was enough experience to consider it safe to use radiation to treat even infants with ringworm.[21]

In the United States ringworm reached epidemic numbers in the 1940s.[22] The U.S. Army's x-ray manual in 1920 described the Kienböck–Adamson

(KA) technique for radiation epilation and noted under the heading "Favus" that "if this contagious disease should gain headway in the Army it would be necessary to treat each individual head with x-ray. There is no other satisfactory treatment, and with a reliable technique the result is certain."[23] Ira Kaplan, one of the pioneers of radiotherapy in the United States, noted in his textbook in 1937 that "because it (*tinea*) is contagious it always requires effective treatment. For this condition x-ray therapy is the method of choice, and when administered properly is not a dangerous procedure."[24] Tinea was considered a public health problem in many large cities in the United States and was considered practically impossible to cure without x-rays.[25] Steves and Lynch found epidemic numbers of children with ringworm in at least 61 cities.[26] They noted that the ringworm epidemic was much more severe in St. Paul, Minnesota, than in its twin city, Minneapolis. In St. Paul, where no radiation facilities were initially in place, only 25% of children were cured. In Minneapolis the epidemic began later than in St. Paul, and the health authorities had prepared adequate x-ray facilities to treat infected children before the epidemic spread. After the introduction of radiation epilation, the cure rate in St. Paul increased to 80%. In the United States many children were successfully treated with the K-A technique.[27] In Canada the increased incidence of ringworm was ascribed to immigration from Poland, and radiation epilation was the recommended treatment.[28]

Following an epidemic of ringworm in Northern Ireland, a specialized clinic with two x-ray machines was set up in the Royal Belfast Hospital. Over 500 children were treated with x-ray epilation, including infants aged 1 to 3 years, who were treated under anesthesia. To make the procedure more efficient they introduced a disc pressed on the scalp at a fixed distance from the x-ray tube. They noted that if pressure was applied to the skin to cause blanching, this area did not epilate.[29] The authors did not realize that this may be the first report of the reduced clinical effect of radiation in hypoxic conditions. A ringworm clinic was established in Morocco by the OSE (Oeuvre de Secours aux Enfants—children's aid society) a charitable organization. More than 9,000 children were treated with the KA technique in one session without side effects. The success rate improved from 60% in 1951, the first year of activity, to 88% in 1954. A systemic examination of 13,020 children examined between 1952 and 1954 who were studying in Jewish schools in Casablanca revealed 3,299 (25%) cases of ringworm. A similar group in a Muslim school showed a 35% incidence of ringworm. A further 500 families (mother and children over 15 years of age) of infected children were examined. Forty percent of the siblings and 13% of the mothers harbored ringworm. Following this campaign the incidence of ringworm at one school followed systematically was reduced from 39% in 1952 to 2.6% in 1954.[30] Similar clinics were established in several European countries, including Yugoslavia and Italy, as well as in North Africa and the Middle East and Australia.[31]

The importance of the problem of ringworm in Israel is shown by the fact that the Israel Society of Dermatology dedicated its inaugural conference in 1927 to the subject. Dostrovsky et al. reported a recurrence rate of 2.5% in a series of 5,904 children with ringworm treated with radiation epilation at Hadassah Hospital in Jerusalem.[32] They discussed the efforts of the national authorities in the fight against tinea capitis, including examining each child before entering kindergarten or school and examining new immigrants on disembarkation or arrival at transition camps, thereby preventing an epidemic of tinea capitis. Alternative treatments were tested in order to avoid radiation, particularly in infants. For example, treatment with systemic thallium was tried but was abandoned due to a high recurrence rate (47%) and toxicity.[33] A group of children in Tel Aviv was treated starting in 1956 with systemic potassium iodide,[34] but compliance was poor and the success rate was only 20%.[35] This study was published in 1961 in the same issue of *Harefuah*, the Israeli medical journal, that reported the successful treatment of ringworm with griseofulvin.[36] An accompanying editorial notes that the classical curative treatment of ringworm with radiation epilation requires a specialist doctor and team and expensive equipment and involves the risks of interfering with the anatomic and physiologic attributes of the skin, thereby placing a high level of responsibility on the medical institutes. The introduction of griseofulvin, the first effective antifungal treatment, removed the need for specialized personnel and equipment involved in the previous methods of cure.[37]

TECHNIQUES OF RADIATION EPILATION AND DOSIMETRY

Kienböck and Adamson improved on Sabouraud's technique and delivered a pastille dose to the center of each of five fields (anterior, posterior, opposing laterals, and vertex) at equidistant points on the scalp. In areas of the scalp where the fields overlapped, the overdose was reduced due to the increased distance between the x-ray source and the skin (SSD). The treatment was delivered in a single 90-minute session.[38] There were usually no permanent side effects to the skin, although there were sometimes areas of prolonged alopecia attributed to overlap between fields and different shapes of the skull. By the 1920s accurate calibration of the x-ray machine using ion chambers replaced the need for pastilles to measure the individual dose delivered to each patient, and studies showed that in places where the fields overlapped there could be an overdose of up to 80%. The success in treating thousands of children without permanent alopecia despite the dose inhomogeneity was attributed to the large margin of error between temporary and permanent epilation. There were attempts to modify the KA technique, such as the use of four or six rather than five fields or the use of a field rotating around the skull, but the KA technique remained the standard method of radiation epilation until the end of the 1950s, when epilation was replaced by medical treatment with griseofulvin. Cipollaro and Crossland, in the fifth edition of their textbook in 1967, reviewed the various techniques of radiation epilation and concluded that the KA method was more easily executed, produced a uniform epilation, and had stood the test of time. In 1967 they still recommended radiation epilation for cases of tinea capitis that did not respond to griseofulvin or in patients who could not tolerate the drug.

As noted, the standard KA technique for x-ray epilation was established early in the 1900s and the pastille was developed to calibrate the correct dose. After the development of stable x-ray machines and independent methods of measuring radiation, several authors published their protocols, all of which included a dose in the range of 300 to 400 Roentgens (R), with a dose energy chosen to penetrate to the depth of the hair follicles. Kaplan recommended an energy of 100 kilovolts (kv), an 8-inch (20-cm) SSD, and no filters.[39] He discussed the possible dangers associated with x-ray treatment of tinea (permanent alopecia and brain injury), but he noted that thousands of cases had been treated in the United States, France, and England without a single record of brain injury, either immediate or remote. Cipollaro had found that with an x-ray energy of 80 kv, which penetrates to an HVL of 0.5 mm aluminum, less than 5% of the dose reached the meninges.[40] Cipollaro and Crossland recommended a dose of 300 to 350 R in air to each focal point and cited other authorities who recommended a dose of 300 to 400 R. They noted that penetration of the x-rays below the bases of the hair follicles is undesirable and may cause nausea and vomiting; therefore, the HVL should not exceed 1 mm aluminum with an x-ray voltage between 60 and 100 kv without a filter (which removes less-penetrating, lower-energy rays).

Strauss and Kligman constructed a model of a scalp using a human skull and with a thimble chamber to measure the x-ray dose delivered with the KA method. They used 100-kv-energy x-rays with an HVL of 1.6 mm aluminum produced from a GE Coolidge tube model KX-10. They noted that under these conditions, around 65% of the dose reached the depth of the hair follicles (3 mm), and some 25% penetrated the skull.[41] With an SSD of 25 cm the maximum measured dose reached 223%, compared to a maximum of 198% with an SSD of 20 cm. They nevertheless recommended using an SSD of 25 cm to achieve greater uniformity. With a prescribed dose of 400 R using radiation of 1.6 mm aluminum HVL, the highest dose point in tissue was still below 1,000 R, less than the dose that would result in permanent alopecia. As noted earlier, there is a large margin between the dose needed for temporary alopecia and the dose causing permanent alopecia. Five children in their series developed post-irradiation headaches and severe nausea. The cerebrospinal fluid was examined in these children and normal cell counts and protein levels were found.

RADIATION PROTECTION

Up to the period of the Second World War, radiation-induced cancer was considered an occupational hazard from repeated exposure to radiation. The main emphasis of radiation safety was therefore on protecting the personnel involved in the use of radiation.[42] In April 1898 the Roentgen Society established a committee on x-ray injuries,[43] but no radiation protection standards were adopted until the 1920s. The basic requirements of radiation protection (limiting the area exposed, limiting the duration of radiation, and increasing the distance from the radiation source) were known within 10 years of Roentgen's discovery but were not fully implemented for another 50 years. In 1915 the British Roentgen Society was the first group to adopt x-ray protection standards, but these were not enforced. In 1922 the American Roentgen Ray Society, together with its British counterparts, issued formal recommendations, including limiting the exposure of personnel involved in radiation to 7 hours per day, 5 days per week, with 4 weeks of annual vacation. At the First International Congress of Radiology in 1925, a tolerance dose or recommended maximum exposure for personnel involved in x-rays was suggested. Sievert and others recommended a cumulative annual dose of one-tenth of the erythema dose. At the Second Congress in 1928, the International Advisory Committee on X-ray and Radium Protection (which later became the International Commission for Radiation Protection [ICRP]) was established, and the roentgen unit was adopted as a measure of radiation that could be independently measured with an ion chamber. The Congress recommended that exposure of workers should not exceed a cumulative dose limit, but there were no recommendations for patients exposed to diagnostic or therapeutic radiation.[44,45] In 1934 Mutscheller recommended that for low-energy radiation (which causes erythema), the limit should be 3.4 R per month, and for higher-energy x-rays (which penetrate deeper but cause less skin damage), the limit should be 7.5 R per month. It was believed that below these dose limits there was a negligible risk of radiation damage. These recommendations were adopted and became the first legally adopted limits. It is notable that at this time there was still more concern for the effect of radiation on the skin than for the effect of deeper radiation on internal organs, probably because almost all radiation-induced toxicities reported until this time involved the skin.

After the end of the Second World War and the use of nuclear weapons, the public's attitude toward radiation changed, and the topic of radiation protection began to receive significant notice. Around this time the carcinogenic risk of radiation to patients (as opposed to personnel who were repeatedly subjected to radiation over many years) began to be appreciated. It was realized that radiation could cause severe harm without visible signs and that even very small doses of radiation could be damaging. The tolerance dose (which was based on visible damage following repeated exposure) was replaced by a maximum permissible dose, and in 1954 the concept of "as low a dose as reasonably achievable" (ALARA) was introduced.

SIDE EFFECTS OF RADIATION FOR TINEA CAPITIS

In the early years it was thought that x-rays, which could not be seen, could not cause any harmful side effects. Temporary skin irritation and burns were noted, but this was often attributed to other causes, including static electricity, oxidation secondary to ozone or nitrous acid and idiosyncrasy, or to sparks from faulty machinery. As noted earlier, the dose of x-rays was measured by the amount of erythema seen on the operator's skin. Some of the early experimenters raised a note of caution after a number of reports of severe damage to personnel repeatedly exposed to radiation. On March 5, 1896, Thomas Edison developed eye irritation and blurred vision from repeated fluoroscopy, and he soon abandoned his plans to market x-ray fluorescent light bulbs. One of his employees developed severe dermatitis requiring amputation and died from metastatic carcinoma several years later at the age of 39 years.[46] To investigate whether radiation did indeed lead to skin irritation, Elihu Thompson, an x-ray pioneer, deliberately exposed his finger to radiation for 30 minutes per day for several days in order to test the effect of repeated radiation exposure. This resulted in erythema, pain, and swelling.[47]

In 1902 Frieden described a technician employed in demonstrating roentgen tubes who developed an epithelioma of the hand with metastases to the regional lymph nodes. Mihran Kassabian, the author of an early textbook of radiotherapy (*Electro-therapeutics and Roentgen Rays*, JB Lippincott Philadelphia & London, 1907) repeatedly exposed his own hand to fluoroscopic x-rays and graphically described the malignant ulcers that developed, requiring amputations of his fingers. He later died of metastatic cancer. The reports of radiation-induced cancer in persons employed in professions associated with radiation commonly followed severe radiation dermatitis and were usually attributed to repeated exposure. In the following years shielding introduced to prevent unnecessary exposure significantly reduced the incidence of acute radiation skin injuries. In addition, the x-ray voltage was increased and the lower-energy ("soft") x-rays were filtered in order to produce more penetrating rays and to reduce the dose to the skin. It was felt that by avoiding acute radiation injury, there was little long-term risk from x-rays. Paradoxically, the more penetrating rays reduced the acute skin toxicity but increased the dose to deeper tissues, thereby increasing the risk of long-term injury to internal organs. This only became apparent some 50 years later. Nevertheless, there were lone voices calling for more caution both within the medical profession and outside of it. William Rollins, a Boston dentist who invented a technique for imaging the back teeth, suggested the use of collimators and lead housing to reduce unnecessary scattering. He experimented on pregnant guinea pigs and was the first to show that radiation could result in fetal death.[48,49] John Dennis, a newspaper reporter, in 1899 called for licensing and control of radiation practitioners. Letters to the *London Times* raised the possible dangers of radiation and called for increased supervision and limiting the use of x-rays, but popular belief was that radiation had many beneficial effects and could not cause long-term harm.[50]

Regarding radiation epilation, a debate at the annual meeting of the British Medical Association in 1909 discussed a proposal for compulsory treatment of ringworm by x-rays. Concerns regarding possible neurocognitive side effects were dismissed based on the clinical experience with hundreds of children.[51] Dore in 1911 raised the issue of radiation damage to normal tissues,[52] but reports of side effects such as chronic x-ray dermatitis were usually vague, and for many years it was believed that as long as adequate care was taken to avoid acute toxicity, there was no long-term risk of radiation epilation, except for permanent alopecia.[53] Cases of malignant skin tumors were rare; they usually occurred in sites of previous x-ray dermatitis and were attributed to overexposure to radiation.[54] The ringworm epidemic in the United States in the 1940s led to several publications. Mottram and Hill reported on the successful treatment of a series of children using a modification of the KA technique. They noted, "We anticipate no damaging effects to the brain or pituitary with our technique, inasmuch as we have seen none and none has been reported to date from the many thousands of cases similarly epilated." Commenting on this report, Newell stated, "in general one should be slow to use x-ray in non-malignant conditions, for it is hard to be sure that no bad effects will follow later, even many years later. However, I do believe that x-ray epilation for intractable ringworm of the scalp is proper treatment, if done right and only once."[55] A case–control study published in 1952 concluded that fractional superficial roentgen radiation to a total dose of up to 1,000 R produced no sequelae. When the dose was over 1,000 R, mild, nonmalignant sequelae occurred in 1 of 87 cases.[56] Brauer in 1959, reviewing the use of radiation in dermatology, concluded, "Safe schedules for the application of ionizing radiation to disorders of the skin have been in existence for more than 30 years. Follow-up studies have verified the lack of harmful sequelae that result from these treatment routines when correctly applied." Among these techniques he included 340 to 360 R for tinea capitis according to the KA technique.[57]

Mackee, in his textbook in 1927, noted that thousands of children of any age had been treated with x-ray epilation with no record of brain damage either immediate or remote. Permanent alopecia was only seen in cases of technical error, in cases where radiodermatitis had been seen from the overdose, or in the rare case of idiosyncrasy. There were few systemic studies of the long-term effects of radiation epilation. Thorpe and Grange contacted 365 children 5 years after treatment with radiation epilation for ringworm. No cases of recurrence or toxicity were noted in the 128 children who returned for follow-up, but the study was limited to evaluation of the skin and hair quality.[58]

The first large study of late complications following radiation epilation for tinea was conducted on a cohort of 1,908 patients treated at New York University (NYU) between 1940 and 1958.[59] These were matched with 1,801 children with tinea capitis not treated by radiotherapy. There were nine cases of cancer in the irradiated group and one in the control group. In the irradiated group there was a 19% incidence of some degree of baldness and a 3% incidence of psychotic or neurotic disorder compared to 1% in the control group. Schultz and Albert built a phantom using the skull of a 7-year-old child to measure the dose delivered to various internal organs with the technique and dose used at NYU. A dose of 300 to 380 R was delivered using a 100-kv unfiltered beam (HVL 0.9 mm aluminum). The dose to the scalp ranged from 500 to 800 R and the surface dose to the brain was 140 R.

During the period of mass immigration to Israel between 1948 and 1958, prior to the introduction of griseofulvin, around 20,000 children with ringworm were treated with radiation epilation in four centers, including Hadassah Hospital in Jerusalem and Tel HaShomer Hospital near Tel Aviv, all using the KA technique delivering a dose of 350 to 400 R to each field with an energy of 90 kv and a 0.5-mm aluminum filter (resulting in a beam HVL of 1.25 mm aluminum) at a distance of 25 to 30 cm from the machine. One of the five fields was treated on each consecutive day, probably to make each treatment shorter and more convenient for the children treated. Following the first reports of possible delayed toxicity of radiation and radiation-induced tumors, Werner in 1968 used the original Picker x-ray machine and techniques employed at Tel HaShomer Hospital and, with the aid of an ionization chamber in an Alderson phantom, measured the dose of radiation delivered to the skull, brain, and thyroid during radiation epilation. They estimated that the surface of the brain received a dose of between 95 and 139 R when an epilating dose of 350 R was delivered to each field. The dose delivered to the outer portion of the skull was significantly higher than the dose absorbed by the skin. The upper part of the brain received a dose between 121 and 139 R.[60]

RADIATION-INDUCED MENINGIOMA

Up to the period of the Second World War, radiation-induced cancer was considered an occupational hazard with a latent period between exposure and the development of cancer of up to 20 years. The main emphasis of radiation safety was therefore on protecting personnel involved in the use of radiation.[61] It was only in the 1950s that the carcinogenic risk of radiation to patients (as opposed to personnel who were repeatedly subject to radiation over many years) began to be appreciated. In 1948 Cahan, Woodard, and Coley reported 11 cases of osteogenic sarcoma following therapeutic radiation.[62] In 1952 Jones reported sarcoma developing many years after radiation for benign diseases (arthritis, tuberculosis, fibrous dysplasia, and bone cysts), but the average dose given in these cases (when known) was between 4,000 and 6,000 R. Cade in 1957 described 34 patients with radiation-induced tumors, most of whom had been treated for benign conditions, and reviewed the cases reported in the literature until then. He described a first period after the discovery of x-rays when radiation-induced cancer was an occupational hazard with a latent period from 7 to 20 years and exclusively affected those employed in the science of radiology. Later, a second period, which he called the era of therapeutic radiation-induced cancer, began, with tumors developing after a latent period of up to 56 years. These tumors developed at sites severely damaged by radiation as a result of gross overexposure.[63] In 1958 Simpson for the first time raised the issue of the possible carcinogenic risk of low doses of radiation and reviewed the literature up to this time. She noted the risk of thyroid cancer after doses of less than 1,000 R and stated that "there is evidence that benign tumors may occur at lower levels of radiation in susceptible persons." She stated that "tumors of the central nervous system have rarely been attributed to radiation in man." Simpson noted that no brain tumors had been reported following therapy for ringworm; however, the only follow-up surveys of groups of children treated for ringworm were inadequate in number and length of follow-up.[64]

Meningiomas had been reported to occur after high-dose irradiation with deep x-rays for brain tumors,[65] but the carcinogenic effect of low-dose scalp radiation was first noted in 1969 when Munk reported a series of five patients who developed meningioma following low-dose scalp irradiation for tinea capitis.[66] Following this report Modan established a cohort of over 10,000 children treated for ringworm in Israel between 1949 and 1960, and in 1974 he published that there was an increased incidence of tumors of the head and neck—in particular thyroid and brain tumors—in this group.[67] Apart from the Israeli series and one Russian series of 62 patients,[68] there have been sporadic case reports of radiation-induced meningioma following low-dose radiation to the scalp. These cases have been reported in the United States[69] and Italy.[70,71,72]

Paulino et al. reviewed the literature on radiation-induced meningiomas reported since 1981. There were 17 meningiomas following low-dose irradiation; 14 of these patients had been treated for tinea capitis. The latent time for development of meningiomas in this group was 32.1 years, compared to 14.9 years in those receiving high-dose radiation.[73]

The use of epilation to treat ringworm was abandoned in the late 1950s after the introduction of effective medical therapy with griseofulvin. This coincided with the appreciation that low-dose radiation used to treat ringworm could induce tumors. Fifty years after the abandonment of this technique for treating ringworm, there is still much controversy regarding its use and possible misuse. In contrast to the numerous cases of radiation-induced meningioma reported in this population in Israel, and the official recognition of these patients as suffering from an iatrogenic disease, there have been only sporadic reports of meningiomas induced by low-dose radiation in other countries, although many thousands of children were treated with radiation epilation for tinea capitis. This may be due to underreporting. With the long lag time (30–60 years) between radiation treatment and the development of meningioma, many patients may not remember receiving radiation to the skull in childhood or do not connect this with the diagnosis of meningioma. For example, in a comment on a report of a patient with multiple skull base meningioma[74] (in this case it was "discovered by chance" that the patient had been irradiated 58 years earlier for tinea capitis), it was noted that "we have observed a number of patients in our institution (George Washington University) with multiple basal meningiomas and a prior history of cranial irradiation for tinea capitis." In addition, magnetic resonance imaging (MRI), which is often needed to diagnose meningioma, has only become widely available in recent years. Other factors, including genetics, as discussed earlier, may also be relevant. It can be expected that since radiation epilation was discontinued almost 60 years ago, the occurrence of tumors induced by radiation epilation will gradually disappear.

NOTES

1. SJR. Some effects of the x-rays on the hands. *Nature.* 1896;54:621.
2. Crocker HR. A case of dermatitis from roentgen rays. *Br Med J.* 1897;8.
3. Daniel J. Depilatory action of x-rays. *Med Rec.* 1896;49:595–596 (quoted by Kogelnik HD. Inauguration of radiotherapy as a new scientific specialty by Leopold Freud 100 years ago. *Radiother Oncol.* 1997;42:203–211).
4. Freund L. Ein mit Roentgen-Strahlen behandelter Fall von Naevus pigmentosus pilferus. *Wien Med Wschr.* 1897;47:428–434 (quoted by Kogelnik HD. Inauguration of radiotherapy as a new scientific specialty by Leopold Freud 100 years ago. *Radiother Oncol.* 1997;42:203–211).
5. Mould RF. Invited review: The early years of radiotherapy with emphasis on x-ray and radium apparatus. *Br J Radiol.* 1995;68:567–582.
6. Shanks SC. Vale epilation. X-ray epilation of the scalp at Goldie Leigh Hospital, Woolwich (1922–1958). *Br J Dermatol.* 1967;79:237–238.
7. Dennis JM. Association of irradiation with neoplasia in children and adolescents. *Ann Intern Med.* 1956;44(3):579–583.
8. McKeown SR, Hatfield P, Prestwich RJ, et al. Radiotherapy for benign disease; assessing the risk of radiation-induced cancer following exposure to intermediate-dose radiation. *Br J Radiol.* 2015;88(1056):20150405.
9. Seegenschmiedt MH, Katalanic A, Makoski H-B, et al. Radiation therapy for benign diseases: Patterns of care study in Germany. *Int J Radiat Oncol Biol Phys.* 2000;47(1):195–202.
10. Milakovic M, Popovic M, Raman S, et al. Radiotherapy for the prophylaxis of heterotopic ossification: A systematic review and meta-analysis of randomized controlled trials. *Radiother Oncol.* 2015;116(1):4–9.

11. Merchant TE, Kiehna EN, Kun LE, et al. Phase II trial of conformal radiation therapy for pediatric patients with craniopharyngioma and correlation of surgical factors and radiation dosimetry with change in cognitive function. *J Neurosurg.* 2006;104(2 Suppl):94–102.
12. Order SB, Donaldson S. *Radiation Therapy of Benign Diseases: A Clinical Guide.* Berlin & New York: Springer Verlag; 1990.
13. Bulkley LC. *Clinical Illustrations of Favus and Its Treatment by a New Method of Depilation.* New York: GP Putnam's Sons; 1881.
14. Alder Smith H. *Ringworm and Alopecia Areata: Their Pathology, Diagnosis, and Treatment.* 4th ed. London: HK Lewis; 1897.
15. Allen CW. Treatment of ringworm of the scalp in institutions. *Pediatrics.* 1896;2(4):1–8.
16. Sabouraud R. *La teigne trichophytique et la teigne spéciale de Gruby.* Paris: Rueff er Cie; 1894.
17. Sabouraud R. *Les teignes.* Paris: Masson, 1910
18. MacKee GM. Diseases due to fungi. In MacKee GM, *X-rays and Radium in the Treatment of Diseases of the Skin.* 2nd ed. Philadelphia: Lea & Febiger; 1927:454–482.
19. The roentgen ray treatment of ringworm. *Lancet.* 1909;173(4472):1339–1400.
20. Lancet Commission on ringworm: Its prevalence, influence and treatment. *Lancet.* 1910;175(4505):51–56.
21. Macleod JMH. Observations on the x-ray treatment of ringworm of the scalp in children under three years of age. *Br J Dermatol.* 1926;38:492–501.
22. Lee RKC. Epidemic tinea capitis: A public health problem. *Public Health Rep.* 1948;63:261–268.
23. *United States Army X-Ray Manual,* authorized by the Surgeon-General of the Army, prepared under the direction of the Division of Roentgenology. New York: Paul B. Hoeber; 1920.
24. Kaplan II. *Clinical Radiation Oncology.* New York: Paul B. Hoeber; 1937.
25. Lee RKC. Epidemic tinea capitis: A public health problem. *Public Health Rep.* 1948;63:261–268.
26. Steves RJ, Lynch FW. Ringworm of the scalp. *JAMA.* 1947;133(5):306–309.
27. Cipollaro AC, Brody A. Control of tinea capitis. *NY State J Med.* 1950;50:1931–1934.
28. Dixon HA, Rolph AH. Favus: A report of 17 cases. *Can Med Assoc J.* 1920;12:235–238.
29. Beare JM, Cheeseman EA. Tinea capitis: Review of 1004 cases. *Br J Dermatol.* 1951;63(5):166–186.
30. Levy-Lebhar G. The treatment of Moroccan ringworm. *Maroc Med.* 1955;360:580–589.
31. Donald GF. The history, clinical features, and treatment of tinea capitis due to trichophyton tonsurans and trichophyton violaceum. *Austral J Dermatol.* 1959;5:90–102.
32. Dostrovsky A, Kallner G, Raubitschek F, Sagher F. Tinea capitis: An epidemiologic, therapeutic and laboratory investigation of 6,390 cases. *J Invest Dermatol.* 1955;24:195–200.
33. Dostrovsky A. The thallium in the treatment of *Trichophytia capitis. Harefuah.* 1927;2:3.

34. Tulchinsky Goldstein S. An attempt of ringworm (tinea) therapy without x-ray. *Harefuah.* 1958;55:291–292.
35. Yair C. The treatment of tinea capitis with potassium iodide. *Harefuah.* 1961;60:116–117.
36. Berlin C, Tajer A, Yair C. The treatment of tinea capitis and selected cases of dermato- and onchomycosis with griseofulvin. *Harefuah.* 1961;60:113–116.
37. Dostrovsky A. The biological war on fungi. *Harefuah.* 1961;60:119–121.
38. Adamson HG. A simplified method of x-ray application for the cure of ringworm of the scalp: Kienböck's method. *Lancet.* 1909;173(4472):1378–1380.
39. Kaplan II. *Practical Radiation Therapy.* Philadelphia and London: WB Saunders; 1931.
40. Cipollaro AC, Crossland PM. *X-Rays and Radium in the Treatment of Diseases of the Skin.* 5th ed. Philadelphia: Lea & Febiger; 1967.
41. Strauss JS, Kligman AM. Distribution of skin doses over scalp in therapy of tinea capitis with superficial x-rays. *AMA Arch Dermatol Syph.* 1954;69:331–341.
42. X-ray and radium protection: International recommendations. *Br Med J.* 1931;2(3695):820.
43. Mould RF. *A Century of X-Rays and Radioactivity in Medicine.* London: Institute of Physics; 1993:21.
44. Steward CG, Sowby FD, Stevens DJ. *The basis of radiological protection.* World Health Organization First Regional Seminar on Radiation Health, Manila, Philippines, 1973.
45. X-ray and radium protection: International recommendations. *Br Med J.* 1931;2(3695):819–820.
46. King K. Clarence Dally—the man who gave Thomas Edison x-ray vision. *Smithsonian Magazine*, March 14, 2012. https://www.smithsonianmag.com/history/clarence-dally-the-man-who-gave-thomas-edison-x-ray-vision-123713565/.
47. Meggitt G. *Taming the Rays: A History of Radiation and Protection.* London: Lulu.com; 2008:13.
48. Kathren RL. William H. Rollins (1852–1929): X-ray protection pioneer. *J Hist Med.* 1964;19:287–295.
49. Kathren RL, Brodsky L. Radiation protection. In Gagliardi R, Almond PR, eds. *A History of the Radiological Sciences: Radiation Physics*, 187–221 (ARRS.org/Arrslive/HRS)..
50. Macleod JMH. The x-ray treatment of ringworm of the scalp: With special reference to the risks of dermatitis and the suggested injury to the brain. *Lancet.* May 15, 1909:1373–1377.
51. Proceedings of the 77th Annual Meeting of the British Medical Association. *Br Med J.* 1909:321–322.
52. Dore SE. The present position of the X-ray treatment of ringworm. *Lancet.* Feb. 18, 1911:432–436.
53. Mitchell W, Hutt CW. Correspondence to the editor. X-ray treatment of ringworm. *Lancet.* Jan. 8, 1921:97–98.
54. Rowntree C. X-ray radiation and cancer. *Br Med J.* March 19, 1921;1(3142):440.

55. Mottram ME, Hill HA. Radiation therapy of ringworm of the scalp. *Calif Med.* 1949;70:183–193.
56. Sulzberger MB, Baer RL, Borota A. Do roentgen ray treatments as given by skin specialists produce cancers or other sequelae? *AMA Arch Dermatol Syph.* 1952;65:639.
57. Brauer EW. X-ray, radium and ultraviolet light therapy in dermatology: With particular reference to safety factors and reduction of depth and gonad doses. *Med Clin North Am.* 1959;43:705–714.
58. Thorpe NA, Grange RV. A survey of tinea capitis five years after treatment by x-ray epilation. *Postgrad Med J.* 1954;30(346):422–424.
59. Albert RE, Omran AR, Brauer EW, et al. Follow-up study of patients treated by x-ray for tinea capitis. *Am J Public Health Nations Health.* 1966;56(12):2114–2120.
60. Werner A, Modan B, Davidoff D. Doses to brain, skull, thyroid following x-ray therapy for tinea capitis. *Phys Med Biol.* 1968;13:247–258.
61. X-ray and radium protection: International recommendations. *Br Med J.* 1931;2(3695):820.
62. Cahan WG. Radiation-induced sarcoma, 50 years later. *Cancer.* 1998;82(1):6–7.
63. Cade S. Radiation-induced cancer in man. *Br J Radiol.* 1957;30:393–402.
64. Simpson CL. Radiation is a carcinogenic agent. *CA Cancer J Clin.* 1958;8:156–163.
65. Mann I, Yates PC, Ainslie JP, et al. Unusual case of double primary orbital tumor. *Br J Ophthalmol.* 1953;37:758–762.
66. Munk J, Peyser E, Gruszkiewicz J. Radiation-induced intracranial meningiomas. *Clin Radiol.* 1969;20(1):90–94.
67. Modan B, Baidatz D, Mart H, et al. Radiation-induced head and neck tumors. *Lancet.* 1974;303(7852):277–279.
68. Gabibov GA, Kuklina AS, Martynov VA, et al. Radiation-induced meningiomas of the brain. *Zh Vopr Neirokhir Im N N Burdenko.* 1983;6:13–18.
69. Harrison MJ, Wolfe DE, Lau T-S, et al. Radiation-induced meningiomas: Experience at the Mount Sinai Hospital and review of the literature. *J Neurosurg.* 1991;75:564–574.
70. Marconi F, Parenti G. Radiation-induced cerebral meningiomas: Case reports. *J Neurosurg Sci.* 1997;41(4):413–417.
71. De Tommassi A, Occhiogross M, De Tommassi C, et al. Radiation-induced intracranial meningiomas: Review of 6 operated cases. *Neurosurg Res.* 2005;28:104–114.
72. Spallone A, Gagliardi FM, Vagnozzi R. Intracranial meningiomas related to external cranial irradiation. *Surg Neurol.* 1979;12:53–59.
73. Paulino AC, Ahmede IM, Mai WY, Teh BS. The influence of pretreatment characteristics and radiotherapy parameters on time interval to development of radiation-associated meningioma. *Int J Radiat Oncol Biol Phys.* 2009;75:1408–1414.
74. Spallone A, Neroni M, Guiffre R. Multiple skull base meningioma: Case report. *Surg Neurol.* 1999;51:274–280.

3

The ringworm children at the Hôpital Saint-Louis, Paris

From medical neglect to biosocial obsession

GÉRARD TILLES

INTRODUCTION

The French Revolution deeply transformed the organization of the Paris hospitals. Emphasizing the innovative role attributed to the hospitals in the teaching of medicine, three of them were specialized in 1801: Hôpital des Vénériens for venereal diseases, Hôpital de la Couche for pregnant women, and Hospice du Nord for chronic and contagious skin diseases like scabies, scrofula, ulcers, and tinea.[1] The ringworm children[2] were then treated in the hospital newly devoted to skin diseases. Thanks to the appointment of a new generation of physicians—Alibert (1768–1837), Biett (1781–1840), Cazenave (1795–1877), Gibert (1797–1866), Devergie (1798–1879) (figure 3.9)—and their successors and to its specialization, the Hôpital Saint-Louis (renamed the Hospice du Nord for reasons related to the French Revolution) became the alma mater of dermatology.[3,4]

WHEN THE PHYSICIANS DISREGARDED THE RINGWORM CHILDREN

Alibert,[5] the first physician lecturing in dermatology at Saint-Louis from 1801, described the diseases of the hair in a unique group, naming all of them tinea capitis (in French *teignes or porrigines*). In fact, only one of them was a true mycosis in the modern sense of the word, namely favus (tinea vera, Porrigo favosa). This was characterized by the presence of favi, little straw- or sulfur-colored crusts that had a peculiarly well-marked cup-shaped appearance (Figure 3.1) and that were easily recognizable, "even for a blind due to its characteristic odour of urine of mice."[6] Regarded as an unavoidable stigma of children living in social misery, the favus stigmatized the patients as bearing "a disease so disgusting that the afflicted people fear to socialize and cannot find any activity anywhere"[7] (Figure 3.2).

As far as the treatment was concerned, the French physicians followed the humoralist doctrine. In this respect, tinea capitis was considered as a safety valve allowing the excretion of bad humors so that the balance between good and vicious humors could remain in the right proportion, therefore protecting the children against more severe diseases.[8] Alibert (figure 3.3) regarded tinea as one of the "depurative diseases of childhood [. . .] Prodest prurigo capitis is an axiom admitted by the physicians."[9] Rayer (1793–1867) (figure 3.4), head of the Hôpital de la Charité, recommended, when treating a favus, to create ways-outs on the skin to avoid the deleterious consequences of its cure.[10] A few decades later, Gibert still advised his students to use leeches to provide the bad humors with a "complementary way of elimination."[11]

When the physicians decided to treat it, tinea capitis was usually cured by the *calotte* (skull cap).[12] The calotte involved applying a plaster on the scalp followed by a brutal pulling up that removed sick and healthy hair alike. It was both dangerous and painful: "The room where the young patients were gathered looked more like a room for punishments than for care. All of them came in like victims presenting their heads. [. . .] Fathers

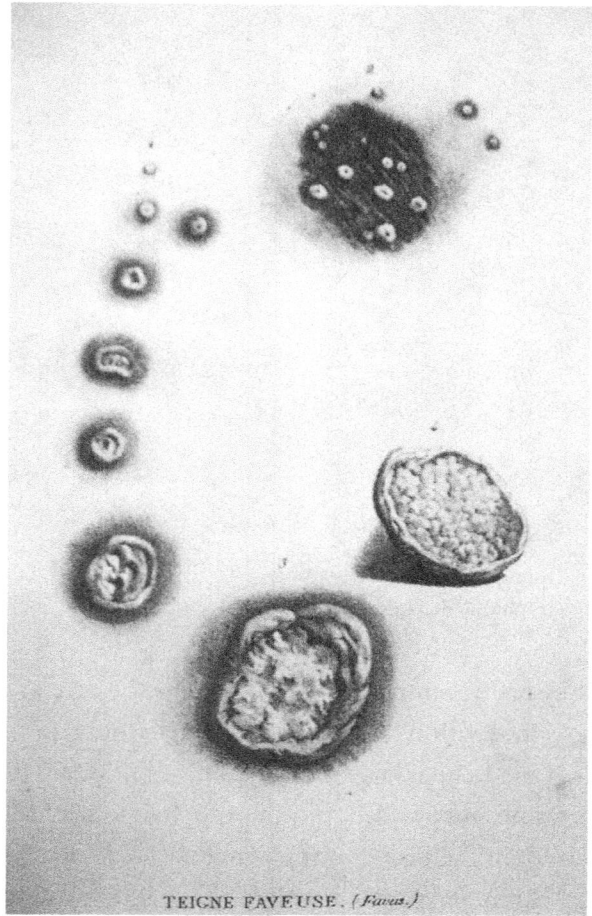

Figure 3.1 Favus, lithographie d'Engelmann
Mahon jeune [1829] *Recherches sur le siège et la nature des teignes*. Baillière, Paris.

and mothers waited for the end of the torture while moaning."[13] Some witnesses reported how horrible the consequences could be:

> On the last 17th February, a man named Abraham, a farmer from Aufranville, brought his two daughters to us, one eight years old and the other twelve. Both had been affected severely with favus from infancy. All previous treatments had failed. We are sorry to say that

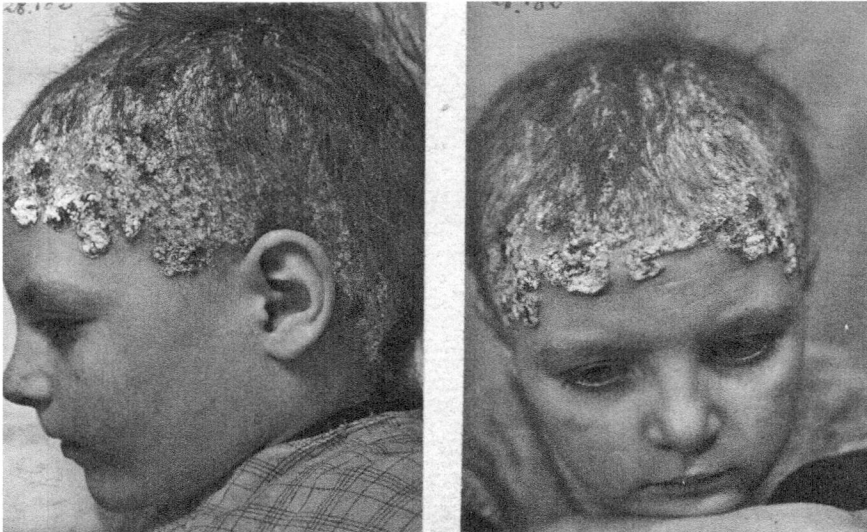

Figure 3.2 Favus, Touraine, October 8, 1946
Coll. Musée photographique de l'hôpital Saint-Louis.

unwisely they had recently been placed under the care of a country practitioner who within a few days reduced them to a frightful scale. He had made up a large plaster from black pitch, Bourgogne pitch, gum arabic and potassium. When applied to the head of these two poor children the plaster immediately became firmly adherent to the scalp. Some days later this large pitiless man wrenched off these caps with all his strength and with great strips of scalp sufficiently to lay bare the skull. As one might expect, haemorrhagy began, and it was so great that the man himself became frightened. Not knowing what else to do to stop the loss of blood, he hurriedly placed the caps back on the scalps. A peasant who was present at this atrocious torment had the presence of mind to mix some vinegar and fresh water and with it to bathe the heads of these deplorable victims of shocking brutality. In that state they were left, no one daring to touch them.

Neither girl survived.[14,15]

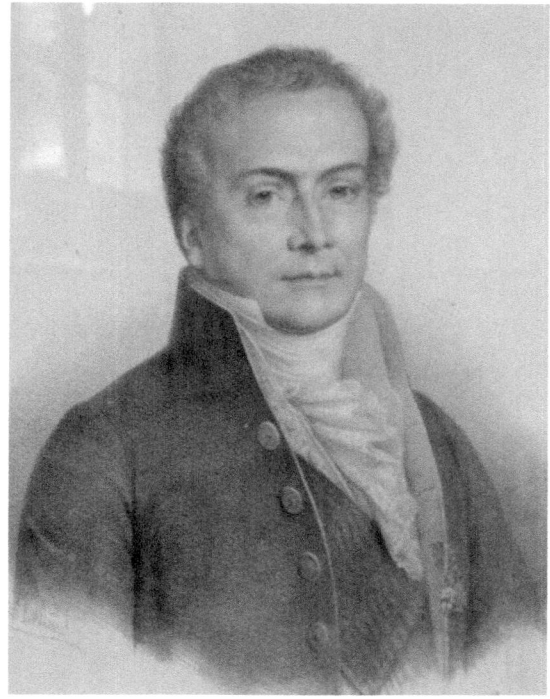

Figure 3.3 Jean-Louis Alibert (1768–1837), first dermatologist at the Hôpital Saint-Louis
Coll. Dr Gérard Tilles.

In this context, the ringworm children disregarded by the society, either victims of horrible methods or not treated or treated with apprehension by the physicians, became a business for medicasters.

THE RINGWORM CHILDREN IN THE HANDS OF EMPIRICS

Until the end of the *ancien régime*,[16] in Paris ringworm children were treated by religious congregations and in a particular hospital (Hôpital des Teigneux, also named Hôpital Sainte-Reine). The treatment was supervised by a layman, neither physician nor surgeon, named Lamartinière, whose

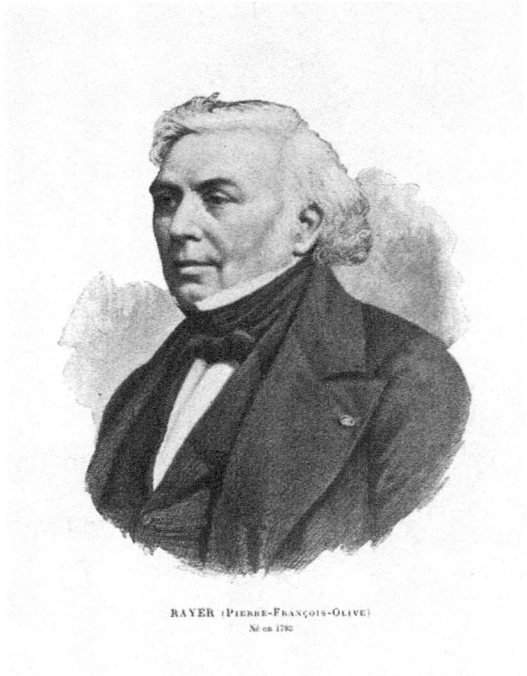

Figure 3.4 Pierre François Olive Rayer (1793–1867)
Coll. BIUM, Paris.

family had been in charge for a century.[17] A few medicasters even tried to obtain an official validation of their "secret remedies" by the Academy of Medicine so that parents would become more confident in their treatment and their job would become more lucrative.[18] Among the empirics involved in the treatment of tinea capitis were the Mahon family (two brothers and their sons-in-law), who on December 31, 1806, were appointed as official healers of ringworm in the Paris hospitals, even though they had no medical education(figure 3.5).[19,20] At Saint-Louis, the Mahons' treatment took place twice a week, Wednesdays and Fridays. The therapeutic effect was actually based on the extraction of the sick hair by the fingers followed by the application of a "secret powder" that was actually used only to facilitate the removal of the hair.[21] The Mahons' treatment was so efficient that several hospitals inside and outside Paris hired them.[22] Compared to

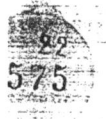
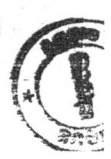

Figure 3.5 Advertisement of the Mahons' medical activity
Coll. musée de l'hôpital Saint-Louis, Paris.

the calotte, the Mahons' method was safe, efficient, and relatively painless to such an extent that the physicians acknowledged it, asserting the method healed almost all the afflicted children.[23] The administrators of the Paris hospitals were so convinced by the results that they encouraged the Mahons to keep on treating the children. The Mahons received a salary and were paid per child; even so, this was far less expensive than a stay in a hospital.[24]

From January 1, 1807, until December 31, 1827, about 20,000 children were treated by the Mahons in the Paris hospitals. Pariset, Secretary General of the Academy of Medicine, acknowledged the merits of the Mahons, who had helped to reduce the expenses of the administration and to put an end to the calotte.[25] In 1812, the Academy of Medicine suggested that a proper evaluation of the Mahons' method be performed. In this respect the Academy thought it would be useful to set aside a special department in a Paris hospital for the Mahons. However, the Conseil Général des Hospices—the administration in charge of the Paris hospitals—rejected the proposition, considering it too expensive. It added that according to the sanitary rules, ringworm did not justify hospitalization. The Mahons' treatment remained the standard, and the family kept on treating ringworm children until 1868 in the Paris hospitals. Few physicians tried to teach their method; none reproduced it with similar success. In fact, the role of the physicians was limited to certifying the healing of the children, which the Mahons needed before they could to be paid.

Outside of Paris, the Mahons' treatment was also successful, and they were officially appointed in the Rouen hospitals, Dieppe, Louviers, and Lyon.[26] In Rouen (in western France), starting in 1819 the Mahon family treated the ringworm children as outpatients 5 days per month. The brothers received 600 francs for their travel from Paris, another 600 francs as an annual fee, and 6 francs per ringworm child whose healing was certified by the chief physician or the chief surgeon.[27] During the first year, 388 children were cured. Starting in 1824 they traveled to Rouen 20 days every other month. They treated between 300 and 400 ringworm children every year and cured half of them.[28]

In other provinces, the ringworm children were treated in a similar way by different medicasters. In Nantes (in western France), nuns took care of them until the 1860s.[29] In Marseille (in southern France) in the early 19th century, Mrs. Hugues was the Mahons' alter ego. Like her Parisian colleagues she extracted the hair with the fingers, used a "secret powder," and was paid per treated child. In 1829, the administration, considering that the expense could be avoided, decided that the treatment should be done by the physicians in charge of the patients. A contract certified by a notary signed in August 1829 allowed the administration to obtain the mysterious powder then produced by the hospitals for the supposed benefit of the children. When Mrs. Hugues died in July 1873, the powder was found to comprise mainly mashed seeds of rye, confirming its uselessness.[30]

TREATING THE RINGWORM CHILDREN, FINALLY A MEDICAL ACTIVITY

Discovered by Schönlein (Berlin, 1839) and Gruby (Paris, 1841–1843) (figure 3.6), the fungal etiology of tinea was strongly debated in Saint-Louis. Cazenave, head of the hospital at the time (figure 3.7), denied the fungi, considering them as "mysterious atoms" and "illusions of microscopy," and finally regarded the "so-called fungi" as "German dreams."[31,32,33] Unlike Cazenave, his colleague Bazin (1807–1878) (figure 3.8), accepted Gruby's discoveries, provided the first modern definition of tinea, and insisted on the need to find a microscopic fungus: "The fungus is the hallmark of tinea [. . .] without it there is no tinea just as there is no scabies without acarus."[34] Moreover, he stressed how the microscopic fungi made the humoralist theories obsolete: "If during the reign of the humoralist theories, few physicians thought it dangerous to treat tinea it would be difficult today to find any practitioner who would accept the responsibility of such an opinion."[35] Bazin enumerated several forms of tinea capitis: favus (porrigo favosa et scutulata), tinea tonsurans (teigne tondante de Mahon, herpes tonsurant de Cazenave), teigne mentagre, teigne décalvante,

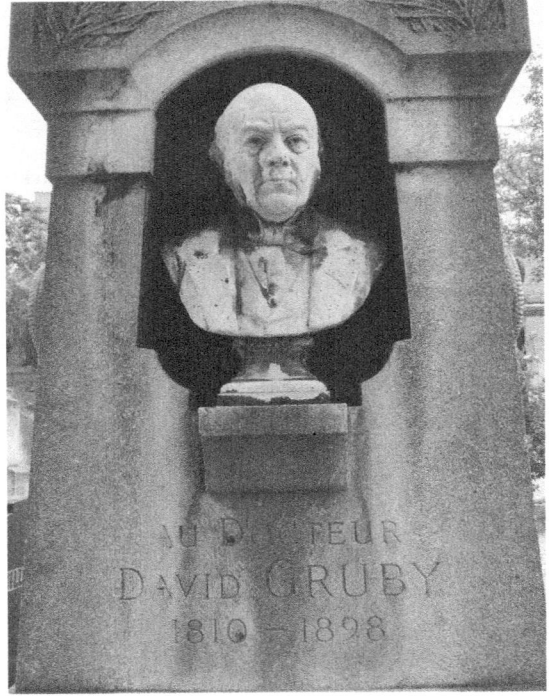

Figure 3.6 David Gruby (1810–1898), St. Vincent's Cemetery, Paris
Coll. Dr Gérard Tilles.

and teigne achromateuse (porrigo decalvans de Bateman), for which he revived the old word *pelade*.[36]

In fact, Bazin confirmed Gruby's misconception on porrigo decalvans, which he erroneously regarded as being of fungal origin. Due to this confusion, the children afflicted with pelade (alopecia areata) were for several decades considered contagious and therefore were isolated from healthy children (see the section on the Ecole des teigneux later in this chapter).

Given Bazin's conclusions, the physicians understood that tinea capitis, which had previously attracted little interest from the medical community, needed attention. The treatment of ringworm children could no longer be left to laypeople.[37] In March 1853, Davenne, the general manager of the Assistance publique (the administration in charge of the Paris hospitals), agreed to establish in the Hôpital Saint-Louis a department

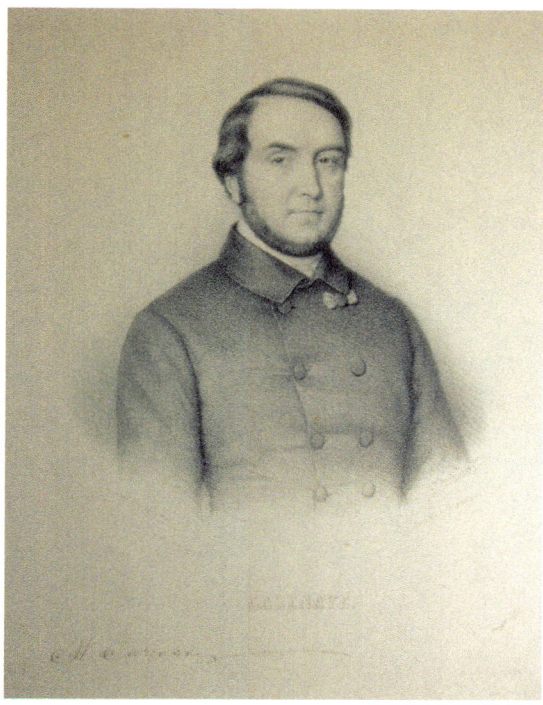

Figure 3.7 Pierre Louis Alphée Cazenave (1796–1877)
Coll. musée de l'hôpital Saint-Louis.

headed by Bazin devoted to inpatients and outpatients with favus and tinea tonsurans. Fifteen boys and 15 girls from ages 4 to 15 years were admitted and treated until they completely recovered. Ringworm children had previously been treated as outpatients to avoid proximity to various contagious patients and for economic reasons but now, under the medical pression, were hospitalized for several weeks.

Bazin's therapeutic procedure involved pulling out infected hair with forceps, as previously used in London by Samuel Plumbe[38] ("without hair removal, the healing is impossible"), and mercurial tonics that were supposed to have an antifungal efficiency. No more aggressive treatment was required, Bazin emphasized.[39] Each session lasted no more than half an hour. The removal of infected hair on the entire scalp required 12 hours. According to Bazin, if the treatment was properly done, favus could be definitively cured in 6 or 8 weeks:

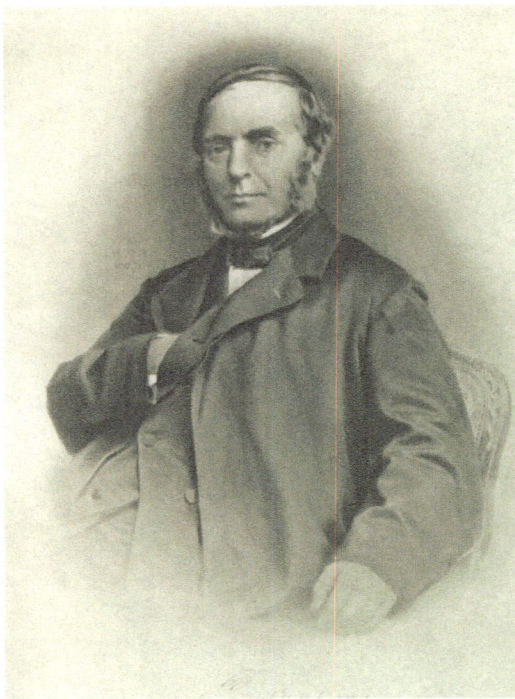

Figure 3.8 Ernest Bazin (1807–1878)
Coll. musée de l'hôpital Saint-Louis.

In 1851 everyone could say that the favus was [...] a serious and everlasting disease that might compromise not only the hair but sometimes the life also [...] Today on the contrary, we can assert that the favus is a slight disease and even the easiest to treat of all tinea.[40]

For tinea tonsurans, the method was slower due to the fragility of the hair. The children also had to remain hospitalized for few months after the last epilation so that the physicians should confirm the absence of recurrence. Emphasizing, like his colleagues, the fragility of the hair afflicted with tinea tonsurans versus favus, Lailler (1822–1893)(figure 3.10) stressed to his pupils the importance of being "extremely prudent before guaranteeing the complete recovery".[41]

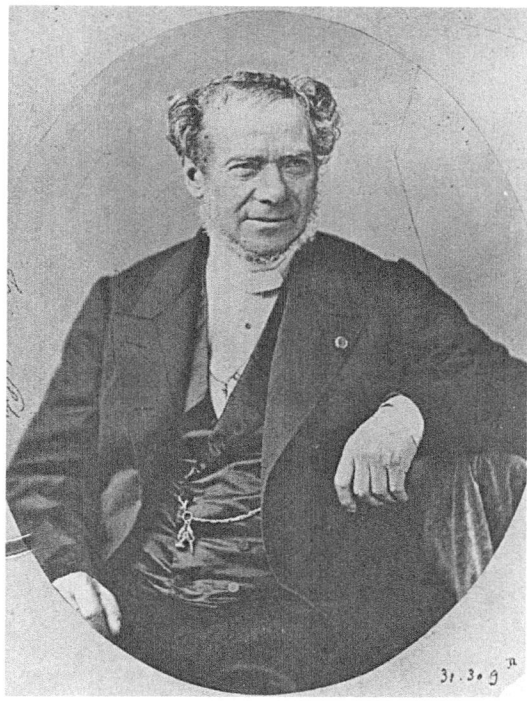

Figure 3.9 Alphonse Devergie (1798–1879)
Coll. musée de l'hôpital Saint-Louis.

Do not forget how great is your responsibility when authorizing a child who may propagate the infection at school. [. . .] You are not allowed to considered him recovered before six weeks have spent without any new pustule [. . .] Clinical examinations are to be organized for one or two months after they are reinserted in the social life.

Consequently, the mean duration of stay at the hospital was longer than the treatment itself.

Regarded as a clinical form of tinea, alopecia areata (porrigo decalvans, pelade) was treated by epilation of healthy hair and topical use of parasiticidal agents also.[42]

The number of patients treated by Bazin increased from 200 in 1853 to 400 in 1868 due to the medical interest in the treatment of tinea capitis and to an actual increase in cases.[43] Apart from Bazin's department, the

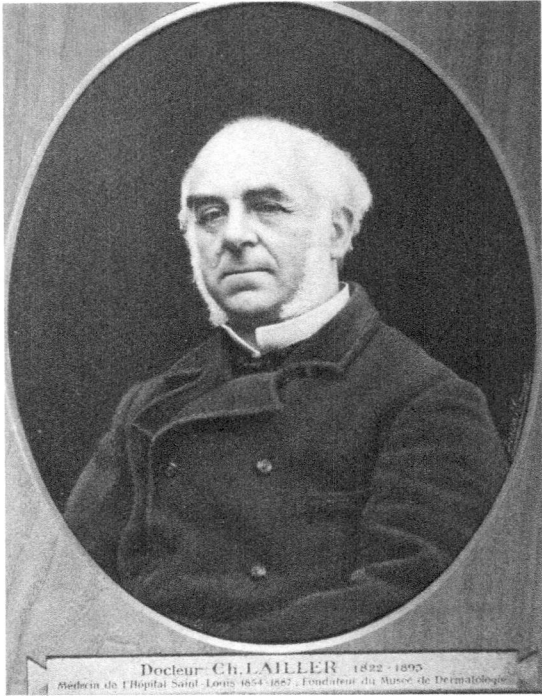

Figure 3.10 Charles Lailler (1822–1893)
Coll. musée de l'hôpital Saint-Louis.

children could be treated as outpatients in the dispensaries annexed to the other medical departments in Saint-Louis or by the Mahon family in their own department. Competing with Bazin's method, the Mahons' method became less and less attractive, to that point that their contribution was officially removed from the Hôpital Saint-Louis in 1868.[44,45,46,47]

In Saint-Louis, every physician set his own procedure to improve the results and to reduce the duration of the treatment. According to Lailler:

> No session [epilation] can last more than one or two hours. After the hair removal, the scalp is rubbed with grease and covered with starched poultices [. . .] In case of favus, three to five epilations may be necessary. [. . .] Complementary general medication such as cod-liver oil and iron iodide syrup may be beneficial. »

Ernest Besnier (1831–1909) (figure 3.11), head of Saint-Louis, proposed four successive steps:

> Cutting the hair very short with scissors, never with razor that might cause an auto inoculation; extracting hair from the afflicted areas and a surrounding zone so that the infected area should be isolated from the healthy ones; then soaping the scalp twice a day; finally applying sulfur ointment and acetic acid sometimes mixed with chloroform to provoke a slight irritation that could accelerate the expulsion of the hair.[48]

The pain provoked by the epilation led a few physicians to use parasiticidal lotions only. Butte proposed the use of iodide protochloride

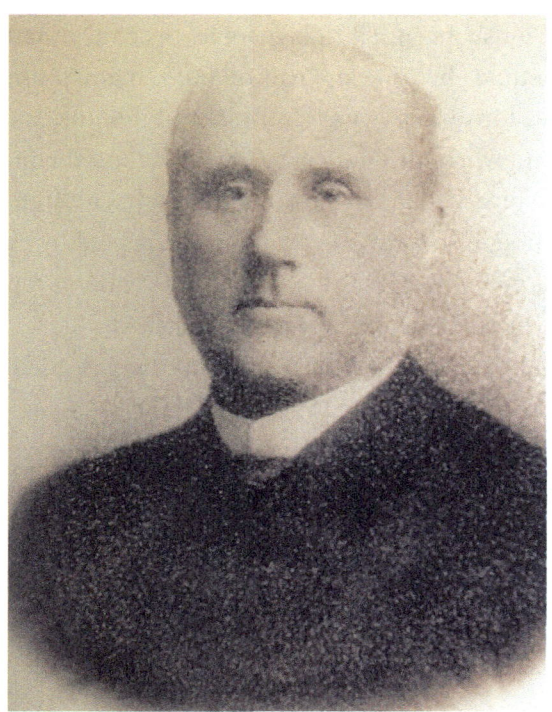

Figure 3.11 Ernest Besnier (1831–1909)
Coll. musée de l'hôpital Saint-Louis.

in an ointment that reduced the duration of stay to between 3 and 5 months instead of a year or more.[49] Despite being less efficient than epilation, the inflammation of the skin caused by scraping or by the application of irritating tonics was considered as a contributing factor. Iron perchloride, croton oil, or salt water was used to facilitate the extraction of hair. Other physicians used different tonics (e.g., chrysophanic acid, salicylic acid, phenic acid, ichthyol, chrysarobin) with or without epilation. Quinquaud (1841–1894), director of the Ecole des teigneux, in 1888 proposed a new method to treat tinea tonsurans using mercurial lotion, with or without epilation, with or without scrubbing the scalp and occlusive dressings.[50] The mean duration of treatment dropped from 17.5 months in 1888 to 5.5 months a few years later thanks to his method. The number of recoveries increased continuously: 14 in 1888, 124 in 1889, and 150 in 1890.[51]

In short, from the 1850s through the 1880s, the treatment of ringworm, which had previously been left to laypeople, became a matter of medical interest. The methods became less painful but remained time consuming, notably for tinea tonsurans (which took several months, sometimes more than a year). Ringworm did not cause any great social concern from the physicians, who regarded it as an ordinary event in children living in poor conditions. Although the mycotic origin was accepted by every physician in the 1880s, the correlation between each type of microscopic fungus and the clinical aspect of ringworm was not established.

Starting in the 1890s, under Sabouraud's influence, medical mycology became a matter for specialists. In this respect, ringworm—even though most cases (tinea tonsurans) spontaneously disappear without scar at puberty—became a matter of medical anxiety, justifying the use of new therapeutics (x-rays) whose adverse effects were unpredictable.

SABOURAUD: THE GOLDEN AGE OF RINGWORM

In the 1870s and 1880s the discoveries of Pasteur and his disciples drastically altered the medical understanding and the social concern about the diseases. Darier (1856–1936), later head of Saint-Louis, summarized the intellectual effects of this new age in medicine:

> Nobody who has not been living these years cannot realize how the medical ideas changed and the enthusiasm they gave rise [. . .] The ancient hypotheses, cosmic and atmospheric causes were swept aside [. . .] One even thought that healing or death and the mysteries of immunity were about to be explained.[52]

The majority of the professors of medicine agreed with the Pastorian doctrines, numerous laboratories were set up in the medical departments of the Paris hospitals, and many scientific papers contributed to spread the spirit of the new medicine.[53,54,55] The role of microbes became so obvious that Emile Duclaux (1840–1904), director of the Pasteur Institute, could wonder whether "diseases may exist without microbes."[56]

In dermatology, the Pastorian doctrines were introduced by Raymond Jacques Adrien Sabouraud (1864–1938). Born on November 24, 1864, in a bourgeois Catholic family, Sabouraud was appointed as an intern at the Hôpitaux de Paris in 1890[57,58] (figures 3.12 and 3.13). Interested in microbiological sciences, he registered for the sixth session of the "Great Course" lectures by Emile Roux (1853–1933) at the Pasteur Institute.[59] Comparing microbiology with a new religion, Sabouraud recalled it as "a fire that invades a single person who communicates it to many others who gather in a church and speak of nothing but microbiology."[60]

In 1892 Sabouraud was an intern in Besnier's department in Hôpital Saint-Louis. Besnier, acknowledged as the leader of French dermatology, encouraged his pupil to study tinea capitis, which he considered a promising matter.[61] Sabouraud received his medical degree on April 24, 1894, writing his thesis on human trichophytia. In 1895 he was appointed head of a laboratory established in Saint-Louis, financially supported by the Paris City Council, that was devoted to microbiology in dermatology, notably to research on ringworm.[62,63]

Thanks to his abilities in mycology, Sabouraud was selected to represent France at the Third International Congress of Dermatology, chaired

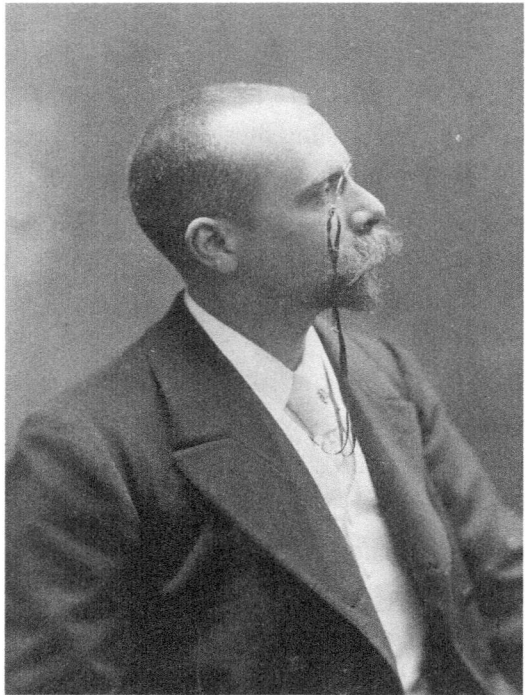

Figure 3.12 Raymond Sabouraud (1868–1938)
Coll. Dr Mathieu de Brunhoff.

by Jonathan Hutchinson, in London in 1896. Lecturing on the "Plurality of Trichophytons," Sabouraud became the international expert in the matter, with many dermatologists sending him samples of microscopic fungi for identification.[64] Within a few years Sabouraud's lab in Saint-Louis had gained worldwide fame. *Les Teignes*, the massive textbook he wrote in 1910, was for several decades the bible of French-speaking mycologists-dermatologists.[65] (Figure 3.3). He was elected president of the French Society for Dermatology and Syphilology in 1925–1926, was president of the Fourth Congress of French-Speaking Dermatologists in 1929, and was named a Commander of the Legion of Honour. He died on Friday, February 4, 1938.

Since Bazin, the various forms of tinea tonsurans were supposed to be caused by a single microscopic trichophyton. Sabouraud regarded this theory as erroneous and summarized it humoristically. "For I, the

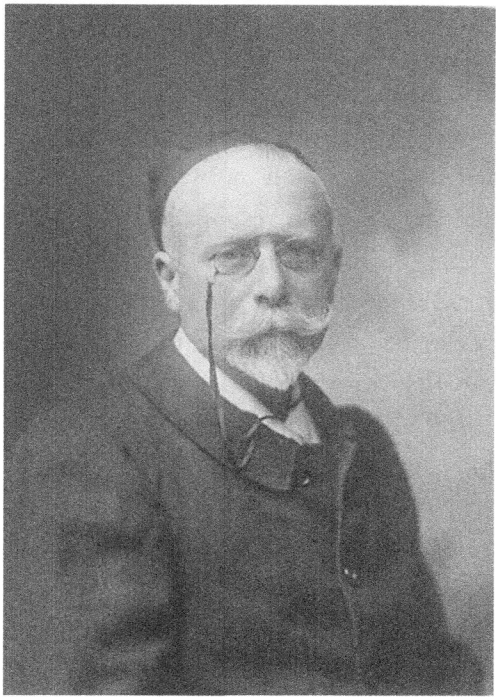

Figure 3.13 Raymond Sabouraud (1868–1938)
Coll. Musée hôpital Saint-louis, Paris.

Trichophyton, am God and there is none else," he stated. "The first problem we have to face is the uniqueness of trichophyton [. . .] This is the fundamental question."[66] His goal was first to "know if, in France, several parasitic agents could cause the trichophytic syndrome, if these parasites were only varieties of a single specie or if several species exist; and finally, if the affections caused by the different parasites had different prognosis."[67]

Sabouraud indicated that in any case the microscopic examination of infected hair was sufficient to make the diagnosis of the trichophytia the tinea belonged to, according to the size of the spores and their location inside or around the hair. In most cases (65%), the spores are small and contiguous, fill the hair, and form a sheath around it. In other cases (35%), the spores are bigger and never surround the hair. Sabouraud stressed that these obvious differences are linked with morphologic differences on the specific culture medium he invented (Sabouraud agar): "A large spore's hair will offer on culture medium an arid, floury aspect, never purely white. When cultivated, the small spores trichophytons will keep the aspect of a perfectly white down."

Sabouraud put an end to the uniqueness of the trichophytons and proved that human tinea is caused by two species of trichophytons: (1) *Trichophyton megalosporon*, often responsible for the ringworm in children (tinea tonsurans) but particularly of the beard trichophytia and of all the circinated trichophytia of the glabrous skin and (2) *Trichophyton microsporon*, responsible for most cases of tinea tonsurans in children. As noted later, "these works got a great echo in the dermatological community, because, for some unknown reasons, the uniqueness of the trichophytons was rooted in the dermatological mind worldwide."[68]

After Sabouraud's works, physicians realized that the microscopic fungi were more numerous than they thought and the identification of the fungi required professional expertise. Medical mycology became a matter for specialists. The creation of a laboratory exclusively devoted to cutaneous fungi mirrored the social anxiety caused by ringworm. In fact, Sabouraud tried to prove how unrealistic was the so-called benignity of tinea capitis: Although "they always heal spontaneously [. . .] these diseases are among the most fearsome of those afflicting our pediatric population." The disease was regarded as all the more worrying because it was "almost invisible to a non-trained eye." When the lesions are easily visible the disease is no longer an epidemic but has become endemic, he insisted.

Given this concern about public health, there was a new emphasis on prevention and screening for early symptoms. Physicians could not lead the fight on their own, and primary school teachers became ideal partners to broaden the battle against ringworm.

PHYSICIANS AND TEACHERS IN PRIMARY SCHOOLS: ACTORS FOR SCREENING AND PREVENTION

Created in 1836 on the initiative of Orfila, the dean of the Paris Faculty of Medicine, the principle of medical supervision of schoolchildren was put into practice in the beginning of the 1870s, when physicians set the elementary rules of school hygiene:

> Every morning when opening the school, the teacher has to inspect the cleanliness not only of the face and hands but particularly of the head and hair. The dirty children will be blamed so that the parents are well aware that the school is a place to respect [...] The inspection of the head requires a special attention; in case of a disease of the scalp, of a parasitic affection or of a general disease [e.g., tinea, impetigo, scrofula] the physician of the school will be visited.[69,70]

The March 28, 1882, law that made primary teaching mandatory reinforced the question of contagion in schools,[71] but the attitude of physicians toward the contagious patients was debated. Some of them declared unambiguously that these patients had to be neutralized:

> The law had to be to the advantage of the public interests against those of a single person[72] ... One has to protect oneself against [them], to consider [them] temporarily as manufacturer of dangerous items or as practicing an unhealthy activity.[73]

Sanitary regulations could even be justified by the "superior interest of the race."[74] In this respect, isolating the contagious patients seemed to be the more appropriate solution,[75] and many pavilions were erected in the Paris hospitals accordingly. By contrast, some other physicians argued the medical secret as a definite obstacle against the reporting of a contagious patient to the public authorities.[76]

Beside these questions, another one arose: Who should be in charge of the inspection of the children and allow or refuse school attendance? Because there were not enough practitioners to allow close examination of the children, a few physicians suggested that primary school teachers could be helpful to screen for the most frequent contagious diseases.[77] The *Hygienic and Medical Guide for the Primary School Teachers* stated:

The law that makes the primary instruction mandatory enforces a double duty on the administration: to instruct every child, to preserve their health against the dangers that may be the consequences of the teaching methods, of the fitting of the rooms, of the gathering of so many children in schools. France must obviously educate citizens aware of their rights and duties; but France must also produce robust men, fit for military service, capable of serving their country thanks to their cleverness and arms.[78]

In this respect the teachers' mission was not only educational but also patriotic. The guidebook listed the main symptoms of whooping cough, diphtheria, epilepsy, scabies, impetigo, pityriasis, and measles. As soon as favus or tinea tonsurans was diagnosed, "the child must be isolated in a separate room; any contact with the playmates must be avoided." A child afflicted with alopecia areata "may be tolerated in the classrooms provided his/her head is constantly covered with a cap."[79]

Charles Lailler, head of Saint-Louis, offered teachers elementary lessons about the hygiene of the hair:

Keeping the head naked [...]
   Giving preference to washable headdresses [...]
   Washing heads once a week in winter, more often in summer
   Every boy or girl should have his or her own hairbrush and comb that must be always clean [...]
   Every child previously afflicted with ringworm who is allowed to attend school will undergo a careful medical examination every second week.[80]

Lailler pleaded for "a medical certificate that guaranteed the child is cleared of any contagious disease [...] I wish no ringworm child could enter a school."[81,82] The Paris Commission for the hygienic inspection of the schools adopted Lailler's views and suggested that the children "will be recommended to have the hair short [...] Any case of abnormality on the scalp, any area of alopecia or crusted zone should be regarded as suspect. Consequently, the children will be dismissed from the school until a complete medical examination is performed."[83,84] However, despite the teaching efforts of the physicians and the involvement of some teachers, many observers deplored that "medical inspection, even limited to its prophylactic role against the spreading of disease, does not exist in France."[85]

There were not enough physicians to examine all the schoolchildren, and primary teachers had no sanitary qualifications, so why not establish a school in a hospital that would offer both sanitary and teaching expertise? The political, social, and biological context favored such a creation. The duration of the treatment required the interruption of schooling or even caused parents to reject the treatment,[86] so combining treatment and teaching seemed sensible. The Hôpital Saint-Louis was a suitable venue for meeting the ringworm children's educational and medical needs.

A SCHOOL FOR RINGWORM CHILDREN: SANITARY IMPROVEMENT OR MODEL FOR EXCLUSION?

The hygiene worries of the Conseil Municipal de Paris and the obligation for primary schooling led to the creation of the Ecole des Teigneux (or Ecole Lailler) in the Hôpital Saint-Louis:

> The administration and Doctor Lailler had the thought to create a department where the children would be admitted at the time they were supposed to go to school. [...] They would be looked after, treated, taught [...] all the day until the evening when their parents come back home.[87,88]

The school opened on August 4, 1886 (Figures 3.14–3.17).[89] The pupils entered the school through a door apart from the hospital's main gate. It was

> divided in two symmetrical parts, one for boys, the other for girls. [...] Nothing is luxurious, the rooms devoted to the medical activities are very small and badly lighted. [...] About 150 children, 100 boys and 50 girls, attend the school. They arrive very early at 6:30

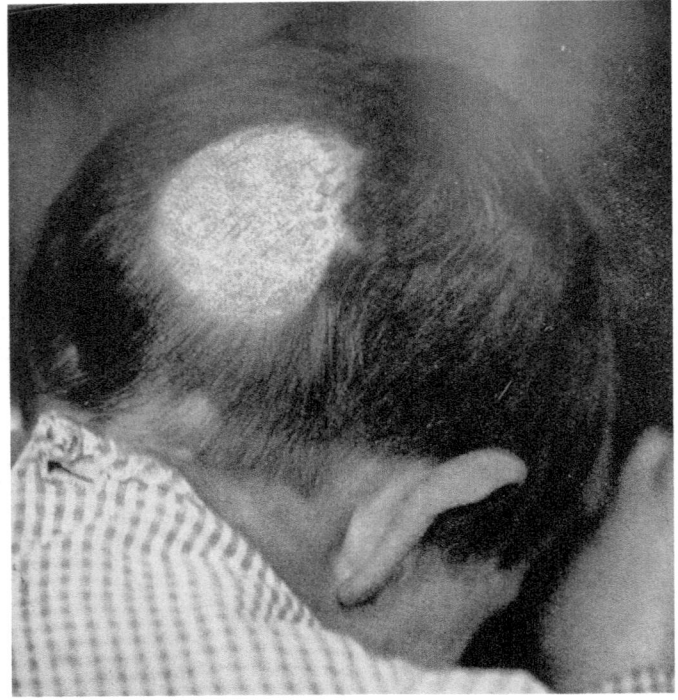

Figure 3.14 Ringworm
Sabouraud R (1936) Les teignes. In Darier J, Sabouraud R, Gougerot H, *Nouvelle Pratique Dermatologique*. Paris, Masson, p. 130.

a.m. or 7 a.m. [. . .] As soon as they come, the nurses wash their heads with antiseptic lotions. Then, they cover the heads with a large gauze that wraps the sick area. [. . .] All the medical procedures are done during the intervals between the times of teaching. The children are served three meals per day: at 8 a.m. a soup, at 11:30 a.m. a complete meal, at 4 p.m. an afternoon snack. Every week they have a bath. [. . .] The teaching took place from 9 to 11 a.m. and from 1 to 4 p.m. [. . .] The school is open every day, except Sunday, from 6 a.m. to 7 p.m.[90]

Roger-Milès, a writer naïvely fascinated by the school, described it as a place where the children, usually poor, found redemption thanks to care,

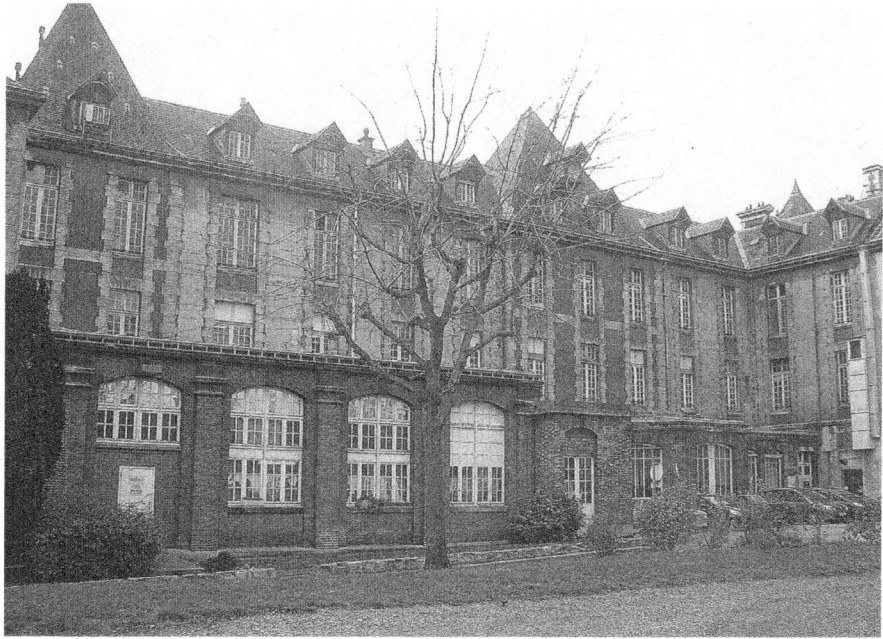

Figure 3.15 Lailler's School, outside view today
Coll. Dr Gérard Tilles.

hygiene, physical exercise, and teaching. Pain and privation seemed absent from their daily life:

> When arriving at school the children are hungry; they know they will be served a good soup in meticulously cleaned plates. When entering the school, they take off their clothes and headdresses [. . .] On the table, in the dining room, flowers, always flowers; happiness is required; open flowers symbolize cheerfulness and youth. [. . .] The doctor and the interns make their rounds. [. . .] The dressings are made carefully, scrubbing, washing, epilation, cutting hair very short with scissors. [. . .] The heads are wrapped with white linen. [. . .] The work may start. [. . .] The children are all happy, cared for, and beloved. [. . .] Listen to them playing! [. . .] When their bodies take exercise freely, when their mind is aroused to learn, how could

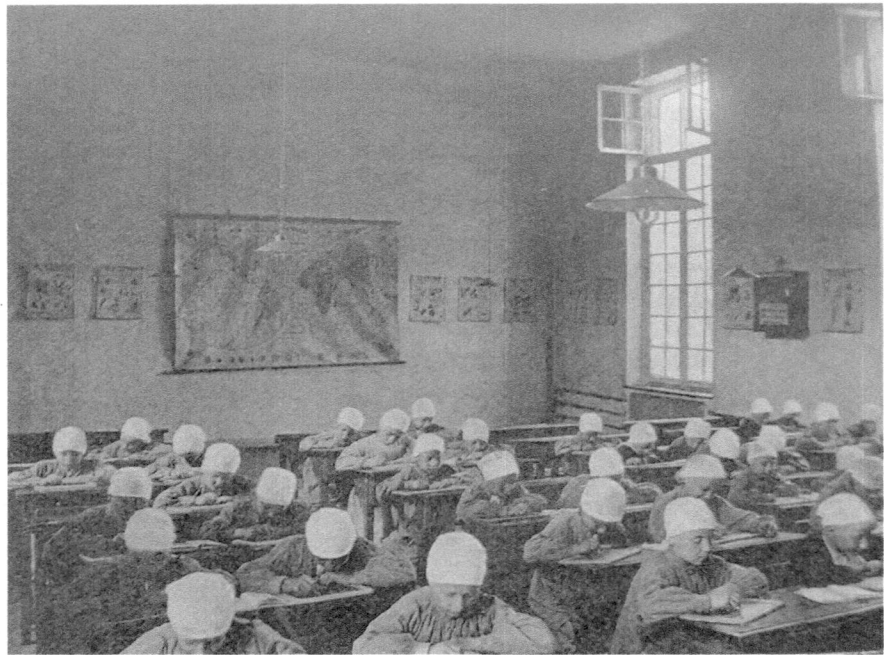

Figure 3.16 Classroom in Lailler's School
In: L'Assistance publique en 1900.

these children be suffering? The pain provoked by the treatment is rapidly fading thanks to the study and play.[91]

More realistically, however, a few years after the construction of the school the physicians did not share Roger-Milès' enthusiasm, objecting to the "awful condition" of the buildings: "They go to ruin; the walls and the ceilings are propped by beams. [. . .] We fear everything will collapse; we will be forced to close the school."[92] Despite these inconveniences, the number of children increased regularly: 66 on November 30, 1886; 94 on January 30, 1887; 163 in October 1888.[93]

In the 1890s, in addition to the Ecole des Teigneux, the department founded by Bazin (40 beds), and the outpatient dispensaries annexed to the medical departments in Saint-Louis, ringworm children could be treated in the Hôpital des Enfants-Malades (100 beds) and in the Hôpital Trousseau (36 beds for girls and 34 beds for boys). In this context about 200 young patients had to wait for several months to be treated.[94] To improve

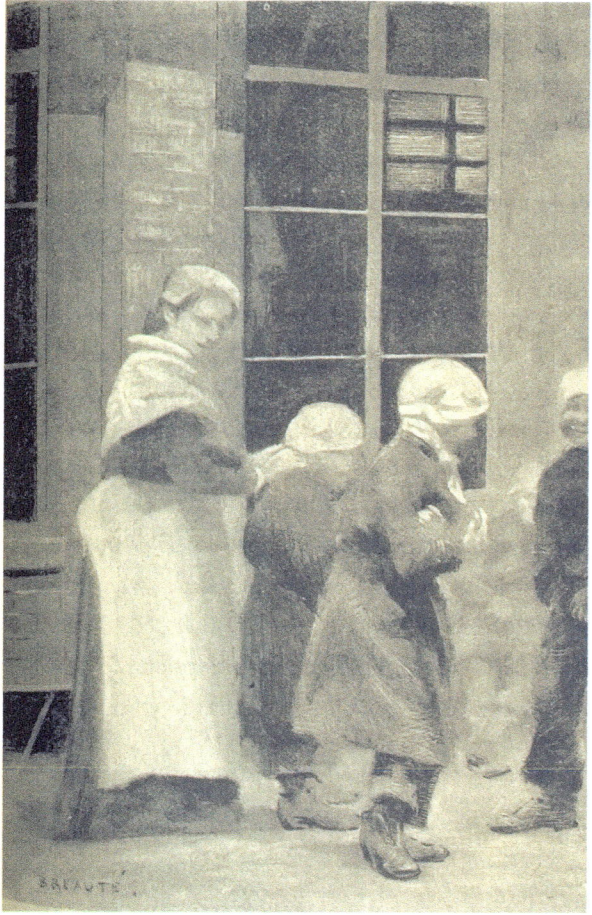

Figure 3.17 Ringworm children in Lailler's School
In: Roger-Milès L (nd) *La Cité de misère*, Marpon et Flammarion, Paris.

the situation, the Assistance publique and the Paris City Council on June 17, 1887, proposed building a ringworm hospital in Créteil in suburban Paris. The Créteil city council protested, fearing contagion, and the Paris city council decided on March 17, 1890, to build a special hospital for children with tinea in the outbuildings of the Hôpital Saint-Louis.[95] Opponents of the project, like Henri Feulard (1858–1897) and Butte, argued that it would be more useful to provide consultations for outpatients in several areas of the city. The waiting periods would be shorter and hospitalization would be restricted to only the most severe cases:

We suggest, before erecting an expensive hospital where only a small number of children will be treated, the treatments for outpatients are reorganized so that more children will be treated, the spreading of the disease will be prevented, and the number of hospitalizations will be reduced.[96,97]

Despite the small amount of opposition, the new school/hospital, "Central Hospital for Ringworm Children," opened at Saint-Louis on July 12, 1897. It was divided into two parts, with the "A" school exclusively devoted to children with tinea tonsurans. The epilation and dressing rooms, the classrooms, and the dining room were on the ground floor. The laboratory for the study and treatment of contagious skin and scalp diseases of childhood and adolescence was in the same section. The dormitories, located in the upper floors, could accommodate 147 boys and 60 girls. The "B" school, accommodating 40 boys and 23 girls, was devoted to children with favus and alopecia areata (pelade) (Figure 3.18); since the days of Gruby and Bazin this had been considered a special form of ringworm, so those afflicted were subject to isolation. In fact, according to the ministerial instructions:

These children will be separated in the classrooms and isolated during the recreation times [...] the immediate contacts will be avoided, the children will be required to keep their heads covered [...] Exchanging headdresses, as a usual cause of contagion, will be strictly prohibited. The toiletries and the bedding of the patients will remain personal.[98,99]

Lailler strongly objected to admitting children with alopecia areata to schools.

Every child was examined by the director of the laboratory (Quinquaud, then Sabouraud), who decided which school (A or B) the patient should be accommodated in. When close to being cured, the children were isolated from those who were still contagious. When cured, the children left

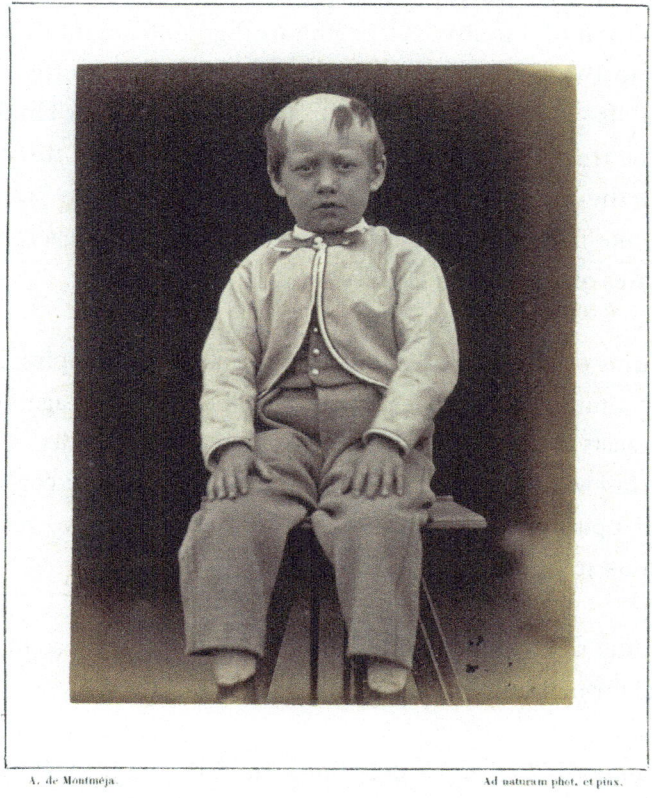

Figure 3.18 Alopecia areata
Hardy A, Montméja A de (1868) *Clinique photographique de l'hôpital Saint-Louis*. Chamerot et Lauwereyns, Paris

the school with a provisory certificate that allowed them to return to regular school. They were required to return to the Ecole Lailler's laboratory a month later. If the cure was considered certain, the children were given a non-contagion certificate. Nevertheless, stating that recovery was definite should be done only with extreme caution, the physicians stressed; medical supervision of the children for several weeks after the end of the treatment was recommended.

Even with the new school/hospital, the medical situation of the children remained unsatisfactory. In 1900, the waiting period for entrance remained around 7 months. According to Pignot, Sabouraud's assistant, from 1897 to 1900 about 10,000 ringworm children were treated in the Paris hospitals—three times more than 15 years earlier. The children who could not be treated in the Lailler School were directed to the provincial hospitals of the Assistance publique, far from Paris.[100]

Pignot, like his master, regarded ringworm as more severe than any other diseases of children:

> Ringworms of the scalp are more contagious than whooping cough, measles or mumps. Moreover, tinea cannot be vaccinated against: The measles lasts a fortnight, whooping cough three months, whereas ringworms will last for years. Several diseases are only contagious in the first part of their evolution; on the contrary, ringworms are as contagious at the end as at the beginning.[101]

Beyond the sanitary necessities, treating tinea capitis was highlighted as essential for maintaining the social order:

> What happen to these untreated ringworm children? [...] They roam. Six months later, their demoralization is complete. [...] During two years or more, these children are outlaws, without schooling, [...] at the age when a primary teacher is necessary [...] We owe them the cure, but one does not treat them; we owe them education, but one does not give it to them.[102]

Whatever the method, epilation or the use of various irritating tonics, it required several months to be efficient. The use of thallium acetate as a depilatory caused severe adverse effects, notably joint pains, drowsiness, irritability, loss of appetite, and albuminuria, which limited its use in children.[103,104,105] Physicians were therefore looking for a "dream solution" to the problem of ringworm.

X-RAYS: INNOVATIVE METHOD FOR A NEW SOCIAL CONSTRUCTION OF RINGWORM

On November 8, 1895, Wilhelm Conrad Roentgen, professor of physics at Würzburg University, discovered an unknown radiation he named "X-ray."[106] A few months later Oudin, Barthélémy, and Darier (Paris) reported about 40 cases of radiodermatitis (Oudin et Barthélémy themselves) in patients treated for various diseases (e.g., lupus, venous thrombosis, deafness).[107,108] In 1897 Leopold Freund (1868–1943) observed hair loss in a 5-year-old girl with a large hairy nevus on her back that had been irradiated 2 hours a day for 10 days.[109] In 1899, Balzer and Monsseaux (Paris) published "a generalized alopecia on every irradiated areas of the body."[110] At the 1900 World Congress of Dermatology in Paris, Schiff and Freund established the first therapeutic indications of x-rays. They focused on "skin diseases in which the hair loss is a major part of the healing."[111] In fact, for the majority of the authors the diseases of the pilosebaceous unit were the main targets.[112]

Unlike the previous painful, long, and restricting methods, radiotherapy promised a rapid, safe, and definitive cure of tinea capitis and was immediately welcomed enthusiastically. In 1902, Gastou and Vieira (Paris) reported the case of an adolescent

> afflicted with favus of the whole scalp. [. . .] He was first treated by the calotte then at the Lailler's School for 8 months by hair removal. Radiotherapy has started February 17, 1902 [. . .] Before the 15th session nothing happened except a slight headache. After the 15th session [. . .] a moderate erythema and edema appeared; the scalp became more sensitive. After the 24th session the hair loss began and a 10-centimeter alopecia occurred [. . .] The result has been therefore quite favourable and has provided the children with a rapid and innocuous effect as a consequence of our cautious method.[113]

In fact, however, the x-ray method was quite hazardous, given the narrow margin between therapeutic effect and cicatricial alopecia. The experimenters became inventors and biophysicists and created ingenious but imprecise devices.

A major actor in the fight against ringworm, Sabouraud praised radiotherapy as the perfect curative method, a *"solution rêvée."* Like Duclaux, Sabouraud conceived his campaign against "parasites" as a fight, following Darwin's thought, which he regarded as definitely " admirable"[114]: "There is no more evidenced cause of diseases but parasitic. Every disease is a duel between two species."[115] In this respect, fungi and microbes were no longer regarded as harmless plants but as enemies threatening the physical integrity of humans. Therefore, any weapon was allowed to win the battle.

Considering the results published by Freund and Schiff, in 1903 Sabouraud and his assistant Henri Noiré (1878–1937) built a new device— the Sabouraud–Noiré radiometer X—using disks of paper coated with barium platinocyanide that turned from green to brown under the influence of x-rays. A disk was placed in a holder between the radiation source and the area to be epilated. Then the color of the disk was compared with a standard brown pastille. When the color of both disks matched, the physician knew the amount of radiation was appropriate to ensure epilation without causing cicatricial alopecia. The technique was more accurate than those previously used (notably Holzknecht's), but reading the disk still required careful attention:[116] It had to be done in darkness to prevent the disc from turning back to green. In fact, in a few cases Sabouraud and Noiré "observed a definite alopecia; therefore [we] felt the method could be quite dangerous."[117]

After a careful examination of the ringworm child, Sabouraud considered two situations: Either the patches on the scalp were few, in which case they were irradiated at once, one after the other; or they were numerous, and manual hair removal of the whole scalp was mandatory prior to the irradiation. Every irradiated area was protected by a lead disc (Figures 3.19–3.24). Using such a method, it became possible to treat a complete head in a single session without any risk or adverse effect, "not even an ordinary headache." In terms of the neurotoxicity that had been suggested by a few authors, Sabouraud declared after treating more than 2,000 children in 5 years that the "action of X ray on the brain is nonexistent

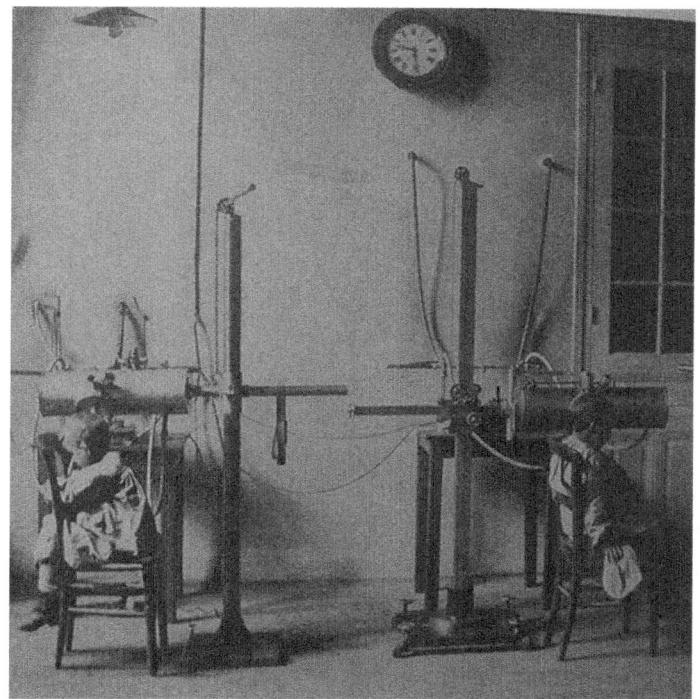

Figure 3.19 Radiotherapy room in the Laboratoire municipal at Saint-Louis
Sabouraud R, *Les teignes*, Paris, Masson, 1910, p. 779.

and should not be feared." In fact, for the physicians who regarded x-rays as a safe method, "the chief risk of the treatment is the danger of overexposure followed by dermatitis and incomplete regrowth of the hair," a risk that could be minimized if the physicians were properly trained.[118]

In fact, the x-rays did not destroy the fungi; they acted as a depilatory. So, after the irradiation, "during thirteen or fourteen days nothing will occur [. . .] But [on] the thirteenth or fourteenth day the hair will fall like those of a fur eaten by worms [. . .] however, the downy hair must remain." From the 18th day, the radiotherapy was completed by soaping and scrubbing the scalp, followed by the removal of the hair that fell out easily. The scalp was rubbed daily with iodine; on the 30th day, baldness was to occur. Four months later, the complete regrowth of new and healthy hair was expected.[119]

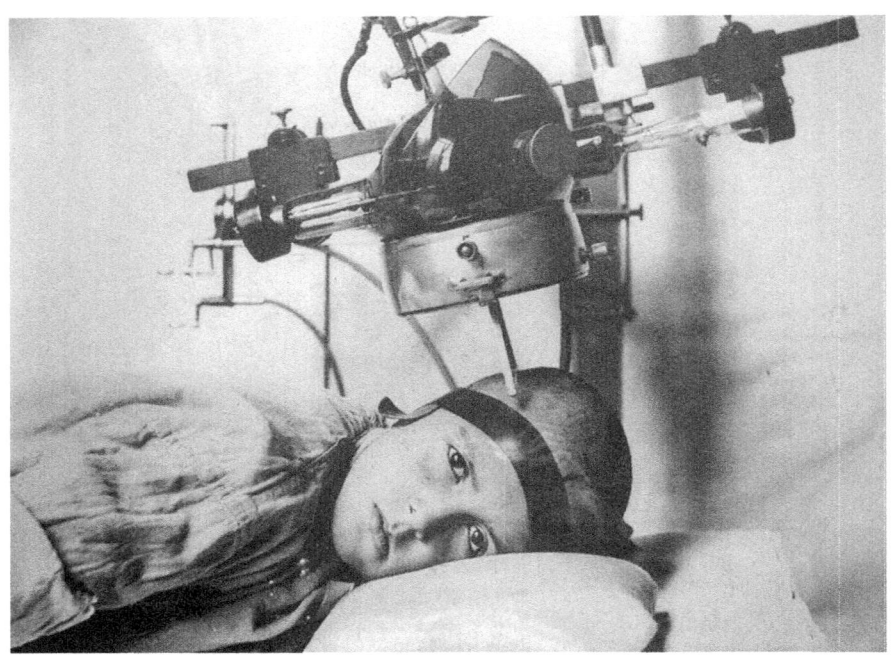

Figure 3.20 Radiotherapy of ringworm
Coll. musée photographique de l'hôpital Saint-Louis.

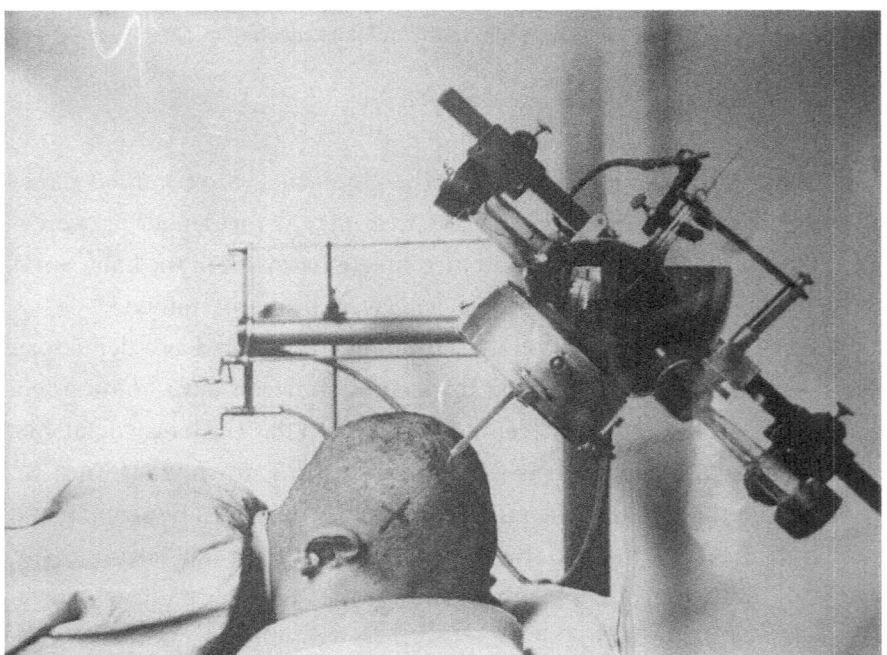

Figure 3.21 Radiotherapy of ringworm
Coll. musée photographique de l'hôpital Saint-Louis.

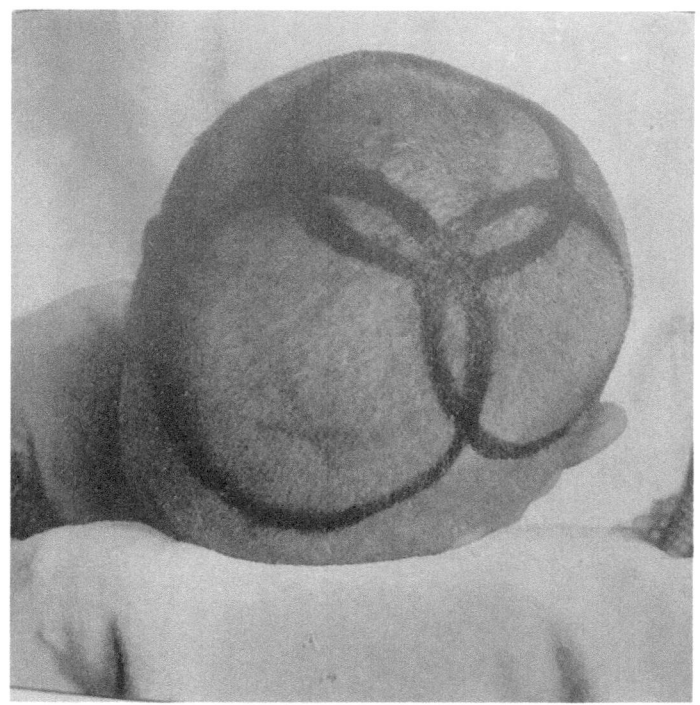

Figure 3.22 Sabouraud R (1910) *Les teignes.* Paris: Masson, p. 787.

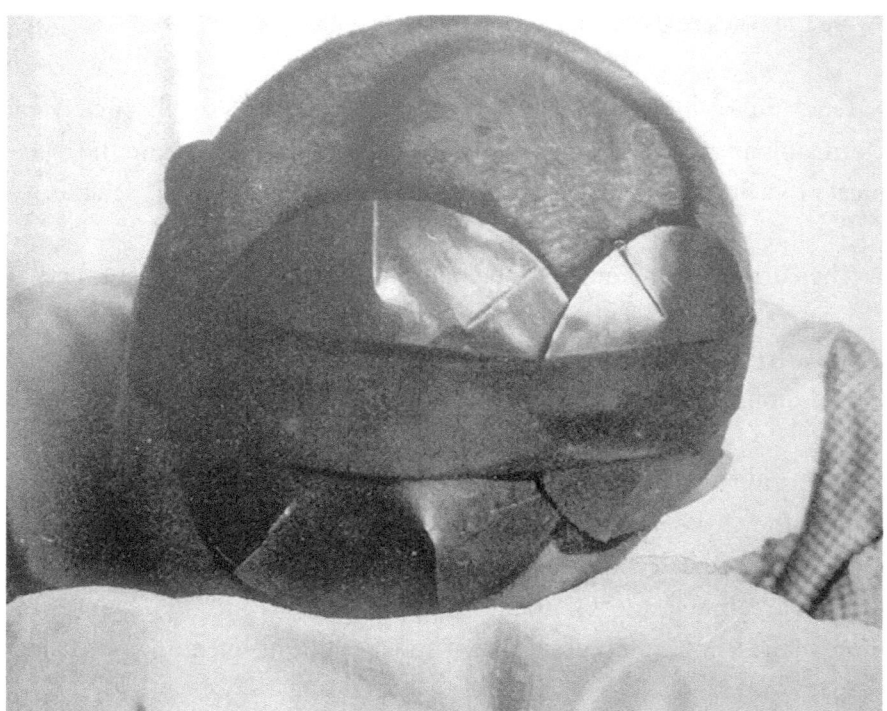

Figure 3.23 Sabouraud R (1910) *Les teignes.* Paris, Masson, 1910, p. 787.

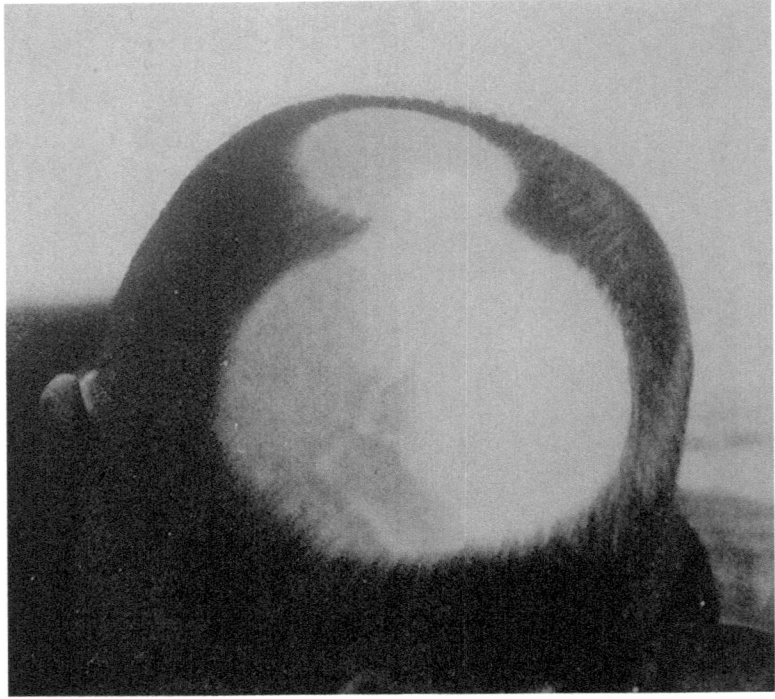

Figure 3.24 Sabouraud R (1910) *Les teignes*. Paris, Masson, 1910, p. 787.

On January 4, 1904, Sabouraud, lecturing at the French Society of Dermatology meeting, discussed the healing of 100 children and the technical procedure used to administer the x-rays safely in a single session:

> Thanks to radiotherapy, 8 to 10 children leave the Ecole Lailler every week; bald but healed, these children leave while waiting for the regrowth of healthy hair [. . .] in 6 months last year we got 57 healings; in 6 months this year we have 134 of them.[120]

"Contrasting with this new treatment," he stated, "the previous ones are as though they have never existed."[121] This new method brought a dramatic reduction in tinea capitis. Moreover, Sabouraud emphasized that thanks to x-ray treatment, the Assistance publique could reduce its expenses by more than 2.5 million francs.[122] The school became obsolete and was taken over by a department of pediatric surgery. Only the laboratory headed by Sabouraud remained active.

In 1909 Robert Kienböck and H.G. Adamson introduced a technique that distributed x-rays evenly on the hemisphere of the scalp by dividing the area into pie-shaped sections.[123] Dewulf, after treating 39 cases, reported on the incidence of accident or failure. According to him, the Kienböck–Adamson method was "absolutely without danger but has to be used with caution and accuracy and without haste."[124] Either method, Sabouraud's or Kienböck's, was used in Saint-Louis until the beginning of the 1950s.

Unlike the previous methods, x-ray epilation changed the medical and social face of tinea capitis. Removing infected hair with forceps or fingers became an anachronism. However, treating tinea capitis with x-rays—the same method used to treat cancers—involved devices with which the physicians had little experience and ignored the possible consequences. After the first reports of adverse effects on physicians, treating tinea capitis became a risky activity.[125,126] Consequently, x-rays provided ringworm children with a more rapid healing while worsening the medical and social face of ringworms.

To the best of our knowledge, Louis Brocq (1856–1928) (Figure 3.25) was the only physician in Saint-Louis to express reservations about the therapeutic use of x-rays for ringworm. He warned dermatologists that "they should be very careful when using this method until the specialists have clearly described the technique." Leredde (Paris) confirmed Brocq's cautious views: "Radiotherapy [cannot be] be regarded as a so easy method [. . .] and I even think it dangerous."[127] Brocq wrote:

> Is it reasonable to risk a cicatricial and definite alopecia to treat a disease that will spontaneously disappear without any alopecia when the child becomes a teenager? [. . .] If one considers the treatment of the ringworms of the scalp, one realizes that these affections have been dramatized. In the near future, the ringworm children will probably be treated by isolation in special schools, their hair cut short, their heads soaped and the lesions topically treated with

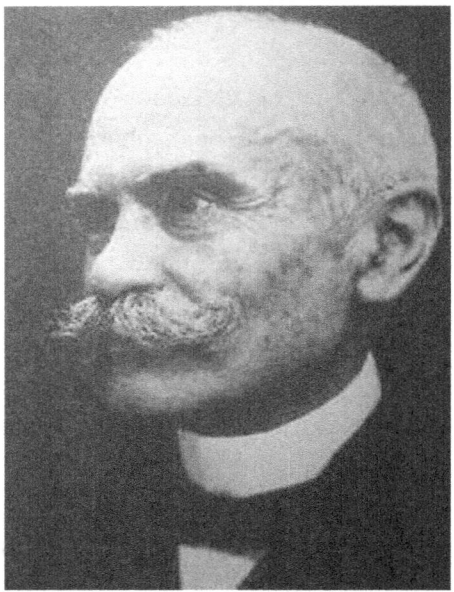

Figure 3.25 Louis Brocq (1856–1928)
Coll musée hôpital Saint-Louis, Paris.

iodine only without inflicting on children distressing and even dangerous methods to treat a disease that should spontaneously heal.

Noting the pressure physicians felt to use treatment methods out of proportion to the true severity of the disease, Brocq regretted that "we have to carry on treating the ringworm children and using X-rays."[128]

In France, the first reports on cutaneous malignancies occurring after radiotherapy for tinea capitis were published in the 1950s.[129] In 1960, Levy-Lebhar published his results on 18,000 children treated by x-rays, some of them under general anesthesia. According to him, the percentage of healing increased from 60% in 1950 up to almost 100% in 1959 without any adverse effects. The author suggested that the discovery of griseofulvin in 1938 (the first clinical trials were published 20 years later) would limit the use of radiotherapy to cases resistant to this new drug.[130] In fact, griseofulvin became the definitive treatment for ringworm.[131,132] In 1960, Degos, a leading authority in dermatology, enthusiastically asserted that griseofulvin was the expected, efficient, and safe treatment of tinea. The therapeutic results, he concluded, "are striking [. . .] Griseofulvin makes useless the hair removal by X-rays and guarantees the quick healing of favus."[133] After centuries of aggressive and hazardous methods imposed on ringworm children, griseofulvin, a safe and efficient treatment, had become the true *solution rêvée* for the disease.

ACKNOWLEDGMENTS

The Henri-Feulard Library and the Wax Moulages Museum at the Hôpital Saint-Louis; Mathieu de Brunhoff, MD, Sabouraud's grandson; the archives department and library of the Pasteur Institute (Paris); and the archives department of the Assistance publique–Hôpitaux de Paris.

NOTES

1. Règlement pour l'admission dans les hospices de maladies (an X). A Paris de l'Imprimerie des Sourds-Muets, p. 6.
2. Reading dermatology treatises published in the early 19th century shows how dermatologic nomenclature was confused. For instance, in London, Bateman described "ringworm of the scalp" in the chapter devoted to "porrigo," in which elementary lesions were pustules named "favi." Bateman T (1817) *A practical treatise of cutaneous diseases*. London: Longman, Hurst, Rees and Brown, p. 159. In the French literature, "favus" was a clinical form of "teigne." The English word "ringworm" could be translated into French as "teigne du cuir chevelu" or "herpes circiné" of the glabrous skin. In fact, before the pre-laboratory era, only favus was easily clinically identifiable and not confused with any other skin disease.
3. The Hôpital Saint-Louis was founded in 1607 under the reign of Henri IV. It was initially devoted to patients afflicted with plague and was named after Louis IX, who may have died from this disease and was sanctified as St. Louis. As the revolutionary actors rejected all symbols that recalled royalty, the hospital's name was changed to Hospice du Nord, as it was located in the north of Paris.
4. For an in-depth account on the history of the Hôpital Saint-Louis see: Tilles G (2002) *L'hôpital Saint-Louis in Dermatology in France under the supervision of Daniel Wallach and Gérard Tilles*. Toulouse: Privat, pp. 381–458; Schnitzler L (2002) *La dermatologie à l'hôpital Saint-Louis de 1945 à nos jours in Dermatology in France under the supervision of Daniel Wallach and Gérard Tilles*. Toulouse: Privat, pp. 459–491. Online: http://www.bium.univ-paris5.fr/histmed/medica/cote?extwa ll00001.

5. Jean-Louis Alibert was the first dermatologist of the Hôpital Saint-Louis. Lecturing on dermatology sometimes in the open air, he attracted physicians and students and founded the French School of Dermatology. The "Tree of Dermatosis" he created to illustrate his views on the classification of dermatoses symbolized the birth of dermatology in Paris.
6. Alibert JL (1832) *Monographie des dermatoses ou précis théorique et pratique des maladies de la peau* (1st ed.). Paris: Daynac, p. 309.
7. Bazin E (1853) *Recherches sur la nature et le traitement des teignes*. Paris: Poussielgue, p. 78.
8. Alibert, 1832, p. 476.
9. Alibert JL (1835) *Monographie des dermatoses ou précis théorique et pratique des maladies de la peau* (2nd ed., Vol. 1). Paris: Germer Baillière.
10. Favus as other oozing dermatoses was supposed to provide the patient with a natural way to evacuate the so-called bad humors. In this respect, any treatment that stops the oozing was regarded as possibly deleterious and must be accompanied by the creation by the physician of other ways-out on the skin. Rayer PFO (1835) *Traité théorique et pratique des maladies de la peau* (2nd ed., Vol. 1). Paris: JB Baillière, pp. 719–720.
11. Gibert CM (1860) *Traité pratique des maladies de la peau*. Paris: Plon, p. 345.
12. As there was no biological evidence of the mycotic origin of these diseases, one can hypothesize that not only true mycoses of the scalp were treated by the calotte.
13. Alibert, 1835, p. 301.
14. Mahon jeune (1829) *Recherches sur la nature et le traitement des teignes*. Paris: Baillière; Crissey JT, Parish LC (1981) *Dermatology and syphilology of the 19th century*. New York: Praeger, pp. 99–100.
15. Richerand A (1815) *Nosographie chirurgicale* (Vol. 1). Paris: Caille et Ravier, p. 270.
16. *Ancien régime* designates the period that preceded the fall of the French royalty; that is, before the 1790s.
17. Tenon (1788) *Mémoires sur les hôpitaux de Paris*. Paris: Ph-D Pierres, pp. 74–75.
18. Académie de Médecine, Commission des remèdes secrets SRM 102 d.39 n°1 (no date, probably circa 1800).
19. Pariset (1828) Rapport de l'Académie de Médecine adressé à M. le Ministre de l'Intérieur, 1er juillet 1828. In Mahon jeune (1868) *Considérations sur le traitement des teignes*. Paris: Baillière, p. 5.
20. Mahon jeune (1829) *Recherches sur le siège et la nature des teignes*. Paris: Baillière, p. 371. Mahon the younger died in 1833. The elder retired circa 1835. They were replaced by their sons-in-law Vaconsin and Swinger, painter of the plates printed in the 1829 Mahon treatise. Swinger died in 1852; he was replaced by the grandson of Mahon the younger, Mignot-Mahon, and Guilbert, second son-in-law of Mahon the elder!
21. Rayer PFO (1835) *Traité des maladies de la peau* (Vol. 1). Paris: Baillière, p. 714
22. The Mahon family was active in Hôpital Saint-Antoine (1844), Hôpital Sainte-Eugénie (1853), and Hôpital Beaujon (1844).
23. Feulard H (1894) Le traitement des teignes à Paris. *Rev Hyg* XVI, 6: 3–15.
24. Arrêté du Conseil général des hospices, 7 juin 1810, n° 9401, Archives de l'Assistance publique.

25. Pariset, in Mahon jeune (1868), pp. 6–7.
26. The Mahon brothers treated only children afflicted with favus, the diagnosis being made by a surgeon named Richard.Richard (1839) *Traité pratique des maladies des enfants*. Paris: Baillière.
27. The surgeon in charge of certifying the definitive cure was Achille Cléophas Flaubert, father of the writer Gustave Flaubert. Feltgen K (2011) Le remède secret des frères Mahon. Quand les médecins abandonnaient la prise en charge hospitalière des teigneux à une famille d'empiriques. *Rev Soc Fran Hist Hop* 141:8–20.
28. Registre des délibérations des hospices civils de Rouen, quoted in Feltgen (2011).
29. Feltgen K (2012) *Histoire de la prise en charge des enfants teigneux dans les hôpitaux rouennais*. Mémoire de la protection sociale en Normandie (to be published).
30. Arnaud F (1888) *Les teignes à Marseille. Notes historiques et statistiques*. Marseille: Barlatier-Freyssat, p. 10.
31. Cazenave PLA (1843) Porrigo decalvans et herpes tonsurans. *Ann Mal Peau Syph* 37–44.
32. Cazenave PLA (1873) *Bibliothèque médicale*. Paris: Delahaye.
33. Cazenave PLA, Schédel HE (1848) *Abrégé pratique des maladies de la peau* (4th ed.). Paris: Labé, pp. 324–325 (translated by G. Tilles).
34. Bazin (1853), p. 11 (translated by G. Tilles).
35. Bazin (1853), p. 78.
36. *Pelade* was previously used in the 16th and 17th centuries to name the syphilitic alopecia.
37. Bazin (1853).
38. Plumbe S (1837) *A practical treatise on diseases of the skin*. London: Underwood, p. 163.
39. Bazin (1853), pp. 76, 83, 92.
40. Bazin E (1858) *Leçons théoriques et cliniques sur les affections cutanées parasitaires*. Paris: Delahaye, Chamerot, pp. 134–135 (translated by G. Tilles).
41. Lailler C (1878) *Leçons cliniques sur les teignes faites à l'hôpital Saint-Louis*. Paris: Delahaye, pp. 53–55 (translated by G. Tilles).
42. Bazin (1858), pp. 189, 192.
43. Bergeron considered that more than 12,000 children were afflicted by tinea of the scalp in the 1860s in France. Bergeron EJ (1865) Etude sur la géographie et la prophylaxie des teignes. *Ann Hyg Pub Med Leg* 2, 23: 5–50.
44. Rapport sur le traitement des teignes à l'hôpital Saint-Louis pendant le cours des années 1852, 1853 et 1854 par le docteur Bazin, Médecin de l'hôpital Saint-Louis, Imp de Simonet-Delaguette, juin 1854.
45. Feulard H (1886) *Teignes et teigneux. Histoire médicale, hygiène publique*. Thèse pour le doctorat en médecine. Paris: G Steinheil, p. 168.
46. Outside Paris, the Bazin model inspired similar medical departments. In Rouen the physician Jules Hélot was appointed in 1853 to treat the ringworm children and put an end to the Mahon treatment. Feltgen (2012).
47. In Marseille the hospital administrators considered the previous method as anachronistic and decided to establish the Bazin method, headed by physicians, from 1857. Arnaud, pp. 26–29.

48. Quoted in Feulard H (1888) *Teignes et teigneux. Histoire médicale. Hygiène publique.* Thèse pour le doctorat en médecine. Paris, p. 154
49. Butte L (1890) *Du trichophyton. Des dermatoses trichophytiques.* In Congrès international de dermatologie et de syphiligraphie tenu à Paris en 1889. Paris: G. Masson, pp. 193–195.
50. Quinquaud E (1890) *Du trichophyton. Des dermatoses trichophytiques.* In Congrès international de dermatologie et de syphiligraphie tenu à Paris en 1889. Paris: G. Masson, pp. 195–197.
51. Quinquaud (1890), pp. 197–212.
52. Darier J (1935) *Historique de la dermatologie pendant les cinquante dernières années.* In Deliberationes Congressus dermatologorum internationalis IX-I, Budapestini, pp. 29–47 (translated by G. Tilles).
53. Léonard J (1981) *La médecine entre les savoirs et les pouvoirs.* Paris: Aubier, pp. 243–258.
54. Léonard J (1986) Comment peut-on être pastorien? In Salomon-Bayet C. *Pasteur et la révolution pastorienne.* Paris: Payot, pp. 145–179.
55. Rapport au nom de la 5ème commission sur la répartition des subventions aux laboratoires de bactériologie et de radiographie, aux bibliothèques et à l'attribution de bourses de voyage présenté par M. d'Andigné, conseiller municipal, Conseil Municipal de Paris, 1908, p. 3.
56. Duclaux E (1886) *Le microbe et la maladie.* Paris: Masson, p. 18 (translated by G. Tilles).
57. Prègre J (1972) *Sabouraud en son temps.* Thèse pour le doctorat en médecine, Paris.
58. Tilles G (2008) *Teignes et teigneux. Histoire médicale et sociale.* Paris: Springer.
59. Sabouraud R (1936). Mes hôpit*aux*. Archives de l'Institut Pasteur, SAB 1–4. The Pasteur Institute was founded in 1888 in Paris.
60. Sabouraud R (1933) *Pêle-Mêle. Regards en moi et autour de moi.* Paris: Plon, pp. 53–55.
61. Thibierge G (1925) Notes sur les successeurs de Bazin à l'hôpital Saint-Louis, Charles Lailler, Emile Vidal, Ernest Besnier. *Bull Soc Hist Med* XIX, 5–6, p. 129–144.
62. Création d'un laboratoire dans le service de M. le docteur Besnier, Procès-Verbal du conseil de surveillance de l'Assistance publique, séance du 7 décembre 1893.
63. Pignot M (1900) *Etude clinique des teignes. Hygiène publique et prophylaxie des teignes tondantes en 1900 à Paris et dans sa banlieue.* Paris: Steinheil.
64. Sabouraud (1936).
65. Sabouraud R (1910) *Les teignes.* Paris: Masson.
66. Sabouraud R (1894) *Les trichophyties humaines.* Thèse pour doctorat en médecine, Paris, p. 3
67. Sabouraud R (1892) Contribution à l'étude de la trichophytie humaine. *Ann Dermatol Syphil* III: 1061–1087 (translated by G. Tilles).
68. Pautrier LM (1938) Raimond Sabouraud. *Ann Dermatol Syphil* 276–297.
69. Riant A (1874) *Hygiène scolaire.* Paris: Hachette, pp. 182–183 (translated by G. Tilles).
70. In Paris, a sanitary rule dating from June 13, 1879, made it clear that every school had to be visited twice a month and the children examined every month. Quoted

in Mangenot (1887) De l'inspection hygiénique et médicale des écoles en France. *Rev Hyg Police sanitaire* 9: 299–314 (translated by G. Tilles).
71. On March 28, 1882, Jules Ferry, minister of the Public Instruction, originated a seminal law under which primary instruction was mandatory and free for all children of both genders from 6 to 13.
72. Widal F (1909) Mesures à prendre contre les maladies épidémiques. Déclaration obligatoire des maladies contagieuses. Résultats obtenus depuis la loi du 15 février 1902. *Ann Hyg Pub Med Leg* 4, 12: 245–264 (translated by G. Tilles).
73. Duclaux E (1902) L'hygiène sociale. In Guillaume P (1996) Le rôle social du médecin depuis deux siècles (1800–1945). Paris: Association pour l'étude de la sécurité sociale, p. 100 (translated by G. Tilles).
74. Brouardel P, Mosny E (1905) Evolution et tendance de l'hygiène contemporaine. *Ann Hyg Pub Med légale* 4: 534–535 (translated by G. Tilles).
75. Nonnis Vigilante S (2005) La construction sociale du malade contagieux. Enjeux scientifiques, politiques et culturels (19ème–20ème siècles). In *Corps, santé, société sous la direction d'Elisabeth Delmas et de Marie-José Michel*. Paris: Nolin, pp. 92–112.
76. Under the November 30, 1892, law, physicians had to report infected patients to the sanitary authorities. For 13 diseases, reporting was mandatory; for nine others, it was optional. Tinea was on the second list, along with with leprosy and tuberculosis, due to the influence of the physicians concerned about the protection of the medical secret. Carvais R (1986) La maladie, la loi et les mœurs. In Salomon-Bayet C, *Pasteur et la révolution pastorienne*. Paris: Payot, pp. 281–330.
77. Du Mesnil O (1880) De la surveillance médicale des écoles. *Ann Hyg Pub Med légale* 3, 3: 76–92.
78. Between 1831 and 1849, 730 men would have been exempted from their military duties yearly due to tinea capitis. Bergeron EJ (1865) Etude sur la géographie et la prophylaxie des teignes. *Ann Hyg Pub Med légale* 2, 23: 5–50.
79. Delvalle, Breucq A (1892) *Guide hygiénique et médical de l'instituteur*. Paris: Librairie classique Fernand Nathan, pp. 5, 8, 9, 57 (translated by G. Tilles).
80. Lailler (1885), *Rev Hyg*, p. 580, quoted in Feulard (1886) (translated by G. Tilles).
81. Lailler (1878), p. 59.
82. In London, Tilbury Fox expressed the same concerns with similar words: "I do not understand that a school is properly managed unless every child admitted is shown to be free from ringworm of the head (tinea tonsurans) and ringworm of the body (tinea circinata) either as certified by a medical practitioner or by a careful examination at the time of admission by some competent person. [. . .] Every week at least, a careful examination of heads should be made in schools." Tilbury Fox W (1873) *Skin Diseases. Their Description, Pathology, Diagnosis and Treatment* (3rd ed.). London: Henry Renshaw, pp. 442–443.
83. L'inspection hygiénique et médicale des écoles. Réorganisation du service (1888). Paris: Imp. Municipale.
84. In contrast, some physicians disagreed with the exclusion of the ringworm children from school. Arnaud, physician in charge of these children in the Marseille hospitals, stressed how useless such an attitude was: "Once the scalp is covered with a plaster and a special cap the child must always keep, there is no danger of

contagion and the child may socialize with mates either in classes or dormitories." Arnaud (1888), p. 33 (translated by G. Tilles). In 1893 the Minister of Public Instruction issued a warning against the rejection of schooling for contagious children, arguing that it could promote the disease in the population instead of restricting it. Hygiène des écoles (1893). *Ann Hyg Pub Med légale* 3, 29: 569–573.

85. Mosny E (1903) Buts de l'inspection médicale hygiénique des écoles publiques et privées. *Ann Hyg Pub Med légale* 3, 50: 313–336 (translated by G. Tilles).
86. From 1869 to 1885, 938 cases of favus, 2,385 cases of tinea tonsurans, and 614 cases of pelades (porrigo decalvans) were treated in Saint-Louis as outpatients, only a quarter of them on a regular basis.
87. Création à l'hôpital Saint-Louis d'un traitement externe avec demi-pensionnat pour les enfants atteints de la teigne (25 février 1886). Procès-verbal du Conseil de surveillance de l'Assistance publique à Paris, pp. 306–312 (translated by G. Tilles).
88. Mathieu A (1893) Charles Lailler. *Ann Dermatol Syphil* IV: 1101–1108; Le docteur Lailler, médecin de l'hôpital Saint-Louis (1822–1893). Bibliothèque Henri-Feulard, Hôpital Saint-Louis, Paris, cote Mb 43.
89. By administrative decision dated January 4, 1894, the school was officially named Ecole Lailler. The inscription is still visible above the school's main entrance. Attribution du nom de Lailler à l'école des teigneux de l'hôpital Saint-Louis (4 janvier 1894). Procès verbal des séances du conseil de surveillance de l'Assistance publique.
90. Carrère J-C (1890) *Etude sur le traitement de la teigne tondante. Résultats obtenus à l'école des teigneux de l'hôpital Saint-Louis*. Paris: Steinheil, p. 26 (translated by G. Tilles).
91. Roger-Milès L (n.d.) *La Cité de misère*. Paris: Marpon et Flammarion, pp. 169–181 (translated by G. Tilles).
92. Butte L (1891) *La teigne à Paris. Les hôpitaux et les écoles de teigneux*. Paris: Publications de la Policlinique de Paris, p. 7.
93. A similar school was created in 1896 in Rouen. Construction d'un pavillon pour les teigneux par décision du 26 février 1896. Compte moral des hospices de Rouen pour 1896.
94. Feulard (1886), pp. 206–207.
95. Hôpital Saint-Louis création d'un hôpital école de teigneux (1er février 1894). Procès-verbal du Conseil de surveillance de l'Assistance publique.
96. Feulard H (1894) Le traitement des teigneux à Paris. *Rev Hyg* XVI: 510–522 (translated by G. Tilles).
97. Feulard (1886).
98. Circulaire relative aux mesures préventives à prendre contre la contagion de la pelade adressée au Recteur par le Ministre de l'Instruction publique (10 octobre 1888). Archives de l'Assistance publique cote B-2652.
99. The supposed contagiousness of alopecia areata allowed the young afflicted adults to be exempted from military service. Feulard H (1893) Le favus et la pelade en France (1887–1892). II. Internationaler Dermatologischer Congress abgehalten in Wien im Jahre 1892, pp. 393–412.

100. Pignot (1900).
101. Ibid. (translated by G. Tilles).
102. Sabouraud R (1895) *Diagnostic et traitement de la pelade et des teignes de l'enfant*. Paris: Rueff, pp. 71–91.
103. Louste M, Rabut R (1934) L'acétate de thallium dans les traitement des teignes à l'école Lailler. *Bull Soc Fr Dermatol Syphil*, pp. 494–496.
104. Dowling GB (1927) The treatment of ringworm of the scalp by thallium depilation. *Br Med J*, pp. 261–263.
105. Still used in the 1950s, thallium acetate failed in more than 50% of cases to cure tinea of the scalp. Some authors considered it as an alternative treatment where x-rays were not available or had failed. Bureau Y, Jarry, Barrière (1957) L'acétate de thallium dans le traitement des teignes scolaires (résultats obtenus à la clinique dermatologique de Nantes). *Bull Soc Fr Dermatol Syphil* 64: 105–106.
106. Pallardy G (1998) Röntgen et sa découverte des rayons X. Les premières applications en France (1896–1914) In: *Les rayons de la vie, une histoire des applications s médicales des rayons X et de la radioactivité en France 1895–1930*. Institut Curie, pp. 22–36.
107. Oudin P, Barthélémy T, Darier J (1898) Accidents cutanés et viscéraux consécutifs à l'emploi des rayons X. *La France Médicale* 8: 113–118.
108. Richer P, Londe A (1897) Sur des cas d'érythème radiographique des mains. *CR Acad Sci* CXXIV: 1256–1257.
109. Freund L (1897) Ein mit Röntgenstrahlen behandelter Fall von Naevus pigmentosus piliferus. *Wiener Med Wochschrft* XLVII: 428–434.
110. Balzer F, Monsseaux (1899) Accidents cutanés causés par les rayons de Röntgen. *Bull Soc Fr Dermatol Syphil*, pp. 3–8.
111. Schiff E, Freund L (1900) Etat actuel de la radiothérapie. In: *4ème Congrès international de dermatologie*, Paris, pp. 173–177.
112. Belot J (1904) *La radiothérapie. Son application aux affections cutanées*. Paris: G. Steinheil.
113. Gastou P, Vieira P (1902) Essai de traitement des dermatoses par la radiothérapie; cas de favus soumis aux rayons X (dépilation et repousse). *Bull Soc Fr Dermatol Syphil*, pp. 283–285 (translated by G. Tilles).
114. Sabouraud: letter to his father, no date (probably in the 1890s), Coll. Dr M. de Brunhoff.
115. Sabouraud (1894), pp. VIII–X.
116. Sabouraud (1936), *Mes hôpitaux*.
117. Sabouraud R (1937) Henri Noiré (1878–1937). *Ann Dermatol Syphil*, pp. 811–812.
118. McLeod JMH (1928) An address on ringworm and its treatment. *Br Med J*, pp. 656–659.
119. Sabouraud (1910) *Les teignes*, p. 787.
120. Sabouraud R (1904) Sur la radiothérapie des teignes, *Ann Dermatol Syphil* 5: 577–587.
121. Sabouraud R (1936) Les teignes. In: Darier F, Sabouraud R, Gougerot H, et al. *Nouvelle Pratique Dermatologique* (Vol. II). Paris: Masson, pp. 202–203.

122. Sabouraud R, Pignot M, Noiré H (1905) La radiothérapie des teignes à l'Ecole Lailler en 1904. *Bull Soc Fr Dermatol Syphil*, pp. 19–23.
123. Adamson HG (1909) A simplified method of X-ray application for the cure of ringworm of the scalp. *Lancet*, p. 1379.
124. Dewulf L (1953) Le traitement par rayons X des mycoses du cuir chevelu et de la barbe. *Arch Belges Dermatol* 9, 12: 155–165.
125. Noiré, Sabouraud's assistant, was described as "a gadget-minded physician with marvellously dexterous fingers." He died of squamous cell carcinoma. Crissey JT, Parish LC (1981) *The Dermatology and Syphilology of the 19th Century*. New York: Praeger, p. 245.
126. Hayter emphasized the fact that radiotherapy restored physicians' threatened sense of identity as healers. Consequently they received renewed authority and greater adulation from the patients. Hayter CRR (1998) The clinic as laboratory: The case of radiation therapy, 1896–1920. *Bull Hist Med* 72: 663–688.
127. Leredde M (1904) Technique et indications de la radiothérapie. *Bull Soc Fr Dermatol Syphil* 5: 153–159.
128. Brocq L (1917) Quelques réflexions pratiques sur la radiothérapie. *Ann Dermatol Syphilol*, pp. 333–356.
129. Nanta P (1953) Epithélioma après épilation radiothérapique pour teigne. *Bull Soc Fr Dermatol Syphil*, p. 200. To the best of our knowledge no follow-up or retrospective study was performed on the children irradiated at the Saint-Louis hospital.
130. Levy-Lebhar G, Levy-Lebhart JP (1960) Rœntgen épilation du cuir chevelu dans le traitement des teignes. Conclusions après 18 000 irradiations dans une collectivité d'enfants marocains. *Maroc Med* 39, 82–84.
131. Oxford AE, Raistrick H, Simonart P (1939) Studies in the biochemistry of microorganisms LX Griseofulvin C17 H17 O6 Cl, a metabolic product of Penicillium griseofulvium Dierckx. *Biochem J* 33: 240–248.
132. Williams DI, Marten RH, Sarkany I (1958) Oral treatment of ringworm with griseofulvin. *Lancet* 2: 1212–1213.
133. Degos R, Rivalier E, Lefort P (1960) La griséofulvine. *Ann Dermatol Syphil* 87: 121–144.

4

Ringworm

A disease of schools and mass schooling in the United Kingdom

AYA HOMEI AND MICHAEL WORBOYS

Education is an almost universally recognized "good" across histories of the modern world, with more and better-quality schooling seen as a progressive social reform and a marker of a modern, civilized society.[1] However, the introduction of mass schooling in Britain and America was the product of a social and political struggle that was not easily won.[2] Few disagreed that education improved the minds of pupils, but many people argued that it was not always good for their bodies; indeed, schools became great centers of contagion. Epidemics of major childhood infections such as measles, diphtheria, and chickenpox periodically affected institutions and in some cases led to school closures.[3] Less recognized then, as now, was that schools were sites of exchange of endemic, social diseases, ranging from serious, typically fatal infections such as tuberculosis to endemic conditions such as ringworm, which had mild symptoms but carried severe social stigma. The term *ringworm* is very old and comes from the circular patches of peeled, inflamed skin that characterize the infection. In medicine, at least, no one understood it to be associated with worms of any description.

In the early part of the 19th century, ringworm was well recognized by doctors and the public as an inflammation of the scalp, associated with reddening of the skin, itching, and circles of peeling skin and hair loss. In children it was also popularly known as *scald-head*, a term derived from "scaled" and "scabby" rather than burns, and in medicine as a form of porrigo—skin complaints associated with the production of pustules. The naming and classification of skin diseases had been hugely contested from the 1790s until the publication of a system proposed by the English physician Robert Willan, who worked at the Carey Street Public Dispensary in London.[4] However, by the 1830s, when serious medical attention first focused on ringworm, the debate was between those who saw the condition as localized in the skin and those who also looked to constitutional, internal factors. Both sides agreed that it was contagious and prevalent in children, especially the poor, who lived in crowded conditions and in orphanages, boarding schools, and other institutions. The exciting cause was mostly talked about as a "fungus," but susceptibility was explained in terms of the child having immature skin, a weak general constitution, dirty skin, poor hygiene, or all of these.

The role of "seed and soil" in the causes, pathology, treatment, and prevention of ringworm was debated throughout the 19th century and beyond. In this chapter, we tell the story of how and why the understanding on the part of doctors and the public about the nature of ringworm changed in the period from 1830 to 1910, focusing on the disease in schoolchildren. We first set the story of ringworm in the context of the emergence of dermatology, a specialty that grew largely in outpatient and dispensary settings. At this time, fungal diseases generally were understood mostly to affect the skin and outer membranes of the body, which was the domain of surgeons and later the new specialists in dermatology. We discuss the role of dermatologists in the development and spread of germ theories of skin diseases, showing that they were pioneers among clinicians in working with these ideas and adopting antiseptic practices. Our narrative then turns to the problem of ringworm in schoolchildren and attempts to manage the disease for sufferers and their families, and we show that the social consequences and stigma of the infection were far worse than the disease itself. Finally, we analyze newer treatments, especially the use of x-rays, and school medical inspections, where children worried about the nurse finding both nits and ringworm.

"SCALD-HEAD"

Robert Willan, London's leading skin specialist in the late 18th and early 19th centuries, reported that in his career he had seen children from over 200 schools and colleges in London affected by ringworm. While its effects on the physical body were localized and relatively mild, in terms of personal development they were serious, as Samuel Plumbe, Willan's successor, explained in 1835:[5]

> In the earlier periods of the lives of children there is no disease, no species of deviation from sound health, if we except scrofula, which operates so perniciously on the future prospects of the individual, as ring-worm, if of long continuance. The moment an unfortunate child is found by the schoolmaster or the schoolmistress with a spot on the head, the latter, very properly (not merely for interest's sake, but as a duty to the parents of all the other children), sends the child home, refuses to readmit until thoroughly cured. The consequence of this is, to the unfortunate child, a loss of time at that period of life when it can be least afforded, the period of early education.[6]

It was not only children who suffered but also their teachers. Plumbe observed that the disease was "destructive of the best instructors of children, for the conductors of establishments of previously high character and reputation found their pupils drop off in large numbers, and many good schools have been utterly ruined by it."[7]

There are no figures for the incidence of ringworm in the 19th century, but every indication is that it was very prevalent.[8] There were, for instance, a huge number of proprietary ointments, lotions, and potions sold by local chemists, and self-treatment advice was offered in popular health manuals and advertisements. The 1790 edition of William Buchan's *Domestic Medicine* recommended "keeping the head very clean, cutting off the hair, combing and brushing away the scabs, & c.," plus the use of ointments.[9] Mrs. Beeton offered several treatment regimens in her *Book of Household Management*, including the application of sulfur and treacle, creosote, or calomel.[10] There were numerous reports of cases and treatments in national and regional medical journals, for all types of infection.[11] At many sites on the body, the characteristic rings were hidden by clothing and hard to see, which meant that sufferers and doctors found it difficult to distinguish ringworm from other inflammatory afflictions, such as favus, eczema, psoriasis, and impetigo. Surgeons considered therapy relatively straightforward on any part of the body except the scalp, where ringworm was typically persistent. Although the disease affected all ages, medical discussion focused on children and on their scalps.[12] It was the most visible form of the disease, both medically and socially, as infected children were stigmatized as unclean and their parents regarded as uncaring.

In Britain, ringworm first attracted national medical and public attention in 1835 following reports of its high prevalence at Christ's Hospital School, one of London's foremost private schools, which included among its alumni Charles Lamb and Samuel Taylor Coleridge.[13] In this outbreak there were two issues: (1) the infection was often said to be an indicator of poor management by the governors and staff, as well as damaging to the reputation of the school, and (2) if children were excluded for weeks on end, their education was suffering and the school was losing income.[14] An editorial in the *Lancet* complained that the governors had been negligent in not drawing upon the expertise of doctors, especially those who had dealt successfully with other serious outbreaks at the London Orphan Asylum and the Royal Naval School.[15] A committee of Christ's governors was appointed to look into the problem, and they invited Plumbe to advise them. His report nicely illustrates medical thinking on the affliction at the time in terms of exciting causes (contagion) and predisposing causes (general health and cleanliness). As was typical of the fractious character of skin specialists at this time, he was dismissive of Robert Willan (whom he saw as no better than a nostrum monger) and of the French dermatologists. He considered ringworm to be both constitutional and contagious:

> The simple circular contagious ringworm is not, as has been supposed by many, produced only by infection or contagion. It arises in a very large portion of cases from the same sources as other diseases of the skin, such as improper diet, producing constipation of the bowels; restraint of the due and healthy exercise of children; repletion from over feeding, or from merely a single indulgence of sweetmeats or cakes, producing acidity. Yet thus originating it is quite as contagious as that which has spread directly in a family, from child to child, by contact, where no derangement of the stomach or system can be traced or suspected.[16]

Plumbe advised surveillance to control the spread of the disease by examining boys on entry, washing bedding regularly, and isolating those infected. This might involve moving those suffering to separate rooms, or simply making them wear protective caps or headwear. He also wanted pupils to have improved diets, both in quantity and in quality. He linked this to the danger of scurvy, writing that "the almost entire privation of vegetables tends to produce, if it be not the sole cause of the eruptive diseases."[17] Plumbe was a "skin doctor" before the era of specialization, so it would be anachronistic to call him a dermatologist (indeed, that term did not gain currency until the 1880s), but he does represent the common situation in the 19th century where surgeons had known areas of specialist expertise.[18]

DERMATOLOGY AND FUNGUS THEORIES OF SKIN DISEASES

Historians of 19th-century British clinical medicine have highlighted that key national characteristic of resistance to specialism in hospital practice among elite physicians and surgeons and the celebration of the virtues of the generalist.[19] "The narrow specialism of dermatology," as it was termed in 1874, was one of a number of organ- or technique-based specialist areas that drew the wrath of critics.[20] For example, a reviewer of Edward Dillon Mapother's *Diseases of the Skin*, published in 1875, was severe on the author's expertise and his claims to special competence:

> It is, indeed, but too true that the great body of specialists is composed largely of those who are intellectually quite incapable of comprehending all the departments for the healing arts. They succeed only by limiting their sphere of action; they triumphantly paddle in pools who would not live a moment in the stream. With the exception of ophthalmologists, specialists cannot, as a rule, be said to be amongst the best educated of the profession; and worse than all, the exclusive practice of some small speciality tends to perpetuate and increase ignorance, if it do not also deprave professional morals.[21]

However, Mapother was no exclusive practitioner.[22] He had been Medical Officer of Health for Dublin in the 1860s, wrote extensively on medical education, and was appointed Professor of Anatomy and Physiology at the Royal College of Surgeons of Ireland, eventually becoming its president. He had special interests in syphilis and gout, as well as in skin diseases.

Why was so much scorn poured on specialists? One explanation was the rivalry between surgeons and physicians, though this was complicated by the emergence of another divide between general practitioners and consultants.[23] Both consultant surgeons and physicians attacked specialization, but many practitioners had niches with particular diseases, and combined general and specialist work. The case of the emergent specialism of dermatology is instructive.[24] It grew from surgical practice after the mid-19th century, with specialist journals being published from the 1870s. The diagnosis and treatment of skin diseases had been a large and important part of surgeons' work and hence income. The future of general surgery seemed to lie in two directions: on the one hand extending the number and range of operations, while on the other hand becoming more "medical." For example, in the treatment of syphilis, the cauterization or excision of primary lesions on the skin was regarded as ineffectual, and surgeons relied more upon constitutional treatment with mercury.[25] Treating syphilis may have been a good source of income for surgeons, but sufferers were stigmatized, and this rubbed off on surgeons. In fact, the term "quack," widely applied to so-called specialists, was a contraction of quacksalver, or quicksilver, one of the most widely used specific treatments for syphilis.

Specialist practice in skin diseases was largely in hospital outpatient departments and dispensaries, the first of which, the Royal London and Westminster Infirmary for the Treatment of Cutaneous Diseases, was opened in 1819.[26] In the capital, a Hospital for Diseases of the Skin (later the Blackfriars Skin Hospital) followed in 1841, with satellite dispensaries opening in 1843, 1844, 1850, 1851, and 1857.[27] A new era in skin hospitals began in 1863 with the opening of the St. John's Hospital for Disease of the Skin, followed by many more such institutions.[28] John Laws Milton founded St. John's initially with the support of leading figures on diseases of the skin, such as Erasmus Wilson, William Tilbury Fox, and J. Mill Frodsham.[29] The new skin hospitals had few beds, and their dispensary work directly challenged the businesses of local general practitioners and elite consultants. In response, many voluntary hospitals set up "skin departments," promising the best of all worlds: specialist, accessible care without hospitalization, available in general hospitals where other specialist and general consultants were available.

Erasmus Wilson was Britain's leading authority on diseases of the skin, and he founded the short-lived *Journal of Cutaneous Medicine* in 1867.[30] A polymath and popularizer, he published books on the skin, food, and Egyptology, and is best known for funding the transportation of Cleopatra's Needle to London in 1878. Wilson popularized the term *dermatology*, first lecturing on the subject in 1840, and publishing *On Diseases of the Skin: Practical and Theoretical Treatise* in 1842. His private practice and investments were so successful that in 1869 he donated monies to the Royal College of Surgeons to establish a professorship of dermatology, which he held from 1869 to 1878, giving an annual series of lectures. In his own clinical practice, Wilson saw no conflict between generalism and specialism, but he was opposed to the exclusive specialist practice of others. Although trained as a surgeon, he claimed that almost all skin diseases were internal and constitutional in origin and required medical as much as external surgical or topical treatments. Thus, skin diseases needed to be diagnosed and treated by someone who understood the workings of the whole body, not just its outer layer. He was an opponent of contagious germ or fungal explanations of skin conditions, believing that any such matter present was a "secondary or adventitious product" rather an exciting cause.[31]

In the 1860s, two teaching hospitals, University College Hospital and the Glasgow Western Infirmary, established dermatology departments and appointed two men who made ringworm a model for germ theories of skin disease: Thomas M'Call (sometimes McCall) Anderson and Tilbury Fox.[32] M'Call Anderson published *On the Parasitic Affections of the Skin* in 1861 and Tilbury Fox published his *Skin Diseases of Parasitic Origin* 2 years later.[33] Like Wilson, Tilbury Fox opposed specialisms, whereas M'Call Anderson argued that this was how progress was being made in medicine in France and Germany and that Britain should follow.[34] Yet M'Call Anderson was another example of someone who combined general and specialist practice. He became Professor of Clinical Medicine at the Glasgow Western Infirmary and then Regius Professor in 1904, and his obituary celebrated how he maintained specialist work and writing on skin diseases, along with clinical teaching and running a large private practice. Tilbury Fox and M'Call Anderson united against Wilson's claim that fungi had no causal role in skin diseases. Given his dominant position, it is unsurprising that Wilson represented what was termed the "British school of dermatology" that saw most skin diseases to be of internal, constitutional origin (mostly forms of eczema) that required internal remedies.

FUNGUS GERMS

From the 1850s, ringworm was regarded as a fungus disease. This made it an early candidate to be a germ disease when debates about the causes of infectious and contagious diseases turned to microorganisms in the 1870s.[35] Some histories of germ theories of disease, anticipating the closure on bacterial causes in the 1880s, have ignored the many types of entity—animal, vegetable, and mineral—that were candidates to be disease germs in 1860s and 1870s. Good examples of such openness were the views of Samuel Wilks, the leading London physician. In his "Address in Medicine" at the British Medical Association in June 1872, he spoke variously of disease being caused by "vegetable germs," "a fungus," "specific organic particles," and "a virus."[36] Wilks also made the point that the "seeds" of disease, its germs, needed to find suitable "soil." Ringworm was one of his examples, and he placed it, no doubt surprisingly for modern readers, alongside cancer as a disease that grew and spread within the body:

> A ringworm grows and grows wherever the soil is propitious; the itch insect spreads over the body and the hydatid often swells until its host is destroyed. Cancer-cells divide and propagate until they have killed their victim which has supplied them with nourishment; and the germs of small-pox will do the same.[37]

Another key issue with fungi (the collective botanical name at the time was the *Mycetes*) was whether they were made up of fixed species, or whether they were so simple that their biology was shaped by the conditions in which they grew. Moreover, if there were fixed species, how could these be differentiated when their forms and modes of reproduction were so variable?

The same question was important in germ theories of diseases, not least with bacterial versions. The scientific name for bacteria at this time was the *Schizomycetes* (literally, "fission fungi").[38] Being surgeons by training, dermatologists were early adopters of antiseptics, if not converts to germ theories of putrefaction and inflammation, and through the promotional activities of Joseph Lister had early and consistent exposure to new ideas on germs. The standard chemical antiseptic, carbolic acid, was tried as a fungicide with ringworm and other skin infections, along with sulfurous acid, acetic acid, iodine, and mercuric chloride.[39] However, the lengthy applications of such caustic substances meant that the treatment was often worse than the cure.

The books of Tilbury Fox and M'Call Anderson, which many read as suggesting that almost all skin diseases were of fungal origin, prompted debates that anticipated many of the issues that divided opinion over bacterial germ theories of disease in the last quarter of the 19th century.[40] First was the question of whether any fungi found in diseased skin were necessary causes of disease or just concomitants.[41] Second, doctors asked whether fungi, when present, could only develop on dead tissue, acting as saprophytes, or whether they could actually invade and colonize living tissue, as infective agents or *contagium viva*. It was in this vein that the cholera fungus controversy in the late 1840s and 1850s had been framed.[42] Third, if fungi were agents of disease, was there one pathogenic fungus that produced different diseases because its effects and form depended on the tissue on which it grew (that is, it was pleomorphic; *pleo* = many + *morphic* = form)? Or, did distinct species of pathogenic fungi produce different diseases? In his volume, Tilbury Fox argued that all pathogenic fungi were forms of *Tinea*, the ringworm fungus, which he made "the generic term for parasitic affections of the surface," echoing the views of Ernst Hallier in Germany on the pleomorphic character of fungi.[43] Against this, M'Call Anderson maintained that different fungi caused distinct and specific diseases, and that they could do so in both dead and living tissue. He classed fungal infections as "vegetable parasitic affections," placing them alongside animal parasitic ones, such as scabies, and those caused by "poisons" or "viruses," such as syphilis.

The impact of bacteriology on the management of skin diseases was to shift treatments to be anti-germ.[44] As noted above, doctors recommended germ-killing antiseptics but also tried to break the passage of germs by "isolating" the infected area by covering it with a dressing or grease of some type. The ringworm caps worn by children combined all of these.

The exclusion of infected children from school became more common, and there were some suggestions of isolating families in their homes. At the same time, most doctors continued to recommend measures that aimed to strengthen the bodily "soil" against the "seeds" of disease. Although it would be wrong to make too much of the conjunction, the Dermatological Society of London was founded in 1882, the very same year in which Koch announced his discovery of the "tubercle bacillus," which could also infect the skin and was associated with leprosy and lupus.[45] From this time, leading dermatologists associated particular germs with specific skin diseases.[46]

RINGWORM IN SCHOOLS: "RINGWORM SCHOOLS"

Outbreaks of ringworm in schools, workhouses, and other institutions were reported throughout the mid-Victorian period, but they attracted little medical or public attention. However, things changed after the introduction of mass schooling following the 1870 Education Act, and the government called on Tilbury Fox in 1875 for advice on control and prevention.[47] School attendance had revealed both the "verminous condition" of many children and created "nurseries of ringworm" as classrooms and playgrounds were ideal for spreading infection.[48] Ringworm was one of a number of health problems that were taken up by medical officers of health, and later school medical officers.[49] The *Lancet* established a Commission on the Sanitary Condition of Our Public Schools, which released a report in 1875 calling for improvements in buildings, diets, and welfare, plus measures to control infectious diseases, especially scabies, scarlet fever, and ringworm.[50] There was broad medical agreement that children with ringworm should be excluded from school, though there was disagreement on remedial action: Some doctors recommended shaving the head and wearing a cap, whereas others preferred the vigorous application of disinfectant ointments and lotions. When children who had been excluded could return was, in fact, more of an issue than when to exclude them.[51] Capped and shaved "ringworm children" represented popular fears of contagion, though doctors often downplayed the link with dirt and insanitary environments, claiming ringworm was simply a "catching," germ disease. Indeed, Robert Liveing, a leading authority on dermatology, noted in 1879 that "gutter children" tended to be exempt from infection, despite being filthy and unkempt. Why? Because they did not attend school, nor did they ever brush their hair, so they were never exposed to the germs.[52]

The leading medical authority on ringworm in the latter part of the 19th century was Herbert Alder Smith, who spent his whole career as a medical officer at Christ's Hospital School at Newgate in London.[53] His book *Ringworm: Its Diagnosis and Treatment* went through four editions between 1880 and 1897.[54] Alder Smith took the view that ringworm was a local infection that had no impact on general health; hence, it should be treated locally, with general remedies only used as an adjunct. He only saw the bodily "soil" in terms of age and diet, making the familiar point that the disease was rarely present after puberty and that children who disliked fat, along with those who were ill nourished, seemed more vulnerable. He gained a readership in part because of his experience and in part because he offered a novel treatment. He claimed that he had identified "nature's method of effecting a cure," a type of inflammation he termed "kerion" that led to hair loss.[55] To produce a localized "kerion" reaction artificially, he applied drops of croton oil, a widely used counter-irritant, to individual hair follicles to make them "tender, swollen, red and infiltrated"; the aim was to produce "a speedy and certain cure" by depilation.[56]

However, this was one was among hundreds, possibly thousands, of formulae that doctors prescribed for ringworm, with new treatments being regularly reported in medical journals.[57] On hairless parts of the body, such as the hands and face, ringworm was readily treatable, with schoolchildren finding ordinary writing ink very effective, probably because it contained "gallic acid and tannin (derived from vegetable galls), ferrous sulphate, mucilage, and haematoxylin (derived from logwood)." However, ringworm on the scalp was often unmovable, hence the attraction of shaving and chemical depilation. In addition to medical remedies, ringworm was included in the conditions purportedly cured by the huge number of proprietary or popular remedies sold by chemists and available from many sources. For example, advertised in the Manchester press in 1889 was the Health Restorer Ointment, which was said to be the "Best, Safest and Speediest Cure in the World for Burns, Scalds, Ulcer, Chilblains, Itch, Ringworm, Scabbed Heads, Eczema, and all Skin Diseases," while Old Doctor Townsend's blood-purifying "Old American Sarsaparilla" offered cleansing from within.[58] Londoners could try Cook's Antiseptic Soap, which had been endorsed in the *Lancet* in May 1888, and Grasshopper Ointment, which also cured "Bad Legs, House-Maids Knee, Ulcerated Joints, Carbuncles, Poisoned Hands, Tumours, Cancers and Abscesses."[59]

The main impact of germ ideas and practices was in public health, with a switch to policies that focused on individuals as carriers of pathogens and practices of disinfection, isolation, and notification.[60] With regard to infectious diseases overall, this change particularly affected children, who were by far the majority of patients in the new isolation hospitals and whose health was targeted by school medical inspections.[61] A prominent example of the new concerns and approaches was in 1891, when the Poor Law North Surrey Board School in Anerley called in a top London dermatologist to advise them on dealing with the large number of children with persistent ringworm.[62] Joseph Payne found that 23 out of 45 children had been in isolation for over 1 year and five had suffered for over 4 years. He found no fault in the "thorough, scientific and conscientious" response of the teachers, the medical officer, or the managers.[63] He made recommendations, but the problem persisted. Two years later, in May 1893, the school turned to another London specialist, Dr. Alfred Eddowes. He found 47 cases and, while agreeing that the medical officer was highly competent, he nevertheless recommended that he took overall control, as with ringworm "detail" was all important.[64] He visited once a fortnight over 4 months, after which he claimed to have cured 25 children and improved the remainder; eventual eradication seemed inevitable.[65]

Policies for ringworm were developed along similar lines to diphtheria and scarlet fever, although it was much less serious, because of its impact on sufferers and their families. It became, quite literally, a social disease. Infected children were given special status and treatment because they seemed manifestly "unclean" and were stigmatized by other children and their families, and by neighbors. In addition, teachers and doctors expressed concerns about the consequences of exclusion for the individuals, their families, and the future mental fitness of the nation. Abraham and Eddowes explained the issues in 1894:

> Now that school attendance is compulsory and that the well-cared-for children of poor but respectable families often have to associate at school with those of the dirtiest and most careless classes of the community it is a moral duty that all reasonable precautions should be insisted on by the authorities in order to minimize the risk of infection from the diseased to the healthy. A skin disease also, contracted at school, may be taken home to the brothers and sisters.[66]

Malcolm Morris, a leading dermatologist and syphilologist, while unwavering on the need for the strict exclusion of affected children, called for a survey to determine the extent of the problem, suggesting that there should be special "ringworm schools" where excluded children could continue their education.[67]

Ringworm was targeted by London's Metropolitan Asylums Board (MAB) when, in 1897, it included specific measures in its plans for a variety of special institutions "to eradicate the physical taints of pauperism and to place them on a fairer level of health for the race of life."[68] Ringworm was included alongside contagious diseases of the eye, convalescence and open-air treatment, mental defectives, the physically disabled, and "young offenders."[69] The first, and as it turned out temporary, special institution for ringworm was the Bridge School in Witham, Essex, started in 1901. It was replaced by the Downs Ringworm School (also known as Banstead Road School) in Sutton, Surrey, in February 1903. Here children were housed in blocks of 70 beds, attended lessons within the institution, and were treated by the daily bathing of their scalp, intensive applications of lotions, and the extraction of diseased hairs.[70] In the first 10 months, 618 children were admitted, of whom 208 were discharged, 153 "cured" and the remainder recalled by local Poor Law Guardians.[71]

Children sent to special schools were the exception; most children with ringworm were excluded from school and treated at home. Some doctors thought exclusion unnecessary and unproductive, as very few parents were able to keep infected children away from their siblings, or from playing with other children after school. Phineas Abraham, surgeon at the Hospital of the Skin at Blackfriars, London, argued in 1900 that when a child's head was "kept greasy with germicidal ointments and always covered with a closely fitted cap," they should be allowed to attend school.[72] Everyone who wrote on the subject agreed that the ringworm caused more social than physical suffering. Infected children had no pain (other than from itching and the caustic lotions) and no general illness, and there were no permanent effects on the skin or hair. Their suffering was "exclusion from school and, to a great extent, banishment from society."[73] Parents endured some degree of stigma and had to manage their child's isolation.[74] Also, while doctors accepted that all social classes were vulnerable and that "dirt" as such was not a factor, ringworm was far less common among the well-to-do, allegedly because they were "less ignorant and gave greater care to their offspring."

Doctors' confidence in their ability to prevent and treat the condition grew as they increasingly believed that they knew their enemy.[75] The French dermatologist Raymond Sabouraud, who had trained at the Institut Pasteur, was a leading doctor at the famous Hôpital Saint-Louis in Paris, and published major works on the biology of ringworm organisms. In 1886, the Saint-Louis had opened its *L'ecole des teigneux* (ringworm school), colloquially known as "a school for the scabby children." A decade later it opened *"le laboratoire municipal des teignes de la Ville de Paris."*[76] Sabouraud was the first director, and his institution became famous for adapting bacteriological methods to working with fungi in the laboratory and for work on *les teignes* (ringworm).[77] He identified three groups of causal organisms, promising closure to the uncertainty over whether there was one ringworm fungus or many, and the degree to which species were pleomorphic.[78] His publications were well received, but it was above all his demonstrations and displays at the 1896 International Congress of Dermatology in London that were decisive in enrolling others to his standpoints.[79] In 1897 Herbert Aldersmith (he changed his name from Alder Smith in the 1890s) wrote that Sabouraud's "new views have completely revolutionised all older ones, and necessitated the separate description of the different forms of ringworm, and their microscopic appearances."[80]

A key finding was distinguishing between ectothrix infections that affected the outside of the hair (e.g., *Microsporon* spp.) and endothrix ones that invaded the hair shaft (e.g., *Trichophyton* spp.). There was some dissent in Britain, notably from two leading London dermatologists, Thomas Colcott Fox and Frank Blaxall, of the Westminster Hospital, who maintained that *Trichophyton* and *Microsporon* were not in separate families, and from Leslie Roberts, who emphasized physiologic over morphologic differences.[81] Nonetheless, Sabouraud's classification framed medical work on ringworm for the next decade, not least in epidemiologic surveys of the incidence of the different organisms.[82] For example, a survey in 1903 found that over 90% of ringworm cases in London hospitals were due to *Microsporon audouinii* and *Microsporon canis*, the latter found in dogs, which compared with 60% in MAB schoolchildren.[83] In Paris the main species were *M. audouinii* and *T. mentagrophytes*, the latter having a reservoir in dogs, cats, and other animals.

Medical interest in ringworm in the United States was much less pronounced than in Britain.[84] The schooling system was more fragmented, being organized at state and local levels across a vast area. While education was regarded as very important and widely available, compulsory schooling in all states arrived around 1900, three decades after Britain.[85] There was no American medical publication dedicated to ringworm until 1921, when John P. Turner's booklet *Ringworm and Its Successful Treatment* was published.[86] Turner was a medical inspector of public schools in Philadelphia, though he wrote as a general practitioner recommending the application of simple chemicals and cleanliness. There were few articles in American medical journals on ringworm, though cases were discussed at dermatology meetings, along with scabies, pediculosis, and impetigo, but as problems of individual hygiene rather than being associated with age or class. The main problem was with *M. canis*, perhaps reflecting the closeness of humans to pets and other animals, even in urban settings, in America at this time.

However, medical and public responses to the related fungal disease of favus were quite different. By the turn of the century, favus had been linked to the fungus *Achorion schoenleinii* and had been found to be the most common skin infection among immigrants from Europe. Favus was characterized as a "loathsome disease" and, after trachoma, a contagious eye infection, was the second largest cause of immigrants being rejected, or sent to isolation for treatment after inspections at Ellis Island.[87] Howard Markel has discussed why trachoma attracted so much attention given its low incidence, and the same argument applies to favus; namely, that it was an easily recognized condition that was made a marker of the person being "unclean" and hence "unfit" for acceptance into the United States.[88] In American cities, schoolchildren with ringworm were sometimes excluded, but there were no special institutions as there were in Paris and London.[89]

THE X-RAY REVOLUTION

In the 1900s, Sabouraud's reputation as the world's leading authority on ringworm was taken to a new level when he pioneered the x-ray treatment of infected scalps.[90] At this time, x-rays were one of the technological wonders of the age as "skiagraphs" revealed the body's internal structure. They promised not just the transformation of medicine but also wider social and cultural progress.[91] Sabouraud's innovation, first reported in 1904, used x-rays not to kill fungi, but to produce depilation. The rationale was to remove the nidus of infection and allow germicides or fungicides to penetrate more easily into hair follicles. As noted already, depilation was accepted as an effective means of treating ringworm; indeed, Aldersmith had written in 1897 that:

> In fact, my chief experiments during the last few years have been an effort to discover something that will always cause disease hairs to

fall out from patches of ringworm, for I fully believe that this troublesome disease will in time be cured by this method and not by the discovery of new parasiticides.[92]

However, attempts to achieve this by chemical and mechanical means had proved fraught with difficulties, not least because the inflammation and skin damage meant that the treatment was irritating and opened the skin to other infections.

The potential of x-rays for the treatment of skin diseases had been explored from the very beginning of their introduction into medicine in the mid-1890s. The ability to "see" inside the body excited contemporaries and has interested historians, but in many hospitals their main use, along with the Finsen lamp, was for the topical treatment of skin diseases.[93] Around 1900, the potency of x-rays was double-edged: They could reveal the inner structure of the body and cure certain diseases, but they could also maim and kill if too high a dose was given. The most immediate and visible damage caused by x-rays was to the skin. Indeed, it was this experience that led doctors to explore their use as counter-irritants, germicides, and fungicides. However, experimental studies quickly showed that x-rays did not readily destroy bacteria or fungi. Hair loss was noticed after incidental exposures and x-rays were said to have cosmetic as well as medical possibilities. Indeed, a report in the *Lancet* even suggested that exposure to x-rays might be a more convenient method of removing a beard than conventional shaving![94] The systematic application of x-rays for depilation was first reported in 1897 by Leopold Freund, who worked at the Medizinische Universität Wien.[95] He used x-rays for cosmetic procedures, removing surplus hair and unsightly features, such as hairy moles. The problem with such work was controlling the dose received by the patient: A dose that was too large could lead to permanent hair loss and skin damage. There is no evidence of similar experimentation among British and American dermatologists; however, they did keep up with the new applications developed by doctors in continental Europe.

Freund and Schiff in Vienna were probably the first to try x-rays to treat ringworm cases, but the treatment was, and still is, identified with

Sabouraud.⁹⁶ He had recognized the therapeutic value of depilation and had tried thallium acetate, otherwise used as a rat poison, but this produced severe side effects. X-ray depilation, therefore, promised to be safer. Sabouraud's key innovations, which he developed in collaboration with Henri Noiré and Maurice Pignot, were methods and materials to control the dosage of x-rays received by patients, which were lower than with skiagraphs.⁹⁷ His first invention was a generator with controllable output that allowed variation in the intensity of x-rays emitted; the second was developing a chemical that changed color on exposure to x-rays in a graded way that enabled monitoring of the dose a patient received.⁹⁸ The latter was crucial to avoid x-ray burns.

The x-ray therapy developed by Sabouraud was cumbersome. It required the patient to remain very still for up to 40 minutes, which was difficult to achieve with children, and much more so if many sessions (the contemporary term was *séances*) were required. Sabouraud claimed that five sessions on different parts of the scalp were safe; most doctors concurred, though one British doctor wrote that this was "criminal."⁹⁹ With large areas of infection there were two problems: First, the convex form of the skull meant that it was difficult to ensure even exposure; and second, it was imperative to avoid overlapping exposures that would produce burns or permanent baldness. The clinical picture reported by Sabouraud was that x-rays produced reddening of the skin and hair loss in 12 to 14 days.¹⁰⁰ He wrote that once the fungi had been carried away with the hair, the doctor's task was to ensure that the treated areas did not become reinfected, which meant instructing patients on the conscientious and thorough application of fungicidal lotions. Hair started to regrow after 6 to 8 weeks, but did so only slowly, allowing for the long-term application of fungicidals (Figures 4.1 and 4.2).

Despite the laborious procedure, x-rays had two advantages when judged against fungicides alone and other treatments: They reduced treatment times from years to months and produced permanent cures.¹⁰¹ Sabouraud reported a 100% increase in his cure rates, including many cases that had previously been intractable; and all this reduced costs eightfold, from 2,000 to 260 francs per patient.

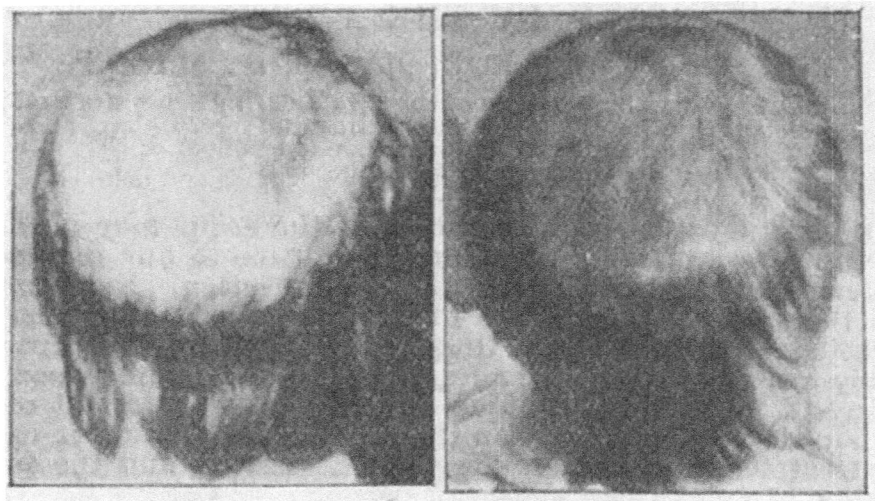

Figure 4.1 Photographs of x-ray depilation treatment of ringworm of the scalp
MacLeod, J. M. H., 'The Treatment of the Scalp by X-rays', *BMJ*, 1905, ii: 14.

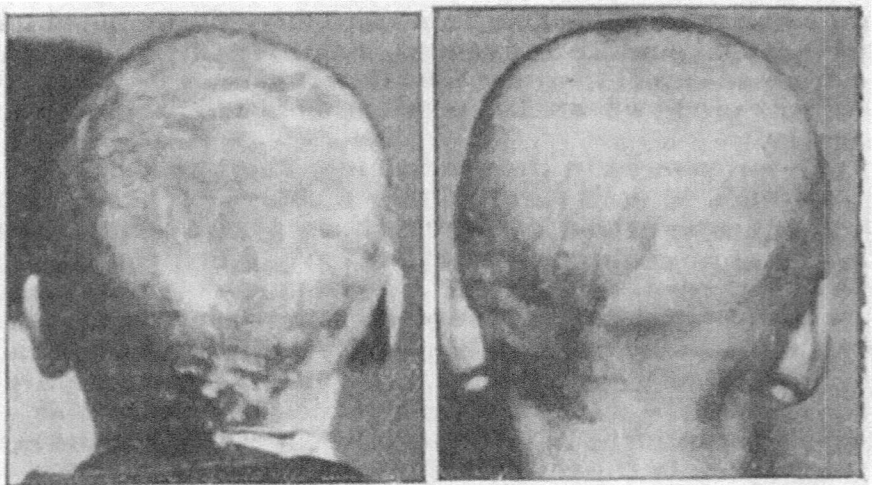

Figure 4.2 Photographs of x-ray depilation treatment of ringworm of the scalp
MacLeod, J. M. H., 'The Treatment of the Scalp by X-rays', *BMJ*, 1905, ii: 14.

In Britain, x-ray treatment was taken up in the outpatient departments of voluntary hospitals and in some of the new radiotherapy clinics. The first, very positive results were published in 1905.[102] The leading dermatologist, Malcolm Morris, confidently claimed that x-rays would mark

> the beginning of a new era in the treatment of an affection which has previously been one of the stumbling blocks of medical practice. It was fitting that we should owe the means of easy victory over a peculiarly rebellious disease to the distinguished man [Sabouraud] who has done so much to dissipate the darkness in which till lately its origin was enshrouded.[103]

The number of published reports of success grew. These were typically of a small number of cases, with doctors cautioning that time was needed to assess whether the cures were permanent. John MacLeod,[104] physician at Charing Cross Hospital and the Victoria Hospital for Children, did not regard x-rays as a panacea:

> It is a treatment, however, which is by no means easy; first there are the difficulties of the technique, second there is the all-important local treatment with the parasiticide remedies, and, third, there is the care which is requisite to avoid mishaps . . . The immediate dangers of the treatment . . . can, as a rule, be avoided, but with regard to the ultimate dangers, if there be any, sufficient time has not yet elapsed to disclose them. It has been suggested that the exposure of the scalp to the rays might have some harmful effect on the underlying brain. Certainly in an infant or a child under 3 years of age, where the scalp is thin and the fontanelles have not closed, one would be timid about submitting the scalp to the X-rays, but with regard to older children no misfortune of that nature has, as far as we are aware, been recorded.[105]

In fact, British dermatologists struggled to obtain results as good as those reported by Sabouraud; however, even a 50% cure rate was regarded as outstanding compared to other methods.[106] Better results were anticipated once doctors developed mastery of the equipment and pastilles, and when patient compliance could be improved[107] (Figure 4.3).

The first systematic use of x-ray treatment in Britain was at the ringworm schools of the MAB; indeed, their success reportedly improved

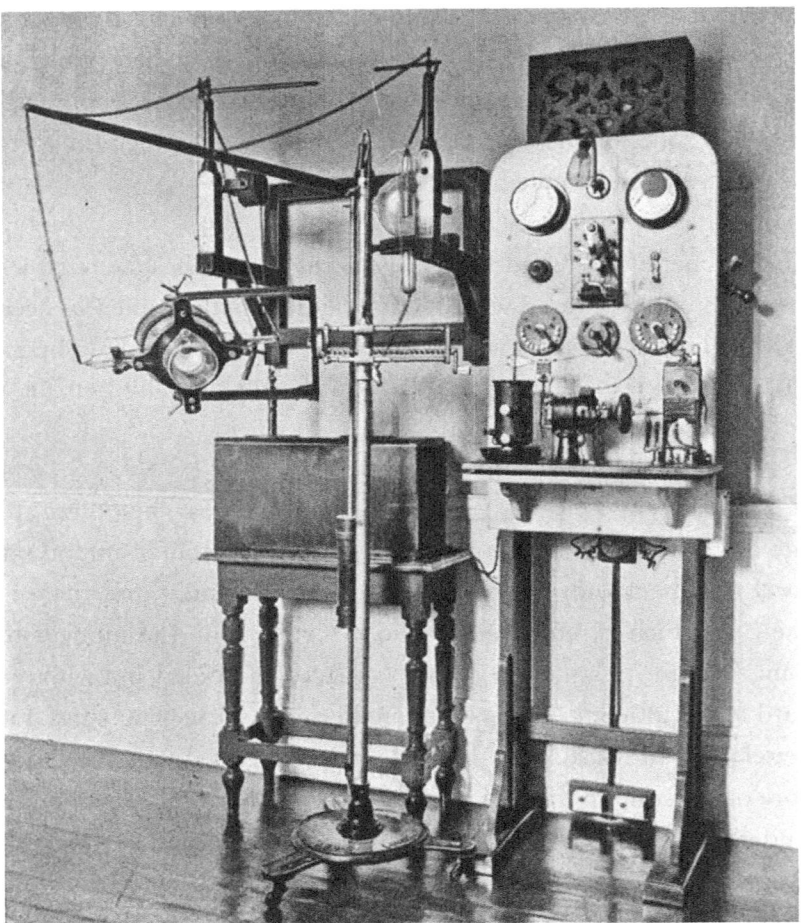

Figure 4.3 X-ray apparatus. Suitable for treatment of ringworm and other cutaneous affections.
Macleod, J. H. M., *Diseases of the Skin: A Text-book for Students and Practitioners*, London, H. K. Lewis, London, 1920. This figure © 2013 Wellcome Images is used under Creative Commons Attribution—Non-commercial licence: http://creativecommons.org/licenses/by-nc/3.0/.

turnover so much that the Bridge School at Witham closed in 1908, saving £500 per year, when the remaining children were transferred to the Downs School.[108] Treatment there was directed by Thomas Colcott Fox, with day-to-day matters in the hands of the school's medical officer, Dr. Sale. Within a year they reported 400 cures.[109] The doctors enjoyed access to a large number of cases and developed facilities for treating many children at once (Figure 4.4). They were treating pauper children, who were in triple isolation: in a special institution, within the Poor Law, and away from their parents. Hence, there were no problems with consent, and compliance with young children was largely a matter of discipline. Colcott Fox and Sale conducted a large "trial," but as was typical for the time there were no controls. Unsurprisingly, when they published their results there was no discussion of the ethics of this "trial," only wonder at its success.[110,111] Indeed, the London County Council's Board of Education

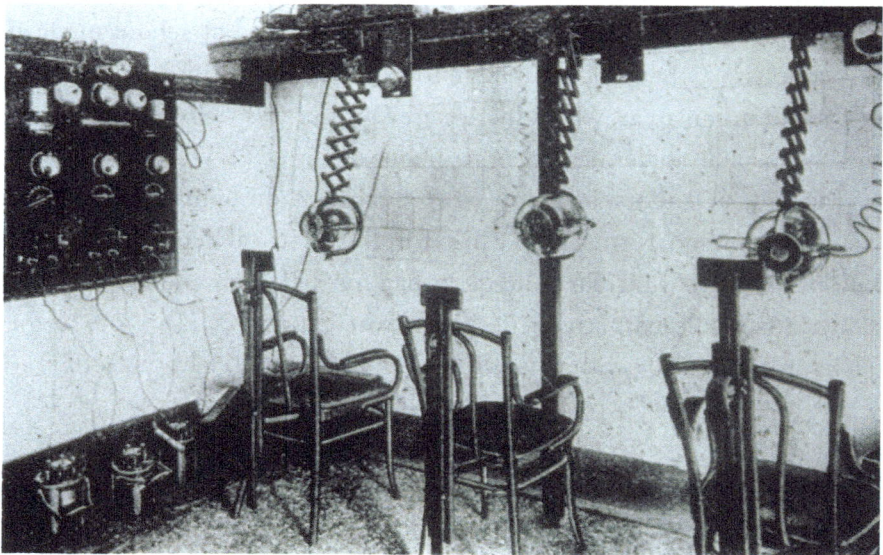

Figure 4.4 Radiotherapy room for ringworm, 1905
This figure is used courtesy of The Royal London Hospital Archives, Wellcome Images. This image is used under Creative Commons Attribution-NonCommercial-NoDerivs license: http://creativecommons.org/licenses/by-nc-nd/2.0/uk/.

was so impressed that in 1907 it considered a program to provide free x-ray treatment for the capital's children at hospitals and special centers.

The Board's program was to be part of a larger plan of school medical inspection and treatment for pupils in elementary schools that aimed to deal with a range of health problems: bad teeth, poor vision, suppurating ears and adenoids, tuberculosis, and general debility.[112] These "conditions" were seen as threats at three levels: to the long-term health and educational development of the child; to the efficient operation of schools; and to the progress of the race. Ringworm was taken up by the school medical service because they saw it being neglected by general practitioners, hospitals, public health authorities, and parents. Proposals were considered in 1908 by a subcommittee of the London County Council (LCC), which had replaced the MAB. They recommended that school clinics deal only with teeth defects, eye defects, skin diseases ("chiefly parasitic, such as, ringworm, scabies, pediculosis & c."), and ear defects.[113] In 1909, this became policy and because of the anticipated high demand, ringworm treatment was contracted out to London voluntary hospitals, with children compelled to attend if ringworm was identified at school medical inspections.[114] Other cities and large towns introduced similar programs; outside of urban areas, where there were fewer or less well-resourced voluntary hospitals, older treatment regimens persisted.[115]

The official endorsement of x-ray treatment brought prompt criticism. Dr. Dawson Turner, who worked in the electrical department at the Edinburgh Royal Infirmary and described himself as an "old worker with x-rays," had suffered permanent injury from exposures. He wrote to the *Times* in March 1909 with what turned out to be a prescient caution:

> The deleterious effects of continuous exposures to X-rays in the case of adults are only too well known to X-ray operators and it is probable that delicate cells of the growing brain of a child may be injuriously affected by much shorter exposures, though the evidence of impairment of function may not become noticeable until development is complete. No helpless child should have the chief centre of its nervous system exposed to the X-rays without the express consent

of its parent, obtained after the possible risks of the treatment have been fully explained.[116]

His plea was answered in a report by two directors of London hospital electro-therapeutic departments. They stated that ordinary precautions had ensured there were no ill effects in their patients, nor did they expect any from other controlled uses of x-rays.[117] However, some parents resisted the use of x-rays, though this was as much about distrust of hospitals and dislike of compulsion as it was about worries over radiation. Mr. Harris, a jeweler from Rotherhithe, on being instructed to take his daughter to Guy's Hospital, wrote back to the LCC's Child Care Branch stating he did not have "much faith in those places" and that his wife, a trained nurse, was treating the child.[118] Walter Longley asserted his independence in similar vein, saying that his boys were already being treated with sassafras oil and that his family would not trouble the LCC, nor the London ratepayer.[119] Henry Carter wrote that the instruction to take his children to the Evelina Hospital was "insulting to my wife and self."[120]

Armed with x-rays and with the backing of the LCC administration, dermatologists and school medical officers were optimistic about the future control of ringworm.[121] Nonetheless, in 1909, the *Lancet* set up an inquiry to address "the grave prevalence" and "the disastrous influence" ringworm was having on the education of children.[122] The *Lancet* Commission on Ringworm, consisting of "two thoroughly competent dermatologists" (who remained anonymous), reported on January 1, 1910. They dealt almost exclusively with the situation in London.[123] The authors opened in eugenic terms, stating that ringworm was more prevalent in the "less educated classes" and that those affected were "really representatives of lower grades of civilisation," where infestation with internal and external parasites was a marker of being left behind by social progress. The authors endorsed x-ray treatment administered by dermatologists and radiotherapists, along with a positive assessment of the capacity of existing facilities to cope with the mass-treatment plan that the LCC was contemplating. However, they were ambivalent about whether to use voluntary and local authority hospitals, or to recommend the creation of special treatment centers, but whatever was decided, they were certain it would be cost effective.

The Commission's report took seriously public concerns about the safety of x-rays, noting that in early years there had been accidents leading to permanent baldness and ulcers. However, burns were said to be a thing of the past as exposures were now well managed. With regard to brain damage, the authors wrote that the experience of thousands of cases, over many years, showed no evidence of any effects: "It is incumbent now on those who imagine that harm does follow the application of X-rays to produce the grounds for the view."[124] Against this backdrop, many parents allowed their children to be treated with x-rays but, as mentioned above, others refused. The manufacturers of popular alternatives, especially antiseptic creams like Germolene and Zambuk ("The Balm that Benefits the Bairns"), also offered their products as direct alternatives to x-rays.[125] However, some medical officers raised the stakes. For example, Dr. Bostock Hill, the Medical Officer of Health for Warwickshire, claimed in 1911 that he instructed parents that "they would be dealt with under the Children's Act for cruelty ... or the case would be referred to the N.S.P.C.C. (National Society for the Protection of Children)" if they refused to allow their children to be treated.[126]

Ernest Dore, a dermatologist at the Evelina Hospital for Sick Children, made a telling observation in his review of x-ray treatment in 1911, a year after the publication of the *Lancet* Commission report.[127] He returned to the issue of stigma, arguing that before x-ray treatments a diagnosis of ringworm was far worse than any physical suffering:

> A trivial complaint as regards the health of the child, tinea tonsurans brings in its train so long a category of ills that I have more than once heard long-suffering mothers say that they dreaded scarlet fever or pneumonia less. The disorganisation of the home that ensues from the isolation of the sufferers; the anxiety of the parents lest other children in the family should become infected; the complications with medical men and schoolmasters; the social ostracism; the loss of schooling; the wearisome process of constantly rubbing on

ointments with little apparent result except the production of sore heads in the children and sore hearts in the parents, these are some of the difficulties which have to be faced under the old *régime*.[128]

Given the reactions of children, family, friends, neighbors, teachers, and doctors to ringworm, and its position as a marker of "low civilization" and social danger, it is clear why a disease that never killed or caused permanent injury attracted such high-profile medical and public attention. Indeed, Dore wanted to up the stakes further, hinting at the possibility of stamping out the disease if compulsion was used: either in prevention, "such as the wearing of some kind of head gear, like the muzzle in the prophylaxis of rabies," or with x-ray treatment.

A national picture of ringworm in schoolchildren was represented in the Reports of the Medical Officer to the Board of Education, Dr. George Newman, the first of which was for 1908.[129] The prevalence of ringworm was around 1% among children inspected in school, much lower than other "defects," which were vision (10%), hearing (3–5%), adenoids and enlarged tonsils (6–8%), tooth decay (40%), and unclean bodies or heads (30–40%).[130] The main issue with ringworm was exclusion and its effects on a child's education—plus, from an administrative perspective, the impact of long absences on a school's grant income. Although the prevalence was low, it still meant that, on average, 3,000 children were absent every day, with a typical absence duration of 9 weeks.[131] Nationally, the longest average exclusion reported, 29 weeks, occurred in Somerset. This finding was seen as surprising for a rural county with few large towns and low population density, and was attributed to poor inspection regimens causing early cases to be missed. Although impetigo, by this time associated with *Staphylococcus aureus* infection, was the most prevalent skin disease found in inspections, ringworm was taken much more seriously.[132] Dr. Ritchie, the School Medical Officer for Manchester, reported that inspections in 1913 had revealed the following: impetigo, 353 cases; ringworm, 187; scabies, 39; and other skin diseases, 110.[133] However, cases reported by doctors and parents led to 2,003 notifications of ringworm in the city, with up to 1,500 children under supervision at any time. The

Manchester containment regimen was strict: "No cases of ringworm of the scalp are allowed to attend school unless the hair over and around the patches is cut and a washable cap worn . . . Children affected with ringworm of the body are not allowed to attend school."[134] In the same year, a ringworm school was established in Edinburgh for long-term absentees, including one boy who allegedly had been excluded for 4 years.[135]

In his annual reports, Newman began to report improvements, particularly in areas where x-ray treatment was available. In London, new cases fell from 5,573 in 1913 to 4,449 a year later, while in Beckenham in Kent, new cases had fallen from 133 in 1911 to just 48 in 1914.[136] However, nationally, the provision of special services was patchy. Only a third of education authorities had made special provision for ringworm treatment, and in many areas, especially outside of cities and large towns, there was still no access to x-ray treatment at all. In addition, many general practitioners chose to continue to recommend topical fungicides and left treatment to "unreliable" parents.[137]

THE DECLINE OF RINGWORM

In Britain, doctors reported that the incidence of ringworm of the scalp in schoolchildren fell during the First World War but increased afterward because of the shortage of school nurses, many of whom continued to work with casualties and invalids.[138] However, this was a minor peak as the incidence fell steadily over the interwar period. In London, the number of new cases had reduced from 6,214 in 1911 to 3,983 in 1920. The number dropped further to 513 in 1930, and by 1936 there were just 89.[139] As early as 1925, the district medical officer for Beckenham reported no new cases, while in Ilford, ringworm was also said to have been "abolished."[140] In his 26th and final report, for the year 1933, Newman observed with satisfaction that "Ringworm is steadily disappearing."[141] This situation was reflected in treatment facilities, the number of which was reduced from 150 clinics in 1923 to 80 in 1938. The London ringworm school, which had moved to the Goldie Leigh Cottage Children's Homes, Woolwich, in 1914, took fewer and fewer residential cases and became instead a center for day treatment with x-rays.[142]

Doctors attributed the decline in the reported incidence of ringworm, in the words of Norman Walker in 1929, not so much to the character of the infection but rather to "the value of cooperation between the scientist, the clinician, and the organiser."[143] Success was said to have come from school inspections spotting early cases, which were followed up by effective treatments such as x-rays. The provision and use of x-rays was variable across the country. In the early 1930s only 20% of diagnosed cases in England were receiving x-rays. The rates of use varied: London was the highest and rural counties were several times lower[144] (Table 1.1).

Chemical and mechanical methods of depilation continued to be used, and there was particular interest again in the 1930s in giving thallium acetate.[145] Some doctors, particularly in the United States, argued that thallium treatment was safer than x-rays; however, critics termed it "A Dangerous Drug" because the margin between achieving effective epilation and poisoning was very small.[146] During the interwar period, dermatologists on both sides of the Atlantic showed less interest in ringworm of the scalp,

Table 1.1 CASES OF RINGWORM IN ENGLAND AND WALES TREATED BY X-RAY OR OTHER METHODS, 1933

	By x-rays	Otherwise	X-ray treatment as percentage of total
England			
Counties	149	2058	6.8
County boroughs	540	2040	20.9
Boroughs	120	597	16.7
Urban districts	22	90	19.6
London	160	18	89.9
Wales			
Counties	20	88	18.5
County boroughs	52	19	73.2
Boroughs	0	24	0.0
Urban districts	7	29	19.4

reflecting its lower incidence and relatively stable therapeutic regimens.[147] Their new areas of interest were ringworm in athletes, college students, soldiers, and miners.

Ringworm, although no doubt a common human infection for centuries, only gained serious medical and public attention in the second half of the 19th century, and then in a specific social group and setting: schoolchildren and schooling. The aggregation of children in crowded classrooms for hours at a time seemed to provide ideal conditions for contagion. Nonetheless, it was as a social rather than a physical disease that ringworm gained medical and public attention. Ringworm epidemics were one of the unintended consequences of the progressive reform of mass schooling, which revealed changing social attitudes to markers of disease and the growing stigmatization of the palpably "unclean." While historians such as Nancy Tomes have detailed public responses to the threat of invisible germs, we have revealed the reactions, some similar and others unique, to conditions where the germs were highly visible. Perhaps the "gospel of germs" won converts more readily for diseases such as ringworm, favus, and trachoma, where the physical and social manifestations of infection were obvious and reinforcing.

From 1905, ringworm was also seen as a pathology that could be remedied by medical progress, and not just any new technology, but by the medical icon of the age, x-rays. The use of x-ray depilation was an innovation that was taken up rapidly, in large measure because it promised so much, but also because the necessary equipment was becoming more readily available and there were opportunities for clinical and organizational innovations. In Britain, major public bodies such as the LCC, having been persuaded to create special ringworm institutions, subsequently invested in the new technologies of treatment. This all seemed to pay off, as the reported incidence of ringworm of the scalp in children declined rapidly in the interwar period.[148] There was debate about the causes of the fall: Was it due to medical inspection regimens and new treatments, or to social factors, such as more bathrooms, better medicated shampoos, or the fashion for shorter hair and grooming with hair creams?

Brylcreem was introduced in 1928 and marketed for better "bounce" in styling and control of dandruff, then said to be caused by a yeast fungus *Pityrosporon*. Whatever the specific reasons, all factors responsible for the decline were seen by contemporary commentators to be due to medical and social progress.

NOTES

1. Homei A, Worboys M. "Ringworm: A disease of schools and mass schooling in the United Kingdom," in *Fungal Disease in Britain and the United States 1850–2000, Mycoses and Modernity, Science, Technology and Medicine in Modern History*. London: Palgrave Macmillan UK; 2013:17–42.
2. Sanderson M. *Education, Economic Change and Society in England 1780—1870*. Cambridge: Cambridge University Press; 1995; Simon B. *Studies in the History of Education*. London: Lawrence and Wishart; 1966; Digby A, Searby P, eds. *Children, School and Society in Nineteenth-Century England*. London: Macmillan; 1981; Nasaw D. *Schooled to Order: A Social History of Public Schooling in the United States*. New York: Oxford University Press; 1979.
3. Richardson N. *Typhoid in Uppingham: Analysis of a Victorian Town and School in Crisis, 1875–7*. London: Pickering & Chatto; 2008.
4. Pusey WA. *The History of Dermatology*. Springfield, IL: C. C. Thomas; 1933; Crissey JT, Parish LC. *The Dermatology and Syphilology of the Nineteenth Century*. New York: Praeger; 1981. On Robert Willan see: Brunton D. Willan, Robert (1757–1812). *Oxford Dictionary of National Biography*. Oxford: Oxford University Press; 2004. http://www.oxforddnb.com/view/article/29438.
5. On Plumbe see: Rosenthal T. Samuel Plumbe. *Arch Derm Syphilol*. 1937;36(2): 348–354.
6. Plumbe S. History, pathology and treatment, of ring-worm and scald-head. *Lancet*. 1835;926.
7. Ibid.
8. Brown H. *Ringworm and Some Other Scalp Affections: Their Cause and Cure*. London: J. R A. Churchill; 1899.
9. Buchan W. *Domestic Medicine: Or, A Treatise on the Prevention and Cure of Diseases* (11th ed.). London; 1790:555–556.
10. Beeton I. *Beeton's Book of Household Management*. London: S. O. Beeton; 1861:2667–2668.
11. Plumbe S. Remarks on the contagious ring-worm of the scalp. *Lancet*. 1835:858.
12. There is an excellent history of ringworm in France; see: Tilles G, Tilles G. *Teignes et Teigneux: Histoire Medicale et Sociale*. Paris: Springer; 2008.
13. Allan GAT. *Christ's Hospital*. London: Town and County; 1984.

14. Plumbe, History, pathology, i:926–928 and ii:50–51; Rosenthal T. Samuel Plumbe. *Arch Dermatol.* 2008;16:36–43.
15. *Lancet.* 1835:683–688.
16. Plumbe, History, pathology, 928.
17. Plumbe S. *An Address to the Governors of Christ's Hospital, on the Causes and Means of Prevention of Ring-Worm in That Establishment, To Which Is Attached, a Few Rules for the Domestic Management of the Scholars during Their Vacations.* London, 1834.
18. Mayne RG. *An Expository Lexicon of the Terms, Ancient and Modern, in Medical and General Science* (Pt. 2). London: J. Churchill; 1854:265.
19. Lawrence C. "Incommunicable knowledge": Science, technology and the clinical "art" in Britain, 1850–1910. *J Contemp History.* 1985;20:503–520.
20. *Lancet.* 1875;i:888.
21. Ibid.
22. *Lancet.* 1908;i:822.
23. Lawrence C. *Medical Theory, Surgical Practice: Studies in the History of Surgery.* London: Routledge; 1992.
24. Rook A. Dermatology in Britain in the late nineteenth century. *Br J Dermatol.* 1979;100(1):3–12.
25. Erichsen JE. *The Science and Art of Surgery.* London: J. Walton; 1869:8.
26. Rook A. James Stratin, Jonathan Hutchinson and the Blackfriars Skin Hospital. *Br J Dermatol.* 1978;99:215–219.
27. Ibid., 216.
28. Russell BF, ed. *St. John's Hospital for Diseases of the Skin, 1863–1963.* Edinburgh: E. A. S. Livingstone; 1963.
29. *Lancet.* 1864;ii:538. The three supporters withdrew their support when they realized Milton's practice was mainly on the treatment of spermatorrhea, the involuntary discharge of semen.
30. Hadley RM. The life and works of Sir William James Erasmus Wilson, 1809–84. *Med History.* 1959;3:215–247; Power D'A. Wilson, Sir (William James) Erasmus (1809—1884), rev. by Aserton GL. *Oxford Dictionary of National Biography.* Oxford: Oxford University Press; 2004. http://www.oxforddnb.com/view/article/29702.].
31. Quoted in Hogg J. *Parasitic or Germ Theory of Disease.* London: Baillière, Tindall and Cox; 1876:33.
32. Asherson GL. Fox, William Tilbury (1836–1879). *Oxford Dictionary of National Biography.* Oxford: Oxford University Press; 2004. http://www.oxforddnb.com/view/article/10048; English MP. William Tilbury Fox and dermatological mycology. *Afr J Dermatol.* 1977;97:100–112; Cooper J. Anderson, Sir Thomas McCall (1836–1908), rev. by Alexander JO'D. *Oxford Dictionary of National Biography.* Oxford: Oxford University Press; 2006. http://www.oxforddnb.com/view/article/30414; Anon. Thomas McCall Anderson, obituary. *Lancet.* 1908;i:468–471.
33. Tilbury Fox G. *Skin Diseases of Parasitic Origin.* London: Robert Hardwicke; 1863; Tilbury Fox G. The true nature and meaning of parasitic diseases of the surface.

Lancet. 1859;ii:5–7, 31–32, 201, 260–261, 283–284, 507–508; M'Call Anderson T. *On the Parasitic Affections of the Skin.* London: Churchill; 1861.
34. Tilbury Fox, *Skin Diseases,* v–vi; Anderson, *On the Parasitic Affections,* 1–2.
35. Hogg J. The vegetable parasites of the human skin. *BMJ.* 1859;i:241; Hillier T. On ringworm and vegetable parasites. *BMJ.* 1861;ii:552 and 577; Worboys M. *Spreading Germs: Disease Theories and Medical Practice in Britain, 1865–1900.* Cambridge: Cambridge University Press; 2000:73–107.
36. Wilks S. Address in medicine. *BMJ.* 1872;ii:146–153.
37. Ibid., 149.
38. Colan T. Parasitic vegetable fungi and the diseases induced by them. *Lancet.* 1874;ii:755–757 and 832–833.
39. Liveing R. Lecture on the peculiarities of ringworm and its treatment. *Lancet.* 1879;ii:642–644, on 643–644.
40. Worboys, *Spreading Germs,* passim; M'Call Anderson T. Introductory lectures to the study of the diseases of the skin. *Lancet.* 1870;i:149–151.
41. *Lancet.* 1861;ii:449–450.
42. Pelling M. *Cholera, Fever and English Medicine, 1830–1865.* Oxford: Clarendon Press; 1976:146–202.
43. Tilbury Fox W. On the identity of parasitic fungi affecting the human surface. *Lancet.* 1880;ii:260–261; *Lancet.* 1867;ii:266–267.
44. *Lancet.* 1889;ii:1232.
45. Stark J. *Industrial Illness in Cultural Context: "La maladie de Bradford" in Local, National and Global Settings, 1878–1919,* Unpublished PhD thesis, University of Leeds, 2011; Jamieson A. *An Intolerable Affliction: A History of Lupus Vulgaris in Late 19th and Early 20th Century Britain,* Unpublished PhD thesis, University of Leeds, 2010.
46. British Association of Dermatologists. *A Biographical History of British Dermatology.* London: British Association of Dermatologists; 1995.
47. Tilbury Fox W. Ringworm in schools. *Lancet.* 1872;i:5–6.
48. Hirst JD. Public health and the public elementary schools, 1870–1907. *History of Education.* 1991;20:107–118.
49. Harris B. *The Health of the Schoolchild: A History of the School Medical Service in England and Wales.* Buckingham: Open University Press; 1995:32–47.
50. Report of the Lancet Sanitary Commission on the Sanitary Condition of Our Public Schools. *Lancet.* 1875,i:795–796, 859–861 and ii:111–112, 314–315, 422–423, 574–575, 682, 785–787.
51. See the case of George Beavis, who, in November 1875, was fined for neglecting to send his daughter to school. *Hansard,* HC Deb 11 February 1876, 227: 227–229; *Times,* 3 February 1876, 5c; 9 March 1876, 6e.
52. Liveing, Lecture on the peculiarities, 643–644.
53. Mansell K. *Christ's Hospital in the Victorian Era.* Whitton: Ashwater Press; 2011.
54. Alder Smith H. *Ringworm: Its Diagnosis and Treatment.* London: H. K. Lewis & Co. Ltd; 1880; 2nd ed., 1882; 3rd ed., 1885; Aldersmith H. *Ringworm and Alopecia Areata* (4th ed.). London: H. K. Lewis & Co. Ltd; 1897.

55. Tilbury Fox W. On ringworm of the head and its management. *Lancet.* 1877;ii:643–644.
56. Alder Smith, *Ringworm*, 1882, vii.
57. Many general patent medicines included ringworm as one of the conditions they cured. Specifically, the most widely advertised topical remedies were Beatson's Ringworm Lotion, Bateson's Specific, and Cuticura Soap. Holloway's Ointment was advised to be used in conjunction with Holloway's Pills, and those seeking a systemic cure could try Orange's Universal Cerate and Vegetable Purifying Pills.
58. *Manchester Times*, 2 February 1889, 2 and 9 February 1889, 8.
59. *Morning Post*, 10 May 1889, 4; *Reynolds's Newspaper*, 26 May 1889, 1.
60. Worboys, *Spreading Germs*, 234–276.
61. Newson Kerr M. *Fevered Metropolis: Epidemic Disease and Isolation in Victorian London*, Unpublished PhD thesis, University of Southern California, 2007; Harris, *Health of the Schoolchild*, passim.
62. On the Ringworm School see: http://www.workhouses.org.uk/index.html? MAB/MAB.shtml.
63. Dr Payne's Report on Ringworm, 1891, London Metropolitan Archives (LMA) MA, NSSD/79.
64. Dr Eddowes' Report on Anerley School, 27 May 1893, LMA, NSSD 80.
65. Ibid., 30 December 1893. It was likely he used an ointment based on chrysophanic acid, ichthyol, and salicylic acid. Eddowes A. Treatment of ringworm. *BMJ.* 1893;i:785–786.
66. Abraham PS, Eddowes A. Contagious skin diseases in schools. *Lancet.* 1894;ii:275.
67. Morris M. Ringworm in elementary schools. *Lancet.* 1891;ii:348.
68. Anon. Enlargement of functions of the Metropolitan Asylums Board. *Lancet.* 1897;i:1483.
69. Baxter Forman E. A lecture on medical London. *Lancet.* 1899;i:213.
70. Downs School Sub-Committee Minutes, 1903, LMA, MAB-5-17, MAB/0509, Sub-Committee Minute Book, pp. 43–44 and 61.
71. Anon. Ringworm and the Metropolitan Asylums Board. *Lancet.* 1904;i:318–319. Also see: Admission and Discharge Registers, 1903–1906, LMA, MAB-22-8, MAB/2326, p. 1, 54, 64, 93 and 133. The first four children admitted on February 26, 1903, were typical, staying respectively 26, 17, 13, and 8 months.
72. Abraham and Eddowes, Contagious skin diseases, 275.
73. Ibid.
74. Morris, Ringworm, 1898:6.
75. Brown, *Ringworm and Some Other Scalp Affections*, 1–3.
76. Tilles and Tilles, *Teignes et Teigneux*, 85–99.
77. Sabouraud R. *Les Trichophyties humaines*. Paris: Rueff and Cie; 1894.
78. Civatte A. Obituary: Raymond Sabouraud. *Br J Dermatol.* 1938;50:206–210.
79. Sabouraud R. La question des teignes (au Congress de Londres). *Annales de dermatologie et syphiligraph.* 1896;7:1333–1357. Also see: Morris M. *Ringworm in the Light of Recent Research*. London: Cassell and Co.; 1898, v; The parasites of ringworm [Editorial]. *Lancet.* 1893;i:1204.

80. Aldersmith, *Ringworm*, 1897, 6.
81. Colcott Fox T, Blaxall FR. An enquiry into the plurality of fungi causing ringworm in human beings, as met with in London. *Br J Dermatol*. 1896;8:241; Roberts L. The present position of the question of vegetable hair parasites. *BMJ*. 1894;ii:685–688.
82. Sabouraud R. X-ray treatment of tinea tonsurans. *International Clinics*. 1904;2:41–49; Sabouraud R et al. La Radiotherapie die teignes a l'ecole Lallier en 1904. *Bulletin de la Société française de dermatologie et de syphiligraphie*. 1905;16:10. Also see: Sabouraud R. *Maladies Cryptogamiques, Les Teigne*. Paris: Masson & Cie; 1910; Tilles and Tilles, *Teignes et Teigneux*, 100–106.
83. *Lancet*. 1903;ii:1102.
84. However, see: Shoemaker JV. Ringworm in public institutions. *Trans Am Med Assoc*. 1878;29:139–147.
85. Pulliam JD, van Patten JJ. *History of Education in America*. New York: Pearson; 2006.
86. Turner JP. *Ringworm and Its Successful Treatment*. Philadelphia: F. A. Davis; 1921; Burnett JC. *Ringworm: Its Constitutional Nature and Cure*. Philadelphia: Boericke & Tafel; 1892.
87. Kraut AM. *Silent Travelers: Germs, Genes, and the Immigrant Menace*. New York: Basic Books; 1994:58–67; Allen SK, Semba RD. The trachoma "menace" in the United States, 1897–1960. *Surv Ophthalmol*. 2002;47(5):500–599.
88. Markel H. "The eyes have it": Trachoma, the perception of disease, the United States Public Health Service, and the American Jewish immigration experience, 1897–1924. *Bull Hist Med*. 2000;74:525–560.
89. Buckley AM. The x-ray treatment of ringworm of the scalp. *JAMA*. 1913;56:1766.
90. Bunch JL. Sabouraud's method of ringworm treatment. *Lancet*. 1905;i:414–416.
91. Natale S. The invisible made visible: X-rays as attraction and visual medium at the end of the nineteenth century. *Media History*. 2011;17(4):345–358; Pamboukian S. "Looking radiant": Science, photography and the x-ray craze of 1896. *Victorian Review*. 2001;27(2):56–74.
92. Aldersmith, *Ringworm*, 1897, 296.
93. Walsh D. *The Roentgen Rays in Medical Work: With an Introductory Section upon Electrical Apparatus and Methods by J. E. Greenhill*. London: Baillière & Co.; 1897.
94. Anon. "X" rays as depilatory. *Lancet*. 1896;i:1296; Daniel J. Depilatory action of x-rays. *Medical Records*. 1896;49:595–596.
95. Report: The roentgen rays as a depilatory. *Lancet*. 1897;i:752; Freund L. Ein mit Röntgen-Strahlen behandelter Fall von Naevus pigmentosus piliferus. *Wien Med Wochenschr*. 1897;47:428–434; Freund L. Nachtrag zu dem Artikel "Ein mit Röntgen-Strahlen behandelter Fall von Naevus pigmentosus piliferus," *Wien Med Wochenschr*. 1897;47:856–860; Report: Depilation by high-tension electric currents. *Lancet*. 1901;i:121; Walsh D. The removal of superfluous hair by a combination of x-ray exposure and electrolysis. *Lancet*. 1901;ii:1191–1192.
96. Pusey WA. Roentgen-ray therapy twenty years ago. *JAMA*. 1923;81(15):1257–1260.
97. Pignot MM. Souvenir sur Raimond Jacques Sabouraud 1864–1938. *Mycopathologia*. 1954;7:348–364.

98. Guido Holzknecht, an Austrian physician, had pioneered the use of chemical monitoring in the 1890s, placing mixtures that were sensitive to radiation in pastilles between the generator and the patient. Doctors calibrated tissue damage against dosage as revealed by color changes, largely by trial and error. Holzknecht created a unit "H" (from his own initial) and an "H-scale" that allowed doctors to quantify the alteration in the "tint" of pastilles by comparison with a painted color chart. However, he kept the formula of his pastilles secret; hence, they were expensive and supplies were limited. Sabouraud introduced a cheaper method using barium platino-cyanide, which was the standard chemical used on x-ray plates before they were fixed photographically. These pastilles were not only cheaper but could also be reused as they returned to their original color after exposure. Sabouraud set out detailed specifications of the distance between machine and patient, the protection of surrounding skin, generator settings, the position of the pastille, and the required degree of color change. For Holzknecht, see: Angetter DC. *Guido Holzknecht: Leben und Werk des österreichischen Pioniers der Röntgenologie*. Wien: Werner Eichbauer; 1998. For more, also see: Paul W. A history of radiation detection instrumentation. *Health Phys.* 2005;88(6):616; Sabouraud R, Noiré H. Traitement des teignes tondantes par les rayons X. *Presse Mèd.* 1904;12:825–827.
99. Walker N. X-rays in the treatment of tinea. *BMJ.* 1904;i:868.
100. Adamson HG. On the treatment of ringworm of the scalp by means of x-rays. *Lancet.* 1905;i:1715.
101. Bunch, Sabouraud's method, 416.
102. Morris M. The Harveian Lecture on some new therapeutic methods in dermatology. *BMJ.* 1905;i:699.
103. Ibid.
104. MacLeod JMH. The treatment of the scalp by x-rays. *BMJ.* 1905;ii:14.
105. Ibid., 13–15. Also see: Higham Cooper R. The supposed risks attending x-ray treatment of ringworm. *BMJ.* 1909;ii:454–457.
106. Sichel G. The x-ray treatment of ringworm. *BMJ.* 1906;i:256–257. Also see: Sequeira JH. The varieties of ringworm and their treatment. *BMJ.* 1906;ii:193–196.
107. See letters in response to Sichel's article in *BMJ*, 1906;i:359–360, 419–420, 539–540, 840, 1018–1020.
108. LMA, Children's Committee Report for 1905, Metropolitan Asylums Board; Ayers GM. *England's First State Hospitals and the Metropolitan Asylums Board, 1867–1930*. London: Wellcome Institute; 1971:171–175 and 207.
109. Report: The Metropolitan Asylums Board. *BMJ.* 1907;i:1314.
110. Bulkley LD. The x-ray treatment of ringworm of the scalp. *JAMA.* 1911;56:1706–1709.
111. Macleod JHM. *Diseases of the Skin: A Text-book for Students and Practitioners*. London: H. K. Lewis; 1920.
112. Report: Children's Committee, Metropolitan Asylums Board. *BMJ.* 1907;i:1314.
113. *Times*, 9 December 1908, 6c.
114. Prior JR. X-ray treatment of ringworm. *Public Health.* 1910–1911;24:153–154.

115. Adam T. The control of ringworm in school. *Public Health*. 1912–1913;26:3–8; Bernard Shaw AF. The diagnosis of ringworm in school children. *Public Health*. 1912–1913;26:366–369.
116. *Times*, 31 March 1909, 12d.
117. *Times*, 1 April 1909, 18e.
118. Letter, H. M. Harris, 18 March 1910, LMA, PH/SHS/2/9.
119. Letter from Walter Longley, 8 April 1910, LMA, PH/SHS/2/9.
120. Letter from Henry Carter, 29 May 1910, LMA, PH/SHS/2/9.
121. Cates J. The administrative control of ringworm. *Public Health*. 1910–1911;24:226–233.
122. On the continuing controversies about the treatment see: Anon. Favus and ringworm among schoolchildren. *Lancet*. 1909;i:1636.
123. Anon. The Lancet Commission of Ringworm: Its prevalence, influence and treatment. *Lancet*. 1910;i:51–56.
124. Ibid., 55.
125. *Daily Mirror*, 5 November 1901, 16; 8 February 1912, 15c–d; 7 December 1922, 14 a–b.
126. Reported in Cates, Administrative control, 232.
127. Ernest Dore S. The present position of the x-ray treatment of ringworm. *Lancet*. 1911;i:432.
128. Ibid.
129. Annual Report for 1908 of the Chief Medical Officer of the Board of Education, BPP, 1910, Cd. 4986, XXIII: 55–57.
130. Health of school children. *Times*, 30 October 1911, 11a.
131. MOH Report for 1912.
132. Payne JF. An address on bacteria in diseases of the skin. *Lancet*. 1896;ii:2–3.
133. MOH Report, Manchester.
134. Manchester and District. *BMJ*. 1913;ii:205.
135. Walker N. Fifty years of dermatology. *Lancet*. 1929;ii:212.
136. LMA.
137. Adam, Control of ringworm, 3–8; Bernard Shaw, Diagnosis of ringworm, 366–369.
138. Report: Medicine in the schools. *BMJ*. 1920;2:826.
139. Report: School health in London in 1934. *Public Health*. 1935;48(12):403; *The Health of the School Child: Annual Report of the Chief Medical Officer of the Board of Education, 1937*. London: HMSO; 1938:87–88.
140. Between 1922 and 1931 2,426 cases were treated there, only 200 or so per year. *The Health of the School Child: The Annual Report of the Chief Medical Officer of the Board of Education for 1925*. London: HMSO; 1926:41.
141. *The Health of the School Child: The Annual Report of the Chief Medical Officer of the Board of Education for 1933*. London: HMSO; 1934:9.
142. Cochrane Shanks S. Vale epilation: X-ray epilation of the scalp at Goldie Leigh Hospital, Woolwich (1922–1958). *Br J Dermatol*. 19;79(4):237–238.
143. Walker, Fifty years, 211.
144. *Health of the School Child*, 1933, 86.

145. Walker, Fifty years, 211; Percival GH. The treatment of ringworm of the scalp with thallium acetate. *Br J Dermatol.* 1930;42(2):59–69.
146. Editorial: Thallium: A dangerous drug. *N Engl J Med.* 1931;204:1117; Lewis DR, Lloyd AW. Treatment of ringworm of the scalp with thallium acetate. *BMJ.* 1933;ii:99–100.
147. *The Health of the School Child: The Annual Report of the Chief Medical Officer of the Board of Education for 1938.* London: HMSO; 1939. Also see: Barber HW. The relationship of dermatology to general medicine. *Lancet.* 1929;ii:363–370, 483–492, 591–599.
148. Underwood EA. National health and physical fitness. *Public Health.* 1937–1938;51:328–333.

5

The JDC-Joint and OSE campaign for eradication of ringworm in the Jewish communities in Eastern Europe and North Africa

SHIFRA SHVARTS, PNINA ROMEM,
ITZHAK ROMEM, AND MORDECHAI SHANI

INTRODUCTION

In 1921,[1] the American Jewish Joint Distribution Committee (JDC-Joint), an apolitical Jewish humanitarian and nonprofit organization,[2] together with the Organization for Safeguarding the Health of Jews (OSE), a union devoted to advancing the health, hygiene, and treatment of Jewish children[3] (and TOZ, its Polish branch),[4] initiated a campaign for the eradication of ringworm among children and youth. This disease was seriously detrimental to the health of Jewish communities in Eastern Europe after the First World War and represented a major barrier to the immigration of Jews to Western countries and to Israel, then under British Mandate. This was part of a comprehensive plan of these organizations to eradicate the contagious infectious diseases tuberculosis, trachoma, and ringworm (tinea capitis or *teigne*), known as TTT for short.[5]

The campaign to eradicate ringworm began in 1921 and continued intermittently until the eve of the Second World War. From 1921 to 1938, 27,760 children in Jewish communities in Eastern Europe (Poland, Lithuania, Latvia, and Romania) were treated with irradiation for ringworm.[6] In the wake of the campaign's success, the JDC-Joint and OSE wanted to carry out a similar program among the Jewish communities of North Africa. The campaign was supposed to commence in 1938 but was delayed by the outbreak of the Second World War in 1939. Following the war, the program was renewed by OSE (which by then had moved its headquarters to Paris), and in 1947 its first center in North Africa was opened in Casablanca, Morocco.

From 1947 to 1960, OSE established centers to treat TTT in Jewish communities in Morocco, Tunisia, Libya, Algeria, and Tangier. These centers operated on a footing similar to the ones that operated successfully in Eastern Europe prior to the war. In these years, some 22,000 children were treated for ringworm: 20,000 in French Morocco and approximately 2,000 in Algeria, Tunisia, Libya, and Tangier.[7]

This chapter describes the health programs for eradicating ringworm that were conducted by OSE and the Joint in Eastern Europe and North Africa as part of these two organizations' joint efforts to advance public health in Jewish communities in these two regions. The chapter will examine the concept upon which embarking on the campaign was based, will describe the key health care entities that took part, and will evaluate the impact of the campaign on similar initiatives by OSE and the Joint in additional Jewish communities around the world and in Israel. The chapter is based on historical archival documentation in Israel and elsewhere and on documents from the private archives of individuals who played a part in these operations.[8]

THE FORGOTTEN OSE-TOZ RINGWORM CAMPAIGN AMONG THE JEWISH COMMUNITY IN EASTERN EUROPE, 1921–1938

In the latter half of 1922, a unique shipment was sent from the Siemens AG plant in Erlangen, Germany. The 12 crates, marked "X-Ray Equipment," were labeled with the name of their final destination: Kovno, Riga, Lodz, Krakhov, Vilna, Bialystok, Rivne, Lemberg (Lvov), Brest-Litovsk, Warsaw (two crates), and Romania. All were for the Jewish communities in these cities, with one objective: to be used in an organized campaign to eradicate ringworm in the Jewish community in Poland and adjacent countries. The ringworm campaign began in 1921 as an initiative of the American Jewish Joint Distribution Committee (henceforth, the Joint) in conjunction with the Jewish health organizations OSE and TOZ.[9] It continued intermittently until the eve of the Second World War. During the campaign some 27,760 children in the Jewish communities of Eastern Europe were treated. Dr. Leon Wulman, one of the heads of OSE, cited that thanks to the intensive operations in Jewish community centers, particularly in educational institutions, ringworm—which had been widespread—disappeared entirely among the children in Jewish communities in Eastern Europe. This chapter covers this unique campaign to eradicate ringworm, which was the first of its kind within the framework of operations to enhance public health among Jewish communities in Eastern Europe during the period between the world wars. It also discusses the concepts behind the campaign, the primary health agents who participated in the campaign, and the long-term impact of the initiative on other health-hygiene initiatives among Jewish communities throughout the world beyond Poland and beyond Europe. The research is based on historical archival material and personal archival material provided by key individuals who took part in this operation. In addition, it seeks to underscore the importance of medical history research as a field of endeavor and its possible contribution to understanding processes and evaluating health and medical operations being carried out in Western countries today.

War, politics, and health: historical background

The end of the First World War in 1918 forged new political realities in Europe, marked by the breakdown of empires, the creation of new-old polities that received independence and national recognition, and the 1917 revolution in Russia, all of which had far-reaching ramifications for the world as a whole. This created a new reality for Jewish communities throughout Eastern and Central Europe. The Jewish community in Russia was cut off from other Jewish communities in Eastern Europe by the revolution, and the hub of Jewish activity shifted to now-independent Poland. Millions of Jewish refugees who had fled eastward during the war into areas of the Russian Empire began to return to their homes in newly established polities such as Lithuania, Latvia, Estonia, Ukraine, and Poland. The return of the refugees over a short period of time, together with the distress experienced by local Jewish communities due to the hardships of the war, led to both economic distress and growing pressure on meager resources, particularly in urban communities. Together with increasing economic straits, immigration restrictions in Western countries were being tightened, and Eastern European Jews found themselves in increasing economic and social distress. Outside assistance became crucial for Jewish communities to survive under such new circumstances. It was against this backdrop that the American-based JDC-Joint and the Berlin-based OSE and its Polish branch TOZ joined forces.

The birth of the campaign

OSE, the Society for the Protection of Jewish Health (*Obshchestvo Zdravookhraneniia Evreev* in Russian), was founded in 1912 in St. Petersburg to bring about a social and health revolution among Russian Jewry. The driving force behind the establishment of the organization was the high level of morbidity and mortality, particularly among mothers and young children, and the low level of hygiene that existed in the Jewish communities. Created by a group of Jewish physicians from St. Petersburg, its mission was to advance the cause of health and hygiene education, eradicate contagious diseases, advance the health of Jewish mothers and children, and develop and nurture physical education as part of Jewish culture, a key to enhancing the overall health and well-being of Jews in Eastern Europe. In 1922, OSE, together with TOZ, established a world federation for organizing health services for Jews, the Union OSE. In 1923 OSE's headquarters moved to Berlin, and in 1933, after the Nazi takeover in Germany, to Paris.

OSE-TOZ's operations expanded across Europe as a whole and, particularly between the two world wars, in Romania, Latvia, Poland, Germany, and France.[10] During the First World War, OSE provided medical assistance to Jewish refugees from areas of Poland and Latvia who fled to Russia, and established a network of maternal and child welfare centers that cared for a quarter of a million Jewish mothers and children. In addition to humanitarian assistance, OSE was dedicated to fighting TTT, the three core diseases that were considered a major detriment to the health status of Jews. These three diseases were a key factor in delaying the immigration of Jews to countries in the West that blocked the entrance of immigrants suspected of suffering from any of them.[11] Already in 1916, OSE had begun operations to treat ringworm, particularly among refugee children in Russia, treatment that included radiation and mass tuberculosis screening.[12] In this framework, ties with the American JDC were first established.

Jewish communities in the United States had founded the JDC-Joint in November 1914 as a vehicle for assisting Jewish refugees in Europe during the First World War. Its primary objective was to provide assistance in times of extreme stress, to assist in material and spiritual rehabilitation, and to be instrumental in enabling Jews to immigrate elsewhere. At the end of the war, the JDC established a special committee headed by the jurist and Zionist leader Bernard Flexner.[13] Flexner was responsible for formulating a list of priorities for assisting the Jews of Eastern Europe. TTT headed the list of health priorities that the JDC-Joint set for itself after the war. The first of the three to be addressed was ringworm, defined as a social-health problem of the first magnitude. This was based on the belief that ringworm was greatly detrimental to the social image of those suffering from this dermatologic ailment, particularly girls, as children suffered social isolation. Due to ringworm entire families were considered ineligible for immigration.[14]

Flexner established close ties with Dr. Ludwig Reichman, a leading authority in public health in the League of Nations and director of the National Institute for Hygiene, established in Warsaw after the First World War to promote public health issues in independent Poland. Reichman had been one of the heads of the typhus epidemic eradication program in Poland.[15] A doctor of Jewish origin, Reichman was an epidemiologist and social activist; he was a pioneer in fighting infectious diseases and an architect of treatment regimens for mass treatment and eradication of ringworm in Jewish communities.[16]

In 1921 a comprehensive working program was formulated by the JDC in conjunction with the heads of OSE for a war on ringworm, to be implemented in two main stages: first, a survey of the extent of ringworm among children in the Jewish communities in Eastern Europe; and second, the establishment of special medical centers to treat sick children, including, where needed, their hospitalization and quarantine (Figures 5.1, 5.2, and 5.6). At the beginning, all treatment of children with ringworm was carried out under JDC administration. Later, management was transferred to OSE-TOZ, while the JDC underwrote the costs and supervised the program though regular reports on its progress from on-site agents (e.g., OSE-TOZ).

The treatment program operated according to prevailing international medical standards at the time: location of children in need of treatment, microscopic diagnosis, hair loss through radiation, manual removal of any remaining hair (plucking), smearing the scalp with medicinal substances (iodine, salves, etc.), covering the head with a cap or kerchief, and quarantine of the child in a clinic or special institution until new hair growth took place.[17] In formulating a working medical program for a war on ringworm, it was specifically stipulated that the final objective was to entirely eradicate ringworm and to advance personal and public hygiene in the

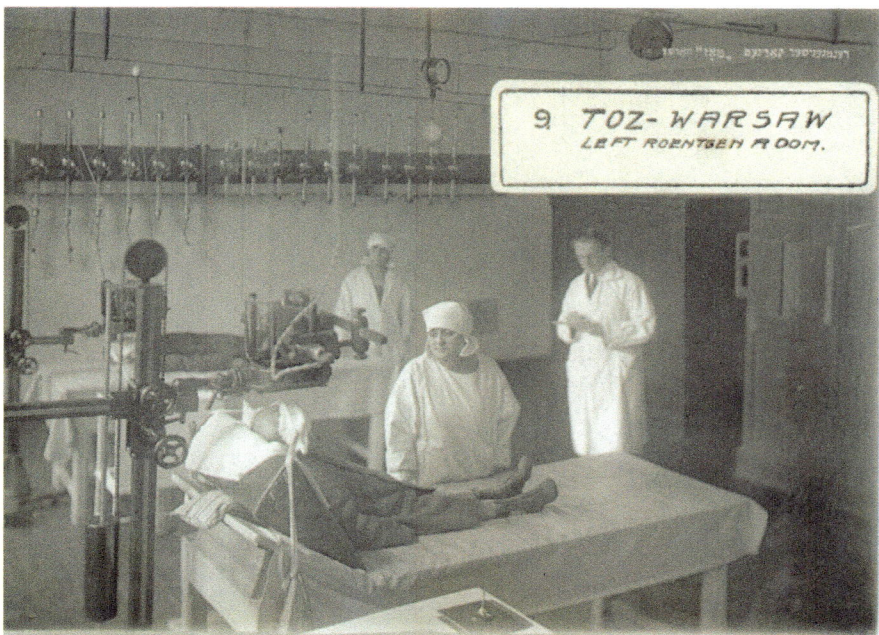

Figure 5.1 "Roentgen room," Warsaw, Poland, 1930s. The radiation dose was determined by a physician radiologist, and the procedure was performed by a radiology technician. The maximum dose given was 400 roentgens (equivalent to $1{,}032 \times 10^{-4}$ C/kg). Courtesy of the JDC Archives, New York City.

Jewish communities of Poland, not just to treat existing ringworm cases (Figures 5.3, 5.4, and 5.5).

The emphasis on eradicating scalp ringworm through treatment of existing cases and health education was repeatedly cited in professional deliberations and was a major motif that impacted the scope, content, and manner of treatment. In one of the first discussions, Dr. Altman, a member of the central ringworm committee, said that "treatment of ringworm without a parallel operation to advance health and health education and achievement of the goal of eradicating the disease would be akin to a Sisyphean exercise and fruitless throwing away of money."[18]

In order to implement the program, members of the JDC and OSE-TOZ established a network of special ringworm clinics, trained nursing and medical personnel in this specialty, and established hospitalization

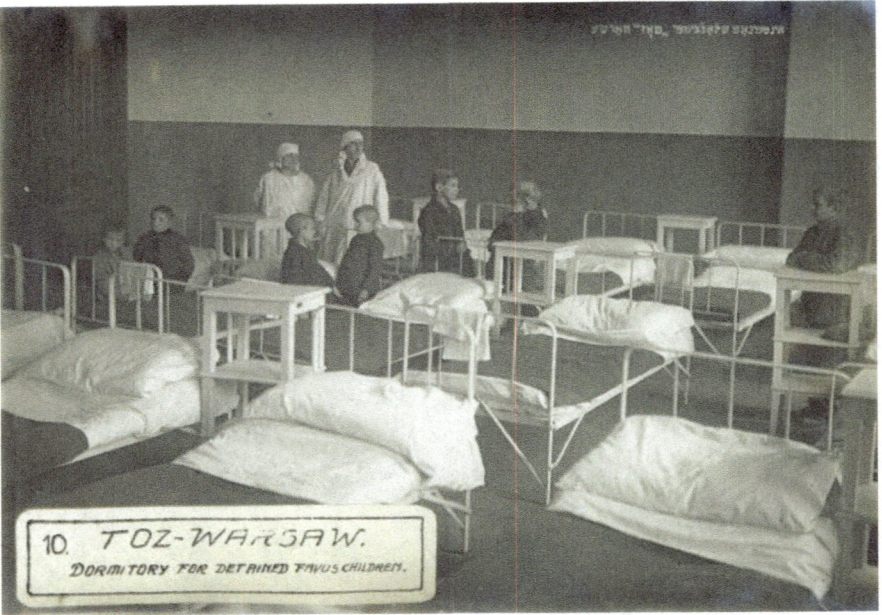

Figure 5.2 Dormitory for detained children with ringworm, Warsaw, Poland, 1930s. All children who received treatment were quarantined during hospitalization. The treatment usually lasted for 21 days.
Courtesy of the JDC Archives, New York City.

and quarantine facilities for the sick. There was to be ongoing supervision of medical work and expenses. The program encompassed all the Jewish communities in Eastern Europe, not just Poland. In 1921, the preliminary survey of the scope of ringworm among Jewish children was completed. According to Dr. Wolman, one out of every six children was infected with ringworm; Gurevitch reported that the number ranged from 10% to 19%.[19] Wolman reported that 80% of the school-age children treated were boys and 20% were girls. He noted that boys' customary head coverings (*kipot* or yarmulkes) created better conditions for the spread of ringworm, and that girls maintained a higher level of personal hygiene; moreover, the number of girls in the school system (where most children were screened) was significantly lower than the number of boys.[20] An educational and propaganda campaign was mounted to raise awareness of family and personal hygiene issues among Jews. In 1922, more than 650,000 pamphlets

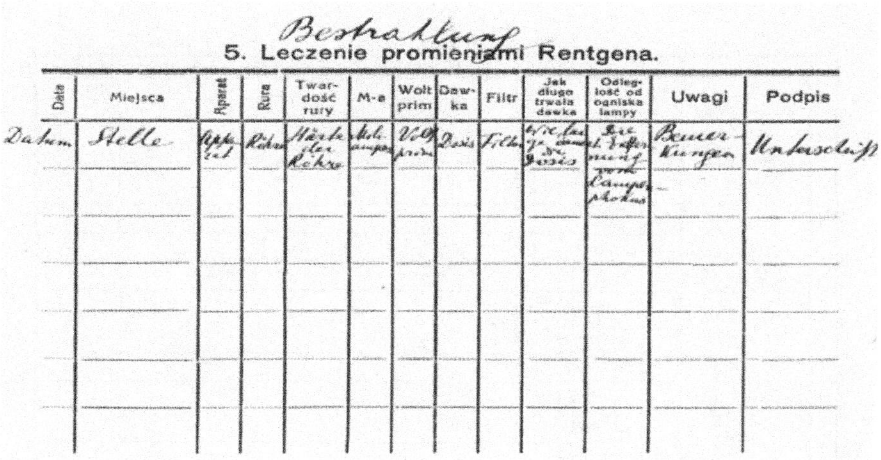

Figure 5.3 Ringworm irradiation patient medical card.

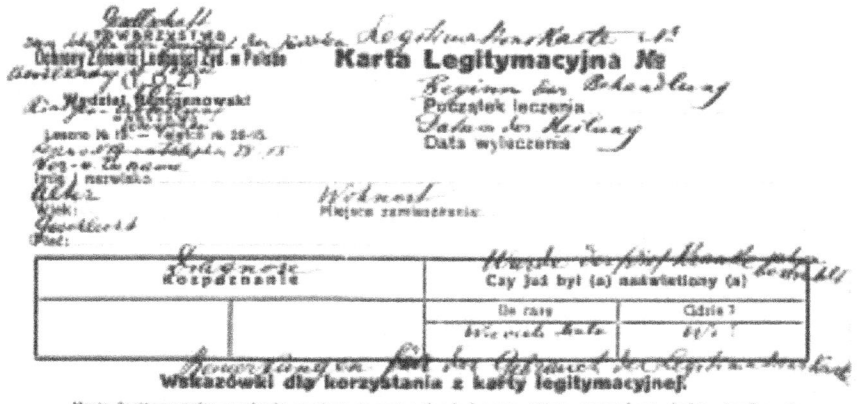

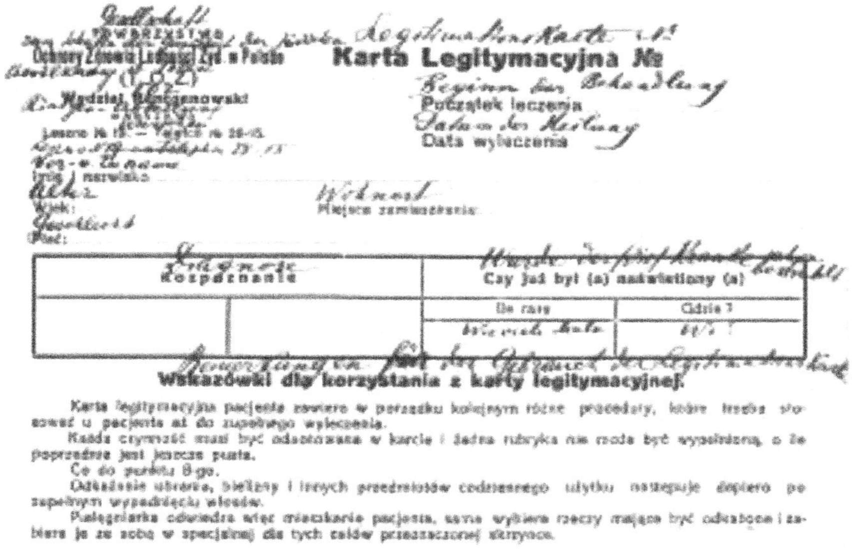

Figure 5.4 Ringworm irradiation patient medical card

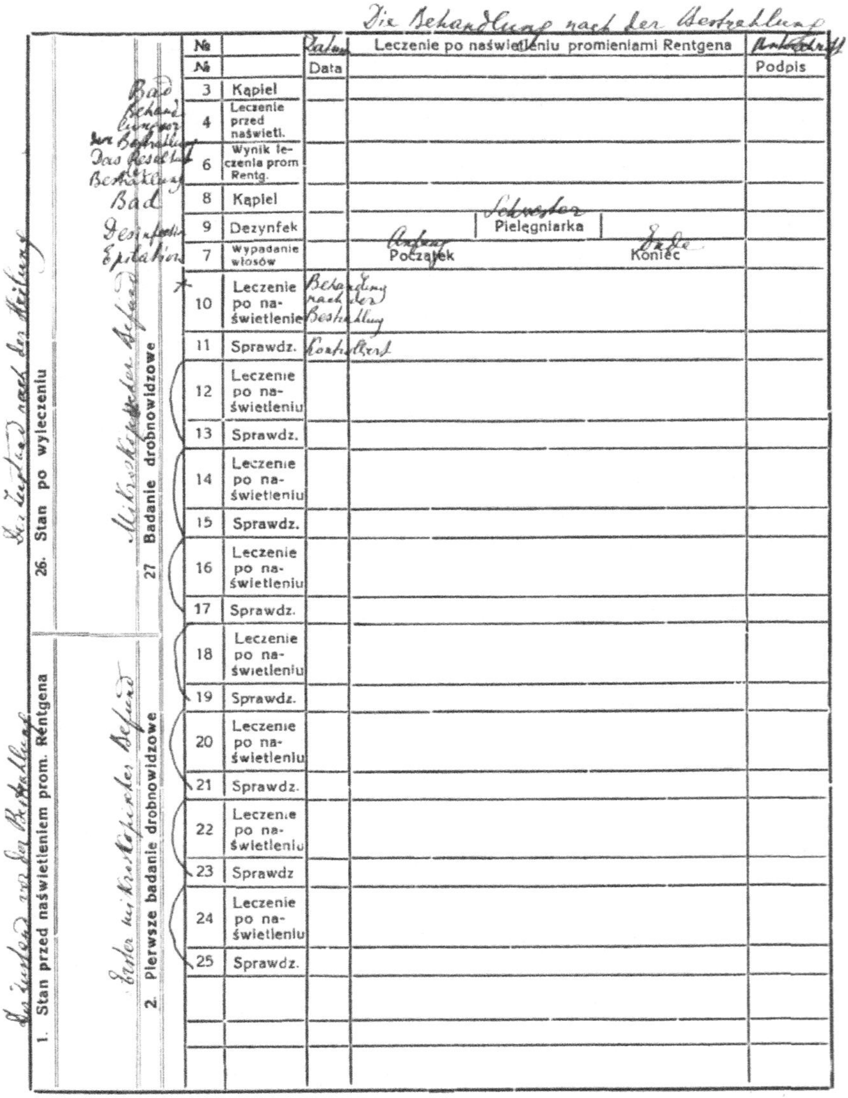

Die Behandlung nach der Bestrahlung

№		Data	Leczenie po naświetleniu promieniami Rentgena	Podpis
3	Kąpiel			
4	Leczenie przed naświetl.			
6	Wynik leczenia prom Rentg.			
8	Kąpiel			
9	Dezynfek		Pielęgniarka	
7	Wypadanie włosów		Początek / Koniec	
10	Leczenie po naświetlenie	Behandlung nach der Bestrahlung		
11	Sprawdz.	Kontrolliert		
12	Leczenie po naświetleniu			
13	Sprawdz.			
14	Leczenie po naświetleniu			
15	Sprawdz.			
16	Leczenie po naświetleniu			
17	Sprawdz.			
18	Leczenie po naświetleniu			
19	Sprawdz.			
20	Leczenie po naświetleniu			
21	Sprawdz.			
22	Leczenie po naświetleniu			
23	Sprawdz			
24	Leczenie po naświetleniu			
25	Sprawdz.			

1. Stan przed naświetleniem prom. Rentgena — Der Zustand vor der Bestrahlung

2. Pierwsze badanie drobnowidzowe — Erster mikroskopisches Befund

26. Stan po wyleczeniu — Der Zustand nach der Heilung

27 Badanie drobnowidzowe — Mikroskopischer Befund

Figure 5.5 Ringworm irradiation patient medical card. The cards included technical information about the irradiation and the names of the patients and treatment received, including details of all stages of treatment, current intensity in milliamps, duration of the treatment, etc.

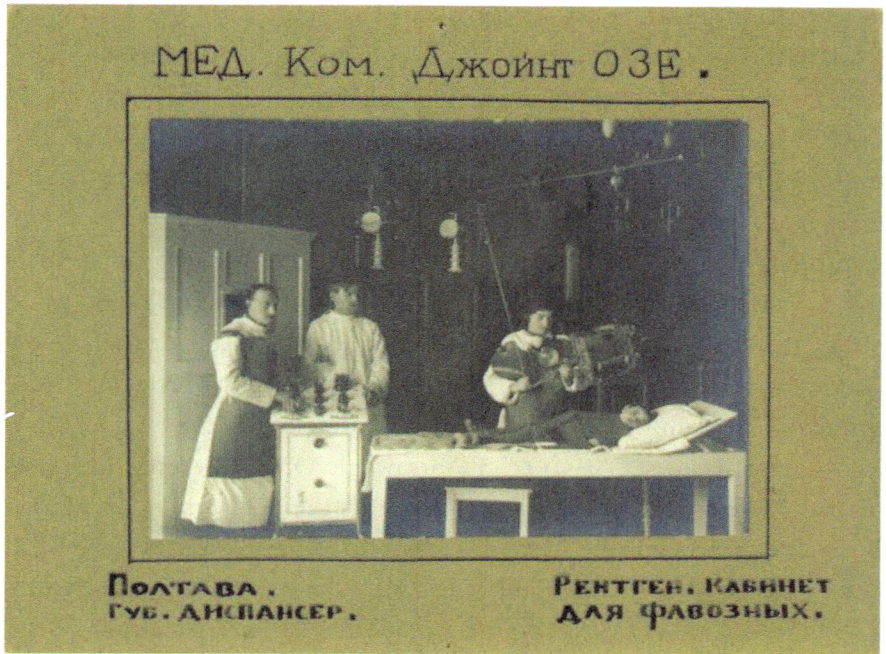

Figure 5.6 "Roentgen room," Poltava, Ukraine, 1930s. The medical personnel and the children receiving treatment wore lead aprons and collars.
Courtesy of the JDC Archives, New York City.

and booklets (in Yiddish and Polish) on contagious diseases, mainly trachoma and ringworm, with guidelines on personal health maintenance were disseminated.[21]

Ringworm care services

Organizing and establishing a network of services for a war on ringworm in all the Jewish communities of Eastern Europe required that the JDC and OSE-TOZ build a comprehensive model that would operate with uniform criteria, but would be flexible enough to accommodate an individual Jewish community being treated. Therefore, it was decided to locate a network of radiation centers (the primary technological agent in ringworm treatment) in Jewish communities in the large cities, parallel to the network of treatment clinics, ringworm diagnostic labs, and sick rooms and youth hostels where children requiring isolation would stay during treatment.[22] The decision to establish this configuration for ringworm treatment was made by a special committee of the JDC and representatives of OSE-TOZ.

In deliberations over the organization of operations, it was decided that a central ringworm committee would be appointed that would work out of Warsaw and would be responsible for the medical administration and logistics of the campaign in each Jewish community included in the program. The committee would submit periodic reports to the program's joint administrators, OSE-TOZ in Warsaw and OSE in Berlin, which had named Professor Albert Einstein as president and Professor Alexander Besredka, director of the Pasteur Institute in Paris, as a member of the board. In addition, it was stipulated that the joint administration (OSE-TOZ in Warsaw and OSE in Berlin) would send periodic medical reports, together with detailed periodic financial reports, to the JDC leadership in the United States. Eight doctors were chosen as the members of the central ringworm committee. Dr. Wolman was appointed medical director of the program.[23] It was also stipulated that each Jewish community would elect a regional ringworm committee headed by either a radiologist or a dermatologist, who would be assisted by a second physician with a specialty in dermatology or radiology. The Jewish communities were divided into seven regions: Warsaw, Brest-Litovsk, Lodz, Bialystok, Vilna, Eastern Galicia, and Western Galicia. Operations in each region were carried out by a local medical-sanitation committee that also served as a regional ringworm committee. The committee was responsible for reporting on operations in the community under its jurisdiction. Coordinating overall activities and solving ongoing problems were in the hands of the regional representatives, who met in Warsaw every few months.

The first meeting took place on September 16, 1922. The meeting protocols document deliberations that set the procedures and organization of the campaign, its operational domains, and the authority and responsibilities of each participating agent. Discussions also established the medical, administrative, and organizational hierarchy. The meeting minutes recorded reports from specific community representatives regarding the state of the equipment (e.g., working order) and its operation. Also present were representatives of the central ringworm committee of OSE-TOZ, the medical administrators of the program, and representatives of the health education departments of the two organizations. An engineer who was responsible for the coordination and operation of technological equipment was also on staff. All in all, 21 physicians and administrators from throughout Eastern Europe were present at this first meeting. The gathering in Warsaw of such a broad spectrum of Jewish community representatives from throughout Eastern Europe, despite the logistical problems such a gathering entailed (transportation, coordination, etc.), reflects the great importance assigned to the war on ringworm; indeed, the regional representatives made great efforts to attend the meeting.

The procedures and work regulations that were hammered out in that meeting, in practice, set the operational framework for the war on ringworm throughout Poland and Eastern Europe, a framework that remained in place until 1938 with only minor changes. At that meeting it was decided that the regional ringworm committees would work to appoint local ringworm committees that would include a dermatologist, an administrator, and two nurses, who would undergo special training in dermatology and radiology to meet the needs of the campaign. These local ringworm committees would follow directives from the regional ringworm committee. It was stipulated that nurses on the local committee would locate children with ringworm; after their needs were assessed, the children would be sent to the regional ringworm center, where they would receive radiation treatment. It was decided unequivocally that all centers would operate according to a unified program of medical protocols. Dr. Wolman noted that the medical protocol was set according to the latest (e.g., "state of the art") medical methods for ringworm treatment to be found in the medical literature, and that a strict framework of medical procedures would be maintained, without any deviations whatsoever.[24] The JDC took it upon itself to transfer the operating funds to the OSE-TOZ administration in Warsaw, which in turn allocated and transferred moneys to the regional agents after the central committee approved their budget proposals. According to the central ringworm committee's recommendation, most of the laboratories and x-ray centers were established adjacent to Jewish hospitals in the regions, and directives for medical collaboration with Jewish community institutions were drawn up. Some members of the central ringworm committee expressed worry that Jewish hospitals would "take over" the x-ray centers or use the facilities without authorization; these fears were addressed and resolved by establishing title to the equipment in an orderly fashion, with a written agreement with the hospitals. In practice, establishment of radiation centers and full collaboration with the heads of the Jewish communities and their institutions in the various cities endowed the ringworm campaign with legitimacy. This helped local promotional campaigns by the community staff of doctors and nurses who collaborated with the regional ringworm committee; made it possible to coordinate the survey of sick children; led the majority of Jewish educational institutions, including Talmud Torahs (yeshivas) from all streams of Judaism, to open their doors to the local ringworm committee to check all the children enrolled; and encouraged the cooperation needed to send sick children for treatment at regional centers. The budget during the first year of operation as set by the JDC was $100,000 (equivalent to $1.5 million in 2018), of which $24,000 ($360,000 in 2018)[25] was earmarked for the workings of the medical administration and the central ringworm committee in Warsaw. In 1922, the Polish Health Ministry approved the program; thus, the war against ringworm received official recognition and legal standing from Polish authorities.[26]

In order to train suitable personnel, the regional committees together with the central committee established special courses. The theoretical course was 2 weeks long; only nurses who had previous experience in similar work were eligible to enroll. Successful completion of a final certification exam was a prerequisite for working in the program. Moreover, it was decided to establish permanent "schools" that would provide training courses for nurses and other health care workers who would take part in the campaign; a special committee was established to formulate a training plan for nurses. As was customary at the time, courses were taught by eight doctors and one engineer, without even one nurse on the teaching staff. Some of the coursework was subsequently adopted as part of the curriculum at Jewish nursing schools in Vilna and Warsaw.[27] Some of the nurses were trained to be "roving nurses" whose role was to visit small communities in the region to locate "hot spots" where there were sick children with ringworm.

It was decided that payment for services would be based on the economic status of the family. Destitute families would bring a receipt from the community leadership authorizing free treatment. In addition to the assessment of the local leadership, ringworm nurses were called upon to carry out home visits to assess the economic status of the children's families. For all Jewish community members, OSE-TOZ conducted a "membership" system of health services that members paid for with graduated income-based fees. The local Jewish committee was the body that assessed this means test, providing certification of the economic status of members that served as the foundation for setting membership fees or receiving exemptions from payment. Confirmation of payment was in the form of "stamps" that were pasted into the membership card as authorization of payment or eligibility for exemption from payment. In articles published about the ringworm campaign, it was unequivocally underscored that the service should be free.

One should note that the families of those treated, primarily the mothers, cooperated fully in medical treatment of their offspring, faithfully fulfilling the doctors' orders. Treatment was carried out with the full assent of the mothers, who were happy their children could be freed of the disease, primarily due to the social stigma ringworm carried.[28] Shame was a core element in attitudes of both children and their families toward ringworm, due to the social stigma it carried and the linkage this stigma made between the disease and poor hygiene. In vintage footage from the period, the heads of children with ringworm were described as "dirty."[29] Just how deep the sham e ran is reflected in the refusal for many years of those treated for ringworm in the past to admit they had contracted the disease. In most cases, family members only discovered that their father or mother had been irradiated for ringworm as a child after they were diagnosed with cancer, usually caused by irradiation. Aharon Weisberg noted that his mother felt a deep embarrassment and refused to talk about her ringworm and treatment in Odessa until her death.[30]

Every ringworm center included the following components: a clinic, a bacteriological laboratory, an x-ray institute, auxiliary service facilities (labeled a "bathhouse" that included central bathing facilities, laundry, and sanitation services), and living quarters for children under treatment. All clinics had telephones, a technological innovation at the time, as reliable communication was essential for coordinating the complex logistics of the campaign. Standardized patient treatment record cards were designed for recording the names of the patients and details of all stages of treatment received.[31] Ongoing operations were managed by the nurses at the local ringworm center, who were responsible for follow-up after treatment in the children's homes and who managed the recordkeeping on children examined and sent for treatment. They were responsible for "sterilizing" the children's clothing to prevent reinfection. They conducted home visits to instruct family members about proper hygiene and evaluated environmental and domestic risk factors to prevent reinfection.

The work of the nurses and the scope of their roles were key issues in deliberations among the regional committees and the central committee. Not all doctors agreed that so much medical responsibility (e.g., authority) and campaign management should be placed in the hands of the nurses. After deliberations in which more than once it was argued that "after all, it is well known that doctors are bad administrators" (Dr. Gershon), it was decided that the nurses would be the ones to administer the campaign on a local level. It was concluded that each of the nurses would receive responsibility for a defined area. Since the patient intake capability of the x-ray institute was finite, it was decided that three children would be treated at one time. Therefore, it was stipulated that each nurse would be charged with bringing a specific "quota" of children to the ringworm center from throughout the region at set intervals to maintain the smooth processing of treatment groups and to prevent delays or downtime at the ringworm centers. The responsibility of each nurse for the children she brought to the center continued after treatment: She was responsible for ongoing follow-up with children who had been treated and for maintaining contact with their families during and after their treatment.

On September 17, 1922, nine nurses completed the first radiology course and a week later another nine completed dermatology training. The two groups were sent to the ringworm centers in Brest-Litovsk and Vilna. The personnel at the ringworm centers were employed on a permanent basis and received monthly paychecks. Wages were set equal to those for Polish government health services at that time. Thus, for example, in the Warsaw branch, which was the largest center, there were 15 nurses, four doctors, three administrative personnel, and a technician. In addition, there were two assistants and another nurse in the x-ray institution. Ongoing recordkeeping was conducted in Polish, German, and Yiddish. According to the record cards, it is clearly evident that the recordkeeping procedure for each sick child was orderly and meticulous, recording the child's particulars; diagnosis; microbiological tests done before, during, and after treatment; the dates radiation was administered; the radiation dosage length and power; and technical details such as use of certain filters during treatment, the distance between the child and the device, and so forth. These specific medical details enabled staff to closely follow all stages of treatment and outcomes.

The regional committee reports more than once noted ongoing problems that delayed work flow, primarily with the medical equipment and operation of the radiation centers, with an absence of suitable electric current input to run the x-ray machines, and with frequent power outages that delayed treatment. Such obstacles were part and parcel of the campaign throughout, but despite these challenges, the entire campaign was carried out according to the original plans without almost any digressions. The 1926 report that summed up 5 years of the OSE-TOZ operations marking the first part of the campaign to eradicate ringworm reported that between 1922 and 1924, 11,642 children were treated; in 1925, 2,139 children were treated; in 1926, 2,526 children were treated; in total, 16,297 children were treated.[32] Wolman, who wrote the report, noted that most of the children treated were from the large cities, and only a portion of the children from towns and villages arrived for treatment. Consequently, Wolman underscored that in the second stage of the war on ringworm, work should focus on communities on the periphery in order to totally eradicate ringworm. According to Wolman, eradication of ringworm on a scale such as this would enable many Jews to immigrate to the West and thus achieve one of the two goals of the program: to bolster Jewish immigration by curing Jewish families of contagious diseases that disqualified them as potential immigrants. In addition to medical treatment, the OSE-TOZ doctors and nurses were required to give thousands of lectures on health and hygiene issues to members of the community. The 1932 report cited, for example, that over the course of 10 years, nurses and doctors treating ringworm gave some 2,000 lectures that reached over a quarter of a million people and held more than 9,000 meetings with schoolchildren.[33]

The OSE-TOZ campaign to eradicate ringworm continued off and on in three stages up until 1937; during this entire period, the working model formulated in 1922 continued to govern operations. In Wolman's and Levine's 1937 summary reports of 15 years of the war on ringworm, they cited that in follow-up studies conducted by the organization, ringworm had disappeared entirely from Jewish communities in Poland and other Eastern European countries.[34] All told, some 250,000 Jewish children were examined in the course of the campaign, and 27,760 children were treated with radiation.[35] This was the largest epidemiologic campaign ever conducted in the first years of the 20th century, and it was extremely successful in eradicating scalp ringworm. In 1938, with receipt of the final statistics on the eradication of ringworm in Eastern Europe, the international leadership of OSE in Paris ended the program and declared the Jewish community of Eastern Europe a ringworm-free community.

Epilogue

The history of the OSE-TOZ operations is the story of a scattered community in Eastern Europe, poor for the most part and underprivileged, that succeeded in garnering the strength and ability to carry out a struggle against a disease that had a negative impact on their lives both physical and psychological, a program based on mutual assistance without the assistance of a third party.

The health campaign's success in eradicating ringworm was cut short by the war, which disrupted other campaigns. At the same time, the extermination of most of the Eastern European Jewry prevented the complications of treatment that would have appeared in adulthood from surfacing, had the children survived the Holocaust. Had these ramifications of irradiation become apparent to the medical community, it is possible that finding alternative treatments would have been accelerated by discovery of the risk, and the irradiation of many children decades later, up until the 1960s, would have been prevented.

THE CAMPAIGN OF THE JOINT AND OSE FOR ERADICATION OF RINGWORM IN THE JEWISH COMMUNITIES OF NORTH AFRICA IN THE YEARS 1947 TO 1960

Health operations in the Jewish community in North Africa

In 1947,[36] OSE embarked on establishing health centers in North Africa and operating a health program in clusters where the Jewish communities there were located. OSE had decided in 1938 to enter this region, but the Second World War and the changes in the world order that came in its wake had a great impact on OSE as well. Its activity in Eastern European countries that ended up as satellites of the USSR behind the Iron Curtain was prohibited, and OSE moved its headquarters to France.

In the framework of OSE's preparations to renew its operations in Jewish communities after the war, its 1938 plans for health initiatives in Jewish communities in North Africa were discussed. The responsibility for examining the feasibility of conducting operations in the Jewish communities of North Africa was placed on the shoulders of Professor

Moshe Prywes.[37] Joe Schwartz (director of Joint internationally) was familiar with Prywes's reputation and success in organizing medical work under difficult conditions in Eastern Europe and therefore asked Prywes to go to North Africa under the auspices of OSE and with JDC-Joint funding in order to evaluate the feasibility of renewing the plans from 1938 into action.

In 1947, Prywes and Dr. Henry Fireman (who had been appointed to direct the program in North Africa along with Prywes) embarked on a tour of the Jewish communities in North Africa. During his first trip (one of three), Prywes concluded that the situation was similar to the health status he had encountered among Jewish communities in Eastern Europe on the eve of the Second World War, although in North Africa he found that three contagious diseases (TTT) were prevalent. In their report to the OSE management, Prywes and Fireman concluded that it was feasible to implement a program to eradicate these diseases on a large scale, in the same manner in which the campaign in Jewish communities of Eastern Europe had been handled two decades earlier.[38] The decision to operate in North Africa and to embark on a TTT eradication campaign in the Jewish communities there was made solely and independently by OSE's and the JDC-Joint's management, without any connection or request to do so on the part of immigration bodies in Israel or of immigration envoys abroad,[39] the Jewish Agency,[40] or agents of the State of Israel (after May 1948).

Carrying out the program required special funding, and this matter was discussed between the Joint and OSE in 1948, based on OSE's assessment of the estimated cost of executing the program in full. On January 1, 1949, a contract was signed between the Joint and OSE regarding funding of the planned medical operations in North Africa, in which it was stated that planning and execution of the campaign would be carried out by OSE, and funding would be provided by the Joint.

The OSE health centers were established in Jewish communities in North Africa with the consent of health agencies in each of the countries and their official approval. It should be noted that the health ministries in Algeria, Morocco, and Tunisia operated under French rule, and the Ministry of Health in Libya operated under British military rule.

The health services initially provided by OSE in the first stage included primary medical services, nutrition assistance, and organization of operations to eradicate tuberculosis (the first priority), trachoma (the second priority), and ringworm (the third priority). The medical services operated in the main cities, while Jews residing in outlying urban centers and villages had to go to the urban center to receive treatment (or settle for local medical services).

Prywes cited that the OSE health team sent to North Africa comprised doctors and nurses who were specialists, most with European medical training.[41] OSE's newsletter, published in each of the Jewish communities in North Africa where it operated, reveals that as in its Eastern European operation, OSE's health teams included Jewish doctors and health and welfare personnel, specialists in pulmonary diseases (primarily due to the high prevalence of tuberculosis), radiologists, ophthalmologists, and dermatologists. The Joint's medical administration, headed by Dr. Alexander Gonik, oversaw OSE's operations and even saw to it that leading world-renowned medical authorities would visit the North African operation, including the chair of the World Health Organization—WHO and key figures in the United Nations Children's Fund—UNICEF

When a problem with a case arose at one of the centers, it was discussed at OSE headquarters, where it was decided whether to continue treatment on site or transfer the case to another center. In addition, there was ongoing monitoring of the doctors, who were required to report regularly on any mishaps and on the quality of treatment.

OSE's operations in North Africa in ringworm eradication were carried out in a manner similar to that employed in Eastern Europe between the world wars. This fact was underscored by Dr. Gonik, who was the president of OSE internationally and the medical director of the Joint in Europe: "One should learn from our experience in Eastern Europe and establish a number of large x-ray centers in order to eradicate the disease."[42]

The arrangements for examining the children in all the Jewish communities of North Africa were similar to those carried out in Eastern Europe. The hub for examinations was schools and other educational institutions. As in Eastern Europe, children in need of treatment were identified by public health nurses who operated in the schools under OSE's auspices. This measure was conducted in full cooperation with the Alliance school network[43] and with the Talmud Torah network.[44] Pupils diagnosed by the nurses as ill were sent for further diagnosis, either x-rays (for tuberculosis) or microbiological examination (for ringworm). If this further examination established that a child was indeed sick, the child was either (1) sent to a treatment center and remained there until cured or (2) sent home to be kept isolated until an OSE nurse approved the child's return to school, after clinical examination to establish the child had indeed been cured. In other cases, topical treatment was provided at local OSE clinics (primarily for trachoma, which did not require hospitalization), and where needed, treatment was provided at other clinics by physicians working under an agreement with OSE.

The operations of OSE and the Joint in the Jewish communities of North Africa were driven by a vision to advance the health of members of the Jewish community per se, with no relation to or dependence whatsoever on Israel's immigration policies or immigration trends in other countries. Both OSE and the Joint viewed themselves as apolitical Jewish philanthropic organizations and repeatedly stressed that they were not Zionist organizations—a position that granted them freedom of action, relatively speaking. While at the request of the Jewish Agency OSE and the Joint took it upon themselves to conduct medical examinations of candidates for immigration to Israel, they zealously safeguarded their organizational independence and did not allow any Israeli entities to intervene in their work.

As a rule, trachoma and ringworm were not grounds for delaying immigration to Israel, and sick children were not required to undergo medical treatment as a proviso to their immigration to Israel. Senior administrators in Israel's Ministry of Health preferred that children with ringworm would come and receive treatment in Israel after their arrival and would not be treated in their communities of departure or in transit camps prior to their immigration to Israel; they argued that treatment in Israel was better. At times, immigration to Israel of persons with tuberculosis was delayed out of fear they could spark an epidemic. They were allowed to immigrate only after they had been treated and their status had improved. In general, tuberculosis testing was also carried out by OSE physicians among Holocaust survivors in displaced persons camps in Europe and in Jewish communities in North Africa, in coordination with the Jewish Agency and the JDC-Joint.[45] Those with tuberculosis were also treated before they were allowed to immigrate to Israel.[46] Thus, for example, in 1951 letters were sent by the Ministry of Health's senior officials to the Joint's staff and to doctors acting on behalf of the Jewish Agency and the Israeli Ministry of Health (henceforth "trustee physicians")[47] operating in Morocco saying that the immigration to Israel of families that included children with ringworm, would not be delayed.[48] Dr. Haim Sheva (director-general of the Ministry of Health in Israel from 1950 to 1953) demanded that the Jewish Agency stop treating children with ringworm or trachoma prior to their immigration to Israel, and demanded they be brought for treatment in Israel. The Jewish Agency administration wrote in December 1951:

> We have emphasized that there is no justification to detain families or even individual children due to ringworm. If we will simply receive notification on the children's arrival, we will treat them immediately... Already during discussion of the immigration of 10,000 children from North Africa, we expressed our opinion that immigration of ringworm children should be permitted **without** [emphasis in the original] any treatment in France on sundry grounds [i.e., whatever the motivation]. We reiterate and underscore that we are prepared to take care of all cases of ringworm that will come... therefore, please give appropriate directives.[49]

And thus, from 1952 to 1960, some 4,000 children with ringworm from North African Jewish communities arrived in Israel, where practically all of them were treated after their arrival. The largest group, numbering 1,840 children with ringworm, immigrated to Israel in 1955 and 1956[50] on the eve of the French withdrawal from Morocco and the establishment of Moroccan independence.

Treatment of ringworm in the Jewish community in Morocco

The Jewish community in Morocco was the largest in North Africa, and most of the Jews lived in French Morocco.[51] From mid-1948 (establishment of the State of Israel) until the late 1960s, close to 250,000 Moroccan Jews immigrated to Israel, the largest group of Jews from Muslim countries to settle in Israel.

OSE-Joint's medical program in North Africa were initiated first in Morocco, where the prevalence of ringworm was particularly high, and only after that in Tunisia, Algeria, and Libya. On the eve of OSE's arrival in Morocco (in 1947), it mobilized a medical team of nurses and technicians; shipped equipment; and in addition to its center operating in Casablanca, also opened community health centers and clinics in Sefrou, Fez, Marrakesh, Salé, and el-Kenitra (Port Lyautey).[52]

Despite the desire of OSE medical director Gonik to begin operations immediately after OSE's arrival in North Africa, in 1947 (its first year of operation) OSE established only one large center to treat ringworm with irradiation (in Casablanca). Jewish communities in smaller cities and on the periphery were also treated there. In communities where the OSE did not operate, children with ringworm, both Jews and Muslims, were treated at the local public clinics, the Santé publique of the Moroccan Ministry of Health, which was under the supervision of the French authorities. These clinics provided primary health care, not only treatments for ringworm.[53] According to Prywes, OSE's operations in Morocco enjoyed the protection and patronage of Dr. Ben Zaken, the private physician of the Moroccan sultan (Figures 5.7, 5.8, and 5.9).[54]

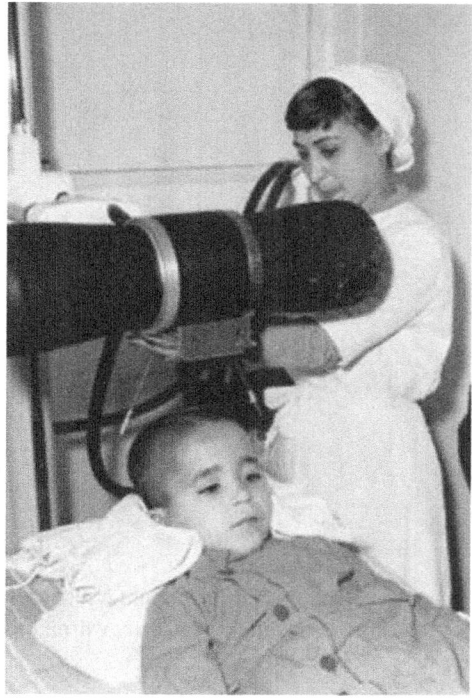

Figure 5.7 Irradiation of a child for ringworm, Morocco, 1950s
Courtesy of the JDC Archives, New York City.

The Casablanca center for ringworm treatment

As noted, ringworm was very prevalent in the Jewish community in Morocco. According to various reports, the percentage of children with ringworm (and also trachoma) was 40% of all Jewish children.[55] For this reason, Morocco was chosen as the first country in North Africa where OSE embarked on its eradication campaign. The first OSE center to treat ringworm was opened in 1947 in Casablanca, where the Jewish population numbered 100,000. In the first stage, the center operated out of the building housing the Jewish community's public clinic, La Maternelle (maternal and child clinic). The clinic had been in operation since the beginning of the 1920s and provided most of the medical services for the Jewish

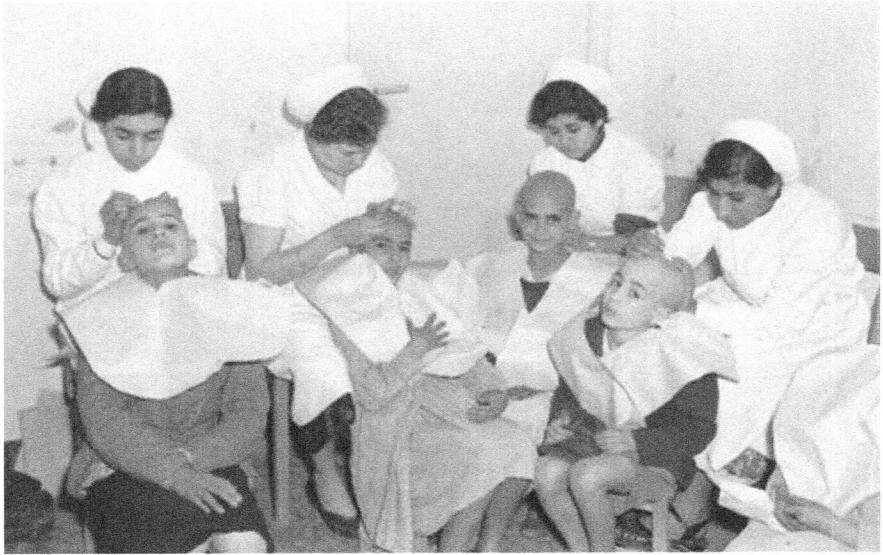

Figure 5.8 Children receiving complementary treatment (epilation) to remove remaining hair with tweezers after irradiation against ringworm, Morocco, 1955 Courtesy of the JDC archives, New York City.

community. Until OSE's arrival in Morocco, the clinic was underwritten jointly by the Jewish community and Jewish organizations abroad.

Under the new framework, the clinic operated in the mornings as a maternal and child clinic and as a primary medical care clinic and in the afternoons as a treatment center primarily for ringworm and trachoma. An x-ray institute was opened on the premises, headed by Dr. Levy-Lebhar,[56] who administered radiation treatment to children. Parallel to this, OSE signed an agreement with the Alliance Jewish school network that enabled OSE to conduct periodic examinations of children at Alliance schools to identify sick children, who were then referred for treatment at the clinic.

According to Dr. Levy-Lebhar, the number of children with ringworm in Casablanca in the Jewish community at the outset of the program was about 10,000. Dr. Levy-Lebhar said that prior to the decision to treat ringworm with irradiation, there was an unsuccessful attempt at the clinic to treat it by chemical means. He stated that the failure of chemical treatment was what prompted OSE's decision to change to irradiation treatment.[57]

The professional staff assigned to treat ringworm in Casablanca included two doctors and 43 nurses and technicians. Due to the large number of sick children, it was impossible to hospitalize them in special dormitories, under isolation throughout the treatment period, as had been customary in Eastern Europe. Therefore, the schools who cooperated with

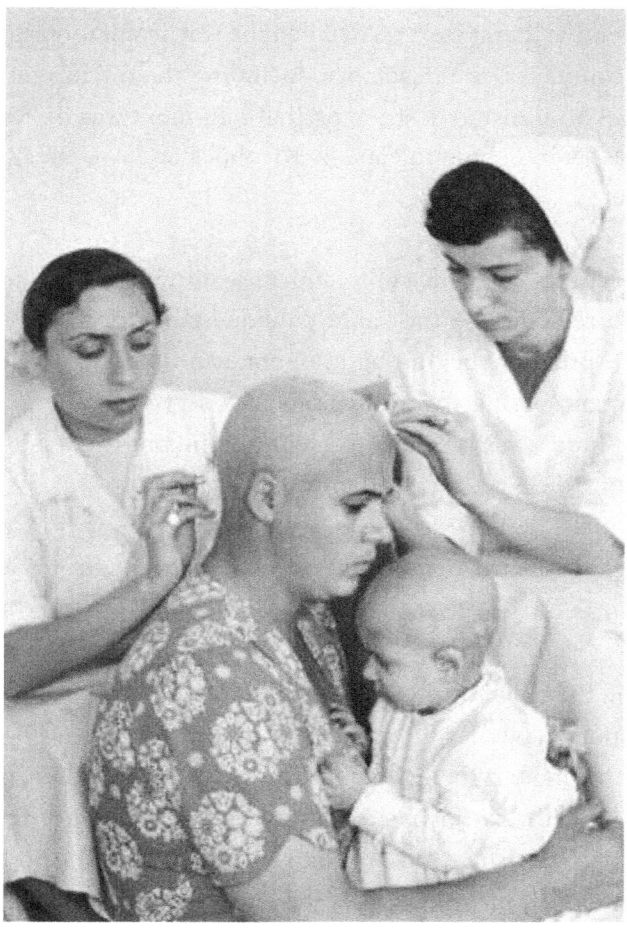

Figure 5.9 Jewish mother and child being treated after irradiation for ringworm, Casablanca, Morocco, 1958
Courtesy of the JDC Archives, New York City.

OSE (primarily those of the Alliance network) decided to establish separate classrooms in the schools—either for children cured of ringworm or for children who were free of ringworm, in order to prevent recurrent infection; this was the classroom configuration for addressing ringworm that was used in France and the United States.

The management of the x-ray setup for ringworm treatment in Casablanca was in the hands of Dr. Levy-Lebhar. He meticulously followed the progress of the ringworm patients and wrote detailed scientific reports on the topic of ringworm treatment.[58] In his articles in the international medical-scientific literature,[59] he detailed the way irradiation against ringworm was conducted in Casablanca, including the intensity of the radiation dosages administered, stressing that treatment was in keeping with the protocols set by Sabouraud and by Kienböck and Adamson, published in the *Lancet*:

> In Morocco, in the OSE clinic and in a number of public health centers [a reference to the Santé publique network run by French authorities] that are beginning to operate and for whom the center for treatment of ringworm in Casablanca serves for them as a department model and a school for staff/administrative personnel, we are applying the Kienböck–Adamson technique.[60]

He compared the treatment used for ringworm in Europe and that required in North Africa:

> In Europe the ringworm more prevalent is *Microsporia* [a strain of ringworm fungus], easy to treat, almost without the need for further complementary epilation. In Morocco, on the other hand, we are dealing with *Trichophytons* [a strain of ringworm fungus] that is particularly resistant, that the hair infected with [Trichophytons] breaks at the hair opening [i.e., at the hairline] or grows from within the hair bulb and there is the need to remove it with a tweezers by experts in epilation, in order to prevent recurrence of the disease. The treatment given initially by the children's families proved

insufficient. In the face of the number of recurrent attacks, we had to establish by ourselves within the OSE clinic a complete setup, thanks to which the children receive as externals [i.e., ambulatory patients] (without hospitalization) all the treatments prior to hair fallout and afterwards, until complete renewed growth.[61]

He noted that recurrent infection with ringworm was one of the key problems in treatment, and several hundred children required additional irradiation treatment due to such recurrence. To prevent reinfection as much as possible, OSE established a ringworm nurses service.[62] The nurses conducted house visits and instructed mothers how to treat their children after epilation had been set in motion by irradiation. Following the success of irradiation treatment, in November 1953 it was announced that schoolchildren in the Alliance network in Casablanca were now ringworm-free.

As for the technical aspect, Dr. Levy-Lebhar noted that "In 1950, we received new devices, and we began new measurements in order to widen the gap between the most effective dosage and the detrimental dosage."[63] According to M.R.,[64] a nurse in a clinic for treating ringworm in Casablanca headed by Dr. Levy-Lebhar, in light of the failure of the conservative ringworm treatment (ointments, mechanical epilation), all the ringworm patients who came for treatment at the Casablanca clinic were treated via irradiation. Until the end of the 1960s, all treatments administered for ringworm included irradiation, and in OSE clinics there was no treatment for ringworm that didn't include irradiation. According to M.R., treatment was as follows:

At the beginning, and for preparation just before irradiation, the hair of the patients was cut off using a barber's appliance. Afterwards, they were taken into the radiation room and a metal frame was put on their head that was in the shape of a X bent and rounded like a hollow *casque* [helmet], for marking 5 fields and different regions of the head that should be irradiated.[65] [They] would mark the two sides of the scalp in the area of the ears, at the back, at the center of the scalp and from the front. This action was carried out while the patient was positioned standing up or sitting. After marking the above areas, the metal cap was removed, and [they] laid the patients down on a kind of table, placed on their bodies pieces of lead, and [they] repeatedly warned and cautioned the patients not to move, and afterwards [they] did the irradiations with a radiation machine in the various regions of the head and in accordance with the markings. The length of time irradiation was given to each region that was marked was between 3 and 3.45 minutes according to the age of the patient and according to the area that was being irradiated. After the irradiation, [they] had to wait 15 days until hair fallout as a result of the irradiation. During these 15 days, [they] would give alkaloid treatment (spreading iodine) on the scalp, and in another 5 days, [they] spread on a white oxide of zinc ointment[66] and the head was wrapped in a bandage, so that hair that fell out and was very contagious would not scatter and infect others. After 5 days, [they] would take off the baggage and the ointment, and remaining hairs that were left [they] would remove by spreading warm wax on the head and tearing out the hair in opposite to the direction of its growth. After the wax, [they] would spread Vaseline ointment in order to cool the head. Afterwards, a dermatologist would examine the patient. For two months after the examination, the patient would come to the Institute once every eight days, and a nurse would extract hair-by-hair with a tweezers, a procedure called epilation. During the 8 days between epilation to epilation, [they] would spread iodine on the head, and it, in essence, was the treatment of the disease itself.[67]

As for the quality of treatment, according to Dr. Levy-Lebhar, "It was what enabled us to treat 15,000 children and to cure them since 1947 without one accident in the OSE clinic in Casablanca."[68] He compared the performance of the treatment against ringworm in Casablanca to other campaigns in Europe, such as UNICEF's ringworm campaign in Yugoslavia (Serbia of today) and programs in Italy and Spain. He even presented his findings at an international conference held in Munich in 1957.

According to Dr. Levy-Lebhar, parallel to OSE's treatment operations against ringworm, there were other private and public centers operating in Casablanca to which parents and children in the Jewish community turned. These centers were not part of OSE's operations. He noted in particular in his reports the Santé publique network of clinics,[69] which treated ringworm with irradiation and constituted the central hub for Casablanca residents (Muslims and Jews alike) receiving this treatment.[70] According to him, OSE's treatment was superior to that provided in public clinics or in local radiology institutes.

In another of his articles, Dr. Levy-Lebhar stated that treatment at the OSE clinic in Casablanca was carried out without any mishaps. He stressed that it was vital to treat ringworm, especially among girls and women. He said that unlike in boys, among most of the women who were not treated for their ringworm, the disease did not disappear spontaneously in adolescence, and they continued to suffer from baldness or bald spots; consequently, after marriage, such women became a contagious agent for their children. Therefore, it was very important to eradicate their ringworm, along with all its contagious agents.[71] The nurses who conducted home visits also stressed that mothers were a core contagious agent, particularly due to their physical proximity to their children, and also due to the low levels of consent among such mothers to receive treatment for their ringworm. As a result, even if their children were treated and cured, the likelihood that such children of untreated mothers would face recurrent infection was high.

The center for irradiation against ringworm in Casablanca also served as an in-service training and consulting clinic for the other centers that were opened by OSE in additional cities in Morocco. The nurses underwent in-service training in Casablanca, and Dr. Levy-Lebhar was also required to oversee the quality of treatment in additional ringworm centers outside the city.

According to M.R., she was invited to instruct nurses in carrying out irradiation at other clinics outside Casablanca, including public clinics run by local authorities: "In Marrakesh I myself gave the irradiations a number of times in order to teach local nurses how to give the irradiations."[72]

At the Eliyahu Jewish Immigration Camp near Casablanca, Jews from throughout Morocco were concentrated in preparation for their immigration to Israel. OSE established a clinic in Casablanca to treat ringworm among children residing in the camp. This action was ceased after the port physician recognized children with ringworm due to their bald heads and detained them in the port on the grounds that under the Naples Convention of the UN's International Labor Organization, the French government was not permitted to allow the emigration of sick people, including children.[73]

Operation and maintenance of the x-ray machines was the key weak point in the ringworm treatment centers in the various cities in Morocco. There weren't enough maintenance technicians or spare parts, and often the machines were out of commission for months on end, halting treatment. In such cases, the children waited until work renewed at the clinic, or were sent in small groups for irradiation treatment in Casablanca. OSE-Joint reports from Morocco stated more than once that maintenance and technical care of the x-ray machines was a core problem for them in the TTT program. A similar problem also existed with regard to chest x-ray equipment used to identify those with tuberculosis.

In the 1950s, additional health centers were opened by OSE in the cities of Sefrou, Fez, Marrakesh, Salé, and el-Kenitra (Port Lyautey), all underwritten as set forth in the OSE-Joint agreement (i.e., by the Joint). These centers were modeled after the Casablanca center—that is, the OSE clinic operated as part of the local clinic of the Jewish community. Ongoing reports from OSE and the Joint reveal that most of the clinics provided mother and child services, primary medical care, treatment for trachoma, and health services for schools (primarily schools in the Alliance network and the Talmud Torah network).

The treatment of ringworm patients in these cities hinged on operation of x-ray machines, accompanied by nurses and trained physicians, but they could not always to be found. Many times, it was reported that for months on end treatment for ringworm could not be conducted, and in other cases children were sent to public clinics in the city or to private doctors in order to receive irradiation, after which they returned to the

OSE clinic for complementary (i.e., post-irradiation) treatment. Also, the supervision of the clinics' work wasn't orderly, and more than once there were reports of improper or unprofessional conduct. Dr. Levy-Lebhar wrote that the treatment at the clinics in other cities was not of the same quality as that given in Casablanca, and he criticized the medical staff in these clinics.

Furthermore, according to the doctors from Israel who visited Morocco and examined the children who were treated for ringworm prior to immigrating to Israel, the treatment in some of the OSE clinics did not meet accepted medical standards. Such assessments played a role in the decision of the Israeli Ministry of Health that it would preferable to treat ringworm patients in Israel rather than in Morocco. Dr. Levy-Lebhar responded that the problem was not just children treated at the OSE clinics, but also those treated at local public health clinics (Santé publique), and OSE had no way to influence the workings of such clinics.

Already by 1950, in correspondence between Dr. Meir (director-general of the Israeli Ministry of Health, 1948–1950) and the Absorption Department of the Jewish Agency, discussion regarding the quality of treatment of ringworm patients in Morocco had begun. This was prompted by dissatisfaction voiced by Professor Druckman, director of the Hadassah Hospital radiology department, concerning the treatment for ringworm being given by OSE-Joint in immigrant camps abroad or by OSE health centers in Morocco. In Druckman's opinion, the children should be treated in Israel under Hadassah's auspices; that way, they would receive optimal treatment and could be monitored afterward to prevent contagion or recurrent infection. However, without a suitable centralized site with x-ray equipment, it wasn't possible to bring all the patients to Israel for treatment. As Dr. Koren, from the Jewish Immigration Department's Medical Supervision Unit, wrote:

> Consequently, the question remains unaltered, whether it isn't more logical to bring to Israel the children sick with these diseases and to cure them here . . . however, the answer always was in the negative,

due to lack of any feasibility to execute treatment such as this on a large scale in Israel.[74]

In additional deliberations between the Joint and the Jewish Agency on this manner, no practical conclusion was reached, and in practice, the situation remained the same, without any uniform treatment policy. Part of the treatment continued to be given abroad, much to Professor Druckman's regret. Rotation of the Ministry of Health's director-general (Dr. Sheba replaced Dr. Meir) changed the situation. Dr. Sheba adopted Professor Druckman's opinion regarding the quality of ringworm treatment, concluding that he preferred irradiation to be done in Israel rather than abroad. He was determined to establish a national center for the treatment of ringworm (primarily children) in order to prevent delay of their immigration to Israel, in addition to his view that the treatment in Israel and its supervision were superior to that customary abroad. On the other hand, Israeli health entities had no ability to intervene in the work of OSE-Joint, since the two organizations operated totally independently and according to policy they set for themselves. In practice, OSE's health centers continued to operate in various cities, providing ringworm treatment through irradiation, with only partial supervision.

OSE-Joint operations to eradicate ringworm in Morocco following independence (1956 to 1960)

In April 1956, a few months after Morocco gained independence, the country announced the closure of its gates and put an end to immigration to Israel. On June 10, all operations in Morocco by Israel or on its behalf were banned, including medical examinations before immigration. The immigrant camp outside Casablanca was also closed. By the end of 1956, all operations on behalf of the State of Israel in Morocco had been shut down. However, OSE and the Joint, which were not Zionist organizations, could continue to provide health services at clinics as they had done previously.

Immigration to Israel was possible only after receipt of permits to emigrate from Morocco to France, and once in France, in an indirect fashion, to quietly immigrate to Israel. Official organized immigration to Israel was only renewed in 1961 after King Hassan II ascended to the throne and allowed Moroccan Jews to leave—in exchange for a ransom paid for every one of the remaining Jews. In a summary report in 1963, Dr. Taville, the medical director of OSE in Morocco, noted that the total number of children who had been irradiated for ringworm at OSE centers in Morocco between 1948 and 1960 was 20,000.[75]

OSE operations in treatment of ringworm in Algeria, Tunisia, and Libya

Algeria

The Jewish community in Algeria in 1948 encompassed approximately 130,000 persons, practically all of them living in the country's three main cities—Algiers, Constantine, and Oran. Unlike the Jewish communities in Morocco and Tunisia, which were also under French rule, the Jews of Algeria had already received French citizenship in 1870. Therefore, their civil status was better than that of their brethren in other North African countries, and they enjoyed public health services that the French operated in Algeria without discrimination. Starting in 1940, the Jewish community operated a central clinic in Algiers. As it had done in Casablanca, OSE sought to integrate its own health work within the community clinic's physical plant and operating schedule. Because the health status of most of the Jewish community's members was better than that of the Jewish communities in Morocco and Tunisia, the initial operating budget of OSE-Joint in Algeria was much lower: $1,500 per year, compared to $30,000 in Morocco and $25,000 in Tunisia.

According to the first health report on the Jewish community in Algiers, only 50 persons with ringworm had been identified; they were treated in private clinics and came to the community's clinic for further complementary treatment. Therefore, the Joint recommended that an irradiation center not be established in the city. Parenthetically, the report cited that a large portion of those with ringworm were the children of refugees from Morocco who arrived in the city and were treated by the Jewish community, which even opened an assistance center in a hotel in Algiers on behalf of Jewish refugees from Morocco.[76]

Reports of the Joint and of OSE, as well as letters sent by Zeev Haklei (a Jewish Agency envoy in North Africa in the 1950s), described a similar situation, where the few children with ringworm were treated by local private physicians and referred for further complementary treatment at the OSE clinic in the city. Other than Algiers, there are no reports from other cities on operations by OSE-Joint in eradication of ringworm.[77]

Because the number of immigrants to Israel from Algeria was very low, the Jewish community there was not included in the agreement the Jewish Agency had signed with OSE-Joint for the latter carrying out medical examinations in North Africa prior to immigration to Israel.[78]

Tunisia

The Jewish community in Tunisia, who lived under the protection of French rule, had a population of 100,000, practically all of them residing in the capital city, Tunis. OSE entered Tunisia in late 1947. It opened community clinics in the cities of Tunis, Gabès, Sfax, and Sousse and on the island of Djerba. OSE's first reports on the health status of Tunisian Jews reveals that no irradiation center was set up under its auspices, and most ringworm children were treated with traditional methods—epilation with thallium acetate (a toxic substance that causes hair to fall out)[79] or mechanically (with tweezers) and application of an antifungal ointment, salicylanilide.[80] The medical staff who treated ringworm children included a part-time doctor, who operated in Tunis. Only in 1953 did treatment with irradiation begin for children with ringworm, and even then only in Tunis on a very partial footing. For this purpose, OSE employed a part-time radiologist. In the rest of the community, treatment with ointments and manual epilation continued, and only in particularly serious cases were the patients sent for irradiation treatment in Tunis.

The scope of ringworm presented in the reports was low: only several hundred children. Reports cite a 90% success rate in eradicating ringworm using conservative treatment methods, without irradiation. Dr. Gonik (the medical director of OSE) remarked that treatment with salicylanilide in children in Gabès was successful and the majority were cured.[81]

From time to time, letters were sent that reveal OSE-Joint in Tunisia vacillated about purchasing an x-ray machine, whose cost was high (about $5,000). In 1953, 1,100 children with ringworm were identified in Tunis, but only 530 of them were treated with irradiation.

It seems that the number of children with ringworm in Tunisia was relatively low. According to Ministry of Health reports, of all the immigrants with ringworm who arrived in the 1950s at the Shaar HaAliyah intake camp (south of Haifa), it appears that the number of ringworm children who arrived from Tunisia was so low that it wasn't even cited in the breakdown by country of origin; in contrast, the number of ringworm children from Morocco, Libya, Iran, Yemen, and Iraq was duly noted.[82]

Libya

The Jewish community in Libya was the smallest among the Jewish communities in North Africa: It numbered approximately 36,000 persons, practically all of them living in Tripoli. Until 1951, Libya was under British military governance, and the situation of the Jews was relatively secure. Since approximately a third of the community immigrated to Israel in the early 1950s, only a relatively small Jewish community remained in Libya. OSE entered Libya in 1949, and the first health survey conducted noted that there were children with ringworm and that they were treated with conservative techniques using salicylanilide and manual epilation. Health services were provided by an Italian physician who had married one of the daughters of the Jewish community and had the full confidence of the community. A physician operating under the auspices of OSE came from time to time to supervise all the medical operations. Further complementary treatment for ringworm among the children was given by an Italian nurse who worked in the Jewish community's clinic.

In practice, the primary health problem was tuberculosis; ringworm was only of secondary importance. Since the community was small, the scope of OSE's operations was partial. Also, the number of immigrating children who had ringworm when they arrived in Israel was not cited in Ministry of Health reports, so one can assume that they were relatively low. Dr. Shmuel Spiro, a Youth Aliyah doctor who visited Tripoli in 1949 on behalf of the Jewish Agency, said that the primary morbidity among the Jews of Libya was trachoma, and ringworm was a secondary issue that was treated successfully with topical treatment.[83] In later reports, out of 1,600 ringworm children mentioned, only 376 were sent for irradiation treatment, practically all of them from the Jewish school in Tripoli. The rest of the children in the Jewish community in Libya were treated with ointments, or antifungal treatment and manual epilation, and only a few were treated with irradiation. Most of the Libyan Jews immigrated to Israel by 1951, the year British control was relinquished and Libya received independence. OSE's operation was subsequently curtailed greatly and came to a close in late 1950.

From North Africa to Israel: ringworm treatment in the transit camps for Jewish immigrants in southern France (Marseille and the vicinity)

The rise in Jewish immigration to Israel at the beginning of the 20th century created a huge logistical problem for the World Zionist Movement and the Jewish Agency. On one hand, the British limited the number of immigration certificates to enter Mandate Israel; on the other hand, masses of immigrants headed for Mediterranean ports in an attempt to find a way to reach Israel. The rise of the Nazis to power in 1933 added greatly to the number of Jews seeking to immigrate. To organize immigration in an orderly fashion, it was decided to establish transit camps for immigrants in the vicinity of Marseille in southern France. Already in the 1940s the Jewish Agency established 15 to 19 transit camps for immigrants to Israel. The majority were old army camps left by the various armies that went through the area beginning with the First World War. From 1945 to 1948 these camps constituted a central juncture where most Holocaust survivors gathered on their way to Israel. Up until the establishment of the state, the camps operated under the administration and organization of Zionist youth movements. With the establishment of the State of Israel, authority was transferred to the Immigration Department of the Jewish Agency, which was the official body handling the immigration of Jews to Israel.

The Marseille camps became the main point of departure for Israel. Due to the lengthy period that immigrants stayed in these camps, it became necessary to establish a broad infrastructure of health services. A large staff of administrators, nurses, and social workers was mobilized to fulfill these functions. The immigrants who arrived in the camps underwent a basic medical exam and received vaccinations, and if they were healthy, sailed for Israel after 2 weeks. The sick and disabled were sent to a special camp for medical treatment, where they stayed until they were well. Among the diseases cited as prevalent among immigrants were trachoma, syphilis, and ringworm.

As in North Africa, the medical treatment at the Marseille camps was provided by OSE and was funded with the assistance of the Joint and the government of Israel. A team of 40 OSE staffers conducted the medical checkups for immigrants who arrived at the camps and sent those who were sick for treatment.

Irradiation was administered at the hospital adjacent to the camp that treated new immigrants in need of hospitalization.[84] The hospital itself received consultation, medical, and academic support on ringworm issues from the Hôpital Saint-Louis in Paris, the leading authority in ringworm research in France.[85] In addition to irradiation treatment at the hospital, OSE established five special clinics specifically for ringworm and one general dermatology clinic. In this manner, ringworm treatment was conducted with full coordination between the hospital and the clinics operating in the framework of the camp.

Children found to have ringworm were hospitalized. Their hair was cut and they were sent for irradiation treatment. Afterwards the scalp was covered with a salve both to prevent infection and to soften the skin prior to manual plucking of the remaining hair (epilation) with tweezers. After treatment was completed, their head was wrapped in a white bandana to prevent hair from falling out and infecting others. During treatment, the child's family waited in the regular camp. After the child was cured, the family was allowed to immigrate to Israel (Figures 5.10 and 5.11).

In a special discussion on this topic on April 18, 1951, it was reported that 80% of the children arriving from North African Jewish communities in the Marseille camps had ringworm, and that the length of treatment for ringworm in the camp prior to immigrating was 5 to 6 weeks. The length of treatment time delayed the immigration of families, placing a heavy economic and organizational burden on the Jewish Agency and the State of Israel.

In 1952, following establishment of a ringworm and trachoma treatment hospital at the intake camp near Haifa, the Israeli Ministry of Health

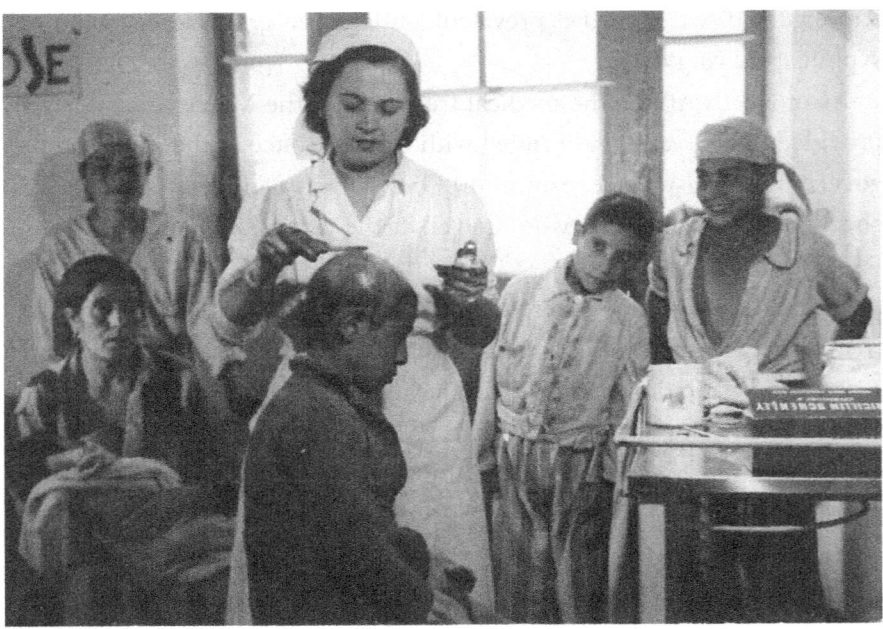

Figure 5.10 Complementary treatment after irradiation for ringworm in the immigrant camp in Marseille
Compliments of Alma Ziv-Goldman, from the estate of Dr. Leon Goldman, physician for *Aliyah B* (clandestine/'illegal' immigration) and the mass *aliyah* immigrant camps.

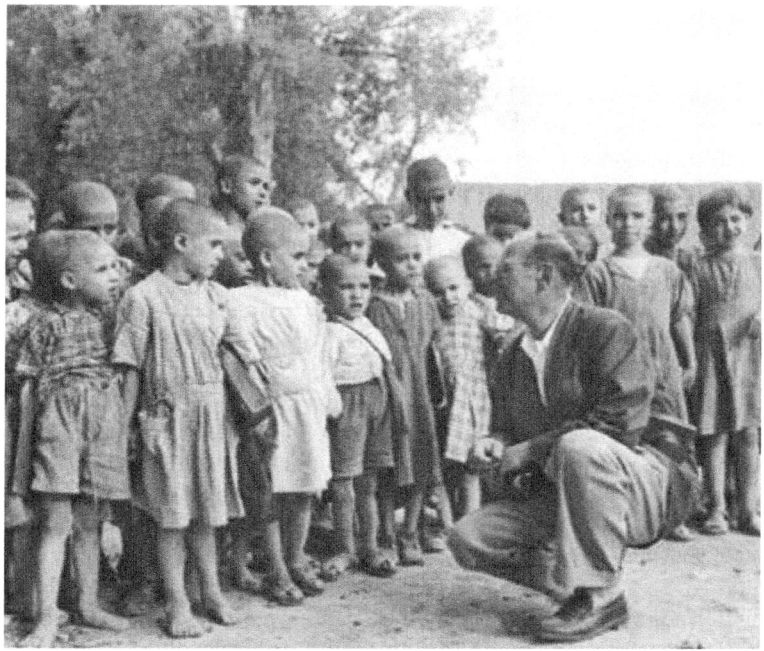

Figure 5.11 Children in the transit camp in Marseille after irradiation treatment for ringworm
Courtesy of the JDC Archives, New York City.

and the Jewish Agency decided to greatly curtail the number of camps in the Marseille area and the number of immigrants residing in them, and to send the children and adults found to have ringworm or trachoma to Israel for treatment. The medical services in the camps were also transferred from OSE to the Jewish Agency in order to reduce the expenditures tied to OSE's operations.

Beginning in the 1960s, after the end of the great wave of immigration and the rehabilitation of some of the Jewish communities in Europe after World War II, the two organizations' close collaboration in the field of health care ended. Since the 1960s, OSE has focused on welfare activities in Jewish communities, mainly in Europe, but still maintains an active social-health center in Casablanca, and the JDC continues to provide comprehensive assistance to Jewish communities around the world.

NOTES

1. This article was presented to the European Society for the History of Medicine and Science, Heidelberg, in 2009. An article on preliminary research for this work focused on Poland was published in Shvarts S, Romem P, Romem I, and Shani M, The mass campaign to eradicate ringworm among the Jewish community in Eastern Europe 1921–1938. *Am J Public Health.* 2013;103(4):e56–e66. Courtesy of the AJPH.
2. The American Jewish Joint Distribution Committee (JDC) is an apolitical Jewish humanitarian nonprofit organization, founded in 1914 in the United States to assist Jews and Jewish communities around the world in times of emergency or crisis. See Romem P. *MALBEN, Mosad le-Tiput b-Olim Nichlashim* [MALBEN, an Institution to Treat Weakened Immigrants]. Bahur Publication, Zichron Yaakov; 2012:12–16.
3. The Organization for Safeguarding the Health of Jews (*Obshchestvo Zdravookhraneniia Evreev* [OZE], today the OSE). OSE was a union devoted to advancing the health, hygiene, and treatment of Jewish children. It was founded on August 7, 1912, in St. Petersburg, Russia (*Obshchestvo okhraneniia zdorov'ia evreiskogo naseleniia*). After the Second World War it established its center in Paris and changed its name to OSE (*Oeuvre de Secours aux Enfants* [Relief Work for Children]). Most of its operations were in the public health and welfare domain for children and youth in Jewish communities.
4. The Union for Safeguarding the Health of the Jewish Population (TOZ = *Towarzystwo Ochrony Zdrowia Ludnos'ci ̇ydowskiej*) was founded in 1921 in Warsaw and operated in Poland prior to the Second World War. In essence, it was a branch of the OSE.
5. In OSE documents they were grouped together under the abbreviation TTT, a term that appears in documents after the Second World War in regard to the work of OSE in the Jewish communities in North Africa. See: Prywes M. *Prisoner of Hope.* Tel Aviv: Zmora Bitan Modan Publishers; 1992:98–209.
6. Shvarts S, Romem P, Romem I. and Shani M, The mass campaign to eradicate ringworm among the Jewish community in Eastern Europe 1921–1938. *Am J Public Health.* 2013;103(4):e56–e66.
7. Not all the children were treated with irradiation for ringworm; most of those in Algeria, Tunisia, and Libya were treated with medicinal remedies. Only in Morocco did most treatment involve irradiation. See "Highlights of the Health Program of OSE Morocco" condensed from a report prepared in July 1963 by Dr. F. Taville, medical director of OSE Morocco, Joint Archives, Morocco portfolio, 1963–1955, Microfilm SS/64:69 ; Levy-Lebhar G, Levy-Lebhar JP, Herman M. Le traitement des teignes par la Griséofulvin. *Maroc Medical.* 1959;38:1603–1608.
8. In the course of the research, documents were surveyed in the following archives: WHO archive (Geneva, Switzerland); Siemens archive (Erlangen, Germany), UNICEF archive (New York); United Nations archive, UNICEF portfolio (Long Island City, NY); YIVO Institute for Jewish Research archive (New York); the American Jewish Joint Distribution Committee archive (Jerusalem and New York); the Alliance Israélite Universelle archive (Paris); the Romanian

Jewry archive (Bar-Ilan University, Ramat Gan, Israel); the Pinchas Lavon Institute for Labour Movement Research archive, Kupat Holim (Sick Fund) portfolio (Efal, Israel); the Israel State Archives & Archive of the Jewish People (Jerusalem); the Sheba archive (Tel Hashomer, Israel); the Yad Yaari Research & Documentation Center archive of Hashomer Hatza'ir (Givat Haviva, Israel); and the Central Zionist Archive (Jerusalem).

9. Ibid. 1 & 2, *Am J Public Health* 2013;103(4): pp. e56–e66; Romem P. MALBEN, *Mosad le-Tiput b-Olim Nichlashim* [MALBEN, an Institution to Treat Weakened Immigrants]. Zichron Yaakov; 2012:12–16.
10. Gurevitch L. *Twenty-Five Years of OSE, 1912–1937.* Paris; 1937:1–12; Ohry-Kossoy K, Ohry A. Dedicated Physicians Facing Adversity: The Polish Jewish Medical Association and the Jewish Health Organization in Poland 1921–1942. *Proceedings of the International Society for the History of Medicine* (Budapest, August 2006), 563–566; Shvarts S. *The Workers' Health Fund in Eretz Israel.* Rochester, NY: University of Rochester Press; 2002:46–47.
11. Gurevitch, 88–101; Prywes, 178–187.
12. Gurevitch, 72.
13. Bernard Flexner (1882–1946), a New York lawyer, was a prominent member of the Zionist Organization of America. He served as counsel for the Zionist delegation to the Paris Peace Conference (1918–1919) and was president of the Palestine Economic Corporation. He was one of the founders of the Council on Foreign Relations.
14. The campaign to eradicate ringworm. *The People's Health*, a monthly journal for public health and sanitation (Yiddish) (January, 1923), 21–24, YIVO Institute for Jewish Research, New York City; Wolman L. Agencies and organizations. *The OSE*, May 1944, 3, 6–8, YIVO Institute for Jewish Research, New York City; Kraut AM. *Silent Travelers: Germs, Genes and the Immigrant Menace.* Baltimore and London: Johns Hopkins University Press; 1994:55, 63, 236, 273–275; Hesse KS. *Letters from Rifka.* NY: Ruffin Books; 1993; Fairchild AL. *Science at the Borders.* Johns Hopkins University Press; Baltimore: 2003.
15. Balinska M. The National Institute of Hygiene and Public Health in Poland 1918–1939. *Social History of Medicine.* 2003;9:433.
16. Reichman was a key figure in the League of Nation's health organization, the founder of UNICEF after the Second World War. Balinska, 433.
17. Steffen C. Dermatopathology in historical perspective: The man behind the eponym: Horatio George Adamson and Adamson's fringe. *Am J Dermatopathol.* 2001;23:485–488.
18. Ringworm Central Committee, "Protocol," November 17, 1922, JDC Archives (New York City), file 371, p. 4.
19. Wolman L. OSE, its achievements and plans for the period after the War. *Hebrew Physician B.* 1944;8; Gurevitch, 106.
20. Wolman L. *Ten Years of Health Activity in Poland, for the Jubilee of TOZ* (Warsaw, 1933), 20–21. New York City: YIVO Institute for Jewish Research.
21. Gurevitch, 100; Levine G. *The Hygiene of the Jews with Introduction by Dr. Z. Bichovski* (Warsaw, 1922) (Yiddish), New York City: YIVO Institute for Jewish Research.

22. The x-rays were sent in 1922 from the Siemens plant in Erlangen, Germany. The shipment included 11 crates marked "X-Ray Equipment," with each crate bearing the name of the crate's final destination: Kovno, Riga, Lodz, Krakhov, Vilna, Bialystok, Rivne, Lemberg (Lvov), Brest-Litovsk, Warsaw (two crates), and Romania. All were for the Jewish communities in these cities, with one objective: to be used in an organized campaign to eradicate ringworm in the Jewish community in Poland and adjacent countries. Dr. Michlin to Dr. Zolchan, head of the Roentgen department in Warsaw, January 10, 1922, JDC Archives, New York City, file 371.
23. OSE-TOZ files, JDC Archives, New York City, file 371.
24. Wolman L. *Medical Welfare Activities Among Jews in Poland 1919–1939* (Warsaw, 1939), 5, YIVO Institute for Jewish Research, New York City; OSE-TOZ files, JDC, New York City, file 371.
25. Letter from the Polish Health Ministry, October 16, 1922. OSE-TOZ files, JDC Archives, New York City, file 373. http://www.measuringworth.com/ppowerus/result.php.
26. Letter from the Polish Health Ministry, October 16, 1922. OSE-TOZ files, JDC Archives, New York City, file 373.
27. *The Jewish Nursing School*, JDC Archives, New York City, file 373, 21/32.
28. "Fighting for Health," Steven Spielberg Jewish Film Archive, Hebrew University of Jerusalem, and the WZO, Central Zionist Archives (short documentary, Yiddish, 1938).
29. *Shmutzik*, a Yiddish term for filthy or smelly, was a common epithet for children with ringworm.
30. "Fighting for Health": Aharon Weisberg interview, September 6, 2008, on his mother's deep embarrassment and refusal to talk about her ringworm and treatment in Odessa until her death; Dr. Gideon Halperin interview, June 19, 2009, about his in-laws, who had been irradiated during the 1920s and never spoke about it until both of them had been diagnosed with cancer; Nelly A., e-mail, March 23, 2010, about her mother and uncle who spoke about it only after they were diagnosed with meningiomas in the mid-1970s.
31. OSE-TOZ Records, JDC Archives, New York City, file 371.
32. Levin G, Wolman L. *Five Years of TOZ, 1922–1926* (Warsaw, 1927), pp. 82–99 (in Yiddish), YIVO Institute for Jewish Research, New York City.
33. Wolman, *Ten Years of Health Work*, 21.
34. Levin G, Wolman L., *Five Years of TOZ*, 9–11.
35. Wolman L. *Fifteen Years of Jewish Public Health* (Warsaw, 1937), 61, YIVO Institute for Jewish Research, New York City.
36. This part of the chapter was written by Shifra Shvarts.
37. An expert in medical education who later in his career served as president of Ben-Gurion University of the Negev, where Prywes founded BGU's Faculty of Health Sciences and served as its first dean. After the Second World War, Prywes was appointed chief physician of OSE. See: Prywes, *Prisoner of Hope*. Tel-Aviv: Zmora bitan Modan Publishers; 1992, quote on the back cover of the volume.
38. Prywes, 226–238; a letter from Dr. William Smith to Dr. Moshe Beckelman, director of Joint in France, 5 December 1951, Joint Archives—New York, JDC 45/54/11.

39. Israelis envoys embedded in Jewish communities worldwide to encourage and direct immigration to Israel.
40. The Jewish Agency for Israel is a Jewish nonprofit organization, established in 1929. It is the primary organization fostering the immigration ("Aliyah") and absorption of Jews and their families from the Jewish diaspora into Israel.
41. Prywes, 202–203.
42. Signed document from Dr. W. Smith (no date) quoting Dr. Gonik. Joint Archives—New York, North African portfolio, file 9, group 6.
43. The Alliance is an Enlightenment-oriented Jewish organization that from 1860, during the 19th and early 20th century, established a network of schools for Jewish children throughout the Mediterranean designed to modernize Jewish life through exposure to French education and culture, parallel to their Jewish education.
44. Traditional Jewish education at the elementary level organized within a community that focused on religious texts with little if any secular education.
45. Urban and rural "holding areas" in proximity to ports of departure where Jews waiting to embark for Israel were concentrated.
46. Clause 8 of the minutes of session 12/309 of the Cabinet on immigration arrangements, Israel State Archives, portfolio Gimel-1/7263 12/309, 3 May 1949 (4 Iyar 5709), a copy of the document in the Ben-Gurion Archive, Sdeh Boker; letter from Dr. Czertok to the Minister of Health, 16 May 1949, Lavon Institute for Labour Movement Research archive IV-243-3-61. The letter was sent with a cc to Kupat Holim central headquarters; Ben-Gurion's diary entry 24 April, 1949, Ben-Gurion Archives—Sde Boker.
47. Such "trustee physicians" were sent to advise, coordinate, monitor, and oversee the health situation in Jewish immigrant camps, in order to prepare for the medical absorption of sick immigrants or, conversely, to treat them onsite in the camps before they immigrated to Israel.
48. It was decided that every month, a maximum of 150 sick children would immigrate to Israel, where they would receive treatment for their illness. Letter from Dr. Haim Sheba, director-general of the Ministry of Health, to the Aliyah Office of the Jewish Agency, 4 November 1951, Sheba Archive—Tel-Hashomer; letter from Dr. Jezierski to Dr. Noach on the pending arrival on the ship *Negba* of a group of children with ringworm, for treatment at the Shaar HaAliyah—the State of Israel's intake and processing center for immigrants, south of Haifa, 15 January 1952, Sheba Archive—Tel-HaShomer.
49. 4 December 1951 letter from Dr. Sheba to the Aliyah [immigration] Department of the Jewish Agency, Sheba Archive—Tel-Hashomer.
50. Statistical Data on Ringworm and Trachoma in 1959, Ministry of Health, the Epidemiology Unit, Israel State Archives Gimel-5088/9.
51. Up until 1956, most of Morocco was a French protectorate. A small area of northeast Morocco, whose capital was Tetouan, was a Spanish protectorate. There was also a small Jewish community of several thousand people in Tangier (adjacent to Spanish Morocco), a city that had special status as an international zone. The operations of the Joint and OSE in Tetouan were tiny, both because of the small size of the community and due to lack of a working relationship with Spanish rulers. Sick

children from the community were usually sent to nearby Tangier for examination and treatment.
52. Highlights of the Health Program of OSE Morocco ; M. Raguet. Prophylaxie des teignes scolaires. *Maroc Medical.* 1956;35:377.
53. France was the first country in the world to employ irradiation treatment for ringworm (from 1904) at public clinics. The French Health Service also operated a network of public clinics (Santé publique) in countries under French rule in North Africa in the early 1920s. These clinics provided free public medical services to all, and many members of the Jewish community who lived in these countries used these services prior to OSE's arrival in these countries.
54. Prywes, 198–209.
55. Highlights of the Health Program of OSE Morocco. M. Raguet. Prophylaxie des teignes scolaires. *Maroc Medical.* 1956;35:377.
56. Dr. Levy-Lebhar, a specialist in radiology, was appointed OSE's chief physician in Casablanca. He published 10 scientific articles in various medical journals on irradiation against ringworm in the 1950s in Casablanca and lectured on this topic at international conferences, including the European Conference for Dermatology and Radiology held in Munich in 1957. https://www.ncbi.nlm.nih.gov/pubmed.
57. Levy-Lebhar G, Levy-Lebhar JP. L'épilation en série des teignes du cuir chevelu par la radiothérapie (A propose de 5600 cas traités de 1947 á 1953) [Serial epilation of teignes of the scalp by radiotherapy with reference to the 5,600 cases treated from 1947 to 1953]. *Radiotherapies.* 1954;35:7–8, 629–631.
58. Levy-Lebhar G, Levy-Lebhar JP. Les teignes du cuir chevelu au Maroc [The treatment of Moroccan ringworm]. *Maroc Medical.* 1956;35:1149–1165; Levy-Lebhar G, Levy-Lebhar JP. Radiotherapie, les épilations en series des teigne par la radiothérapie, Étude Physique. Dosimétrie. Résultats. *Société française d'electroradiologie médicale (p.752) filiale d'Alger et d'Afrique du Nord,* 4 décembre 1954; Levy-Lebhar G, Levy-Lebhar JP. L'épilation en serie des teigne du cuir chevelu par la radiothérapie. *Journal de radiologie, de lectrologie & archives de lectricite medicale.* 1953:629–631.
59. His published work can be found among studies archived in PubMed, an international digital professional medical library of scientific articles from recognized literature, a repository sponsored by NIH.
60. Levy-Lebhar and Levy-Lebhar, Les teignes; Levy-Lebhar and Levy-Lebhar, Radiothérapie.
61. Levy-Lebhar and Levy-Lebhar, L'épilation, 630. Dr. Levy-Lebhar's diagnosis of two different strains of fungi that caused ringworm, between children in Europe and children in North Africa, explains the use waxing to complement epilation by irradiation in North Africa, in contrast to the treatment of children with ringworm in Europe, where this step in treatment following irradiation was omitted. This aspect of treatment is a core issue in discourse associated with children in North Africa and Israel treated for ringworm.
62. Training of nurses to treat children with ringworm and instruction for mothers to conduct further complementary treatment was carried out with great success by OSE in Eastern Europe.

63. Levy-Lebhar and Levy-Lebhar, Radiothérapie; Levy-Lebhar and Levy-Lebhar, L'épilation, 630.
64. M.R., Deposition submitted to the court December 24, 2001. The testimony was a part of a claim by an Israeli citizen to receive compensation for medical damage caused to him by the irradiation he received as a child in Morocco.
65. The description is in keeping with the prescribed Kienböck–Adamson method in the medical literature for irradiation against ringworm.
66. Similar treatment, with the exception of the stage of hair removal by waxing, but with full usage of iodine and zinc ointment after irradiation and complementary epilation using tweezers, was customary for ringworm children in Yugoslavia (see details in Chapter 6 of this volume).
67. M.R., Deposition.
68. Levy-Lebhar and Levy-Lebhar, Les teignes, 1149–1165.
69. After the 1956 independence of Morocco, this public medical service established by the French was continued by the Moroccan government under its own auspices.
70. Levy-Lebhar G. Le traitement des teignes marocaines. *Maroc Medical.* 1955;34(360):583.
71. M.R., Deposition.
72. Ibid.
73. Resolution on basic principles and criteria for medical examination of migrant, adopted on 15 October 1951 by the migration conference of the International Labour Organization, Naples 2–16 October 1951, UN Archives CMig/I/11/1951.
74. Letter from Dr. Koren to Dr. Meir, 13 July 1951, Israel State Archives, Gimel-5087/8.
75. Highlights of the Health Program of OSE Morocco.
76. OSE-Joint Report, 20 April, 1949, pp. 1–4, Joint Archive, portfolio 029, AR45/54.
77. Memorandum Dr. Herman, member of the executive of OSE, 12 June 1957, on the topic of operation in Algeria, Joint Archive, portfolio 029, AR45/54.
78. Eighty-five percent of Algerian Jews immigrated to France in the years 1951 to 1960, and only several thousand chose to go to Israel. See: Tzur Y. Ha-Aliyah me-Artzot ha-Islam [The Immigration from Islamic Countries]. In Tzameret T, Yablonka H, eds. *Ha-Asor ha-Rishon* [The First Decade]. Jerusalem, 1998:57–82; letter from Baruch Duvdevani—the Office for Europe and North Africa, to Dr. Shimon Batish, director-general of the Ministry of Health, 1 June 1954, Central Zionist Archives, Gimel-4247/3.
79. The Joint opposed the use of thallium acetate, which was dangerous due to its toxicity, but despite this health personnel in Tunisia continued to employ it. This issue became a source of controversy in correspondence between individuals from the Joint and individuals from the community engaged in health work. Joint Archive—New York, 494/79/1868.
80. Document Case Box SM 67. Joint Archive—Jerusalem.
81. Letter from Dr. Golink to the Joint management in Tunisia, 15 February 1954, Joint Archive—Jerusalem, in correspondence—Geneva collection, 1954-1955, document 2566713.
82. Cohen Y. Ha-Gazezet b-Israel, Tamtzit Seker al ha-Gazezet b-Israel she-Ne'erach al adei Dr. Yaakov Cohen min ha-Epidemalogia b-Misrad Habri'ut [Synopsis

of a Survey of Ringworm in Israel Carried Out by Dr. Yaakov Cohen from the Epidemiology Unit of the Ministry of Health]. *Briut Hatzibur.* 1958;1:19–21; Ha-Tipul b-Mikrei Gazezet al yadei Hakranot b-Shaar ha-Aliyah [Treatment of Cases of Ringworm through Irradiation at Shaar HaAliyah], Epidemiology Unit, Ministry of Health, 1955.

83. Doch Bikur Dr, Sh. Spiro b-Tripoli, August–September 1949 [Report of the Visit of Dr. Sh. Spiro in Tripoli August–September 1949]. Lavon Institute for Labor Movement Research—Efal,IV 243-3-.

84. The immigrants called the hospital the English Hospital ("Hôpital Anglais" in French), since the building in the past had served as an English hospital that had been founded in Marseille in the 1920s. Consequently, the use of the term "the English Hospital" was quite prevalent in medical reports of the period.

85. On Hôpital Saint-Louis see: Tilles G. *Teignes et teigneux: Histoire médicale et sociale.* Paris: Springer-Verlag; 2009.

6

The ringworm campaign in Serbia (former Yugoslavia) in the 1950s

SHIFRA SHVARTS, GORAN SEVO, MARIJA TASIC,
MORDECHAI SHANI, AND SIEGAL SADETZKI-JACKOBSON

INTRODUCTION

Until the 1960s, tinea capitis, also known as ringworm, was one of the most widespread fungal diseases in children.[1] This superficial fungal infection of the scalp is caused by three ecological groups of dermatophytes that use keratin as a nutrient source: anthropophilic species transmitted from person to person, zoophilic species transmitted from animals, and geophilic species that inhabit the soil but occasionally infect human beings. The exact incidence of tinea capitis epidemics throughout the world is not known because the disease is rarely reported to public health agencies. Reports of tinea capitis infections in the United States date back to 1900, with several documents describing a high prevalence of the disease among children on Ellis Island, an immigrant station in New York.[2] Individuals with severe disease were refused entry into the United States and sent back to their home countries. Despite such measures to control the spread of tinea capitis, reports issued by New York City claimed that by 1944, several thousand children were infected. Other U.S. cities also reported a large number of cases around the same time. Between the 1930s and 1950s, tinea capitis was so widespread that in France, Russia, and some central and southern European countries, separate schools were established for infected children.

During the 1950s, both Spain and Italy reported many cases, and medical reports from North Africa suggested that there were more than 500,000 active cases, mainly in Morocco.[3] The high incidence of infected children necessitated the creation of separate classes in Moroccan schools to minimize the spread of tinea capitis. Also, during the 1950s, after the mass immigration to Israel from North Africa, reports from Israel suggested that there were as many as 20,000 children with tinea capitis, caused by the anthropophilic dermatophyte *Trichophyton violaceum*, which also caused the tinea capitis outbreak in Yugoslavia.

During tinea capitis infection, dermatophytes infect hair follicles. Before the advent of antimycotic treatments powerful enough to penetrate the follicle, hair was removed manually by shaving or waxing before the application of topical antimycotic ointments such as wood tar, sulfur, plaster (wax), iodine, thallium salts, and nitrate of mercury.

Shortly after Roentgen discovered x-rays, people observed that exposure to this radiation caused human hair to fall out together with its follicle, thus proving an attractive means of hair removal for treatment of tinea capitis. Sabouraud[4] introduced a method for treating tinea capitis with x-ray radiation in 1904. The protocol was standardized by Kienböck in 1907 and Adamson in 1910, by which time x-ray epilation had been widely adopted as an efficient method for complete epilation within roughly 2 to 3 weeks of exposure.[5] The use of x-ray radiation to remove hair followed by application of topical antimycotic ointments was the standard treatment for tinea capitis until the introduction of the antifungal oral medication griseofulvin in 1959.

Between 1946 and 1960, Israel undertook a mass tinea capitis elimination campaign. The campaign received financial assistance from UNICEF—the United Nations Children's Fund and used ionizing radiation to treat about 17,000 children, mainly newly arrived immigrants from North Africa and the Middle East.

During treatment, patients' heads were shaved and any remaining hair was removed through a waxing process. Subsequently, the scalp area was divided into sections, each irradiated on one of 3 to 5 consecutive days.[6] Following irradiation, treatment included manual epilation of any remaining hair and application of iodine or other antimycotic ointments.

Since the first half of the 20th century, and before the potential for long-term damage from exposure to x-rays was known, radiation was widely used to treat various benign diseases such as tonsillitis and acne.[7] Data from an Israeli cohort study, along with data from other sources, provided some of the first evidence that exposure to low and medium doses of ionizing radiation was associated with an increased risk for leukemia and solid tumors.[8] In 1965, to assess the delayed effects of ionizing radiation, Baruch Modan recruited a cohort consisting of 10,834 children who had received irradiation as part of the Israeli tinea capitis elimination campaign during the 1950s, as well as two matched groups (one sibling, the other non-sibling) who had not received irradiation. The first follow-up report, published in the *Lancet* in 1974,[9] showed an increased risk for both malignant and benign head and neck tumors in the irradiated group. These results were confirmed in analyses with up to 45 years of follow-up.[10] In 1994, on the basis of these findings, a law was passed in Israel that provided compensation to people who had developed diseases or other late health effects caused by exposure to x-ray radiation.[11] In 2004, during research into the tinea capitis campaign in Israel, several documents came to light that noted the assistance of UNICEF, including provision of x-ray machines.[12] Examination of UNICEF documents from 1948 to 1960 revealed that Israel was not the only country in which tinea capitis elimination campaigns took place; in particular, UNICEF was involved in similar campaigns in both Syria and the former Yugoslavia (Figure 6.1).[13]

In this chapter we review the campaign to eliminate tinea capitis in Yugoslavia during the 1950s and discuss the possible health implications for people treated during the campaign.

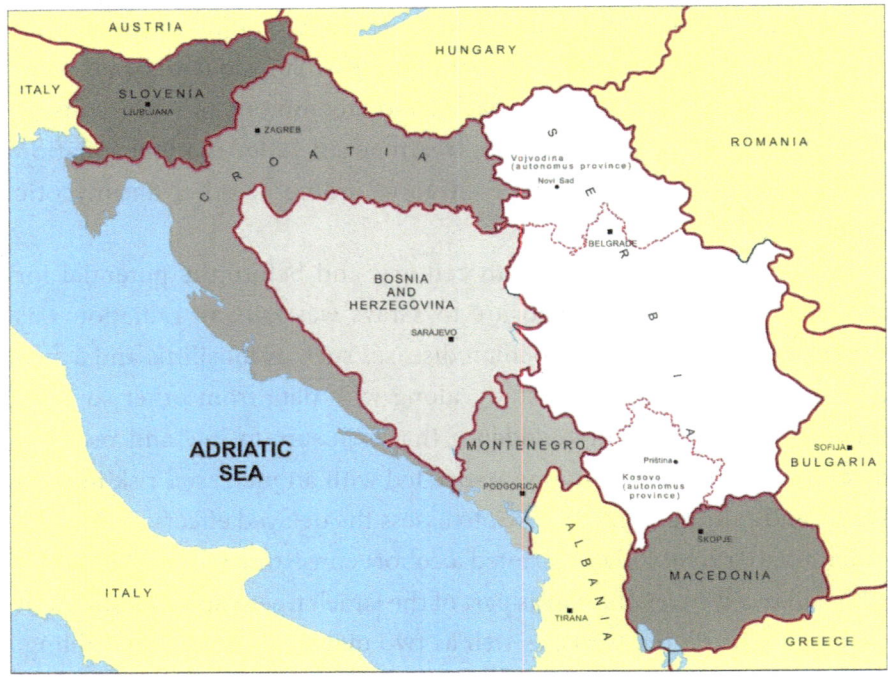

Figure 6.1 Map of former Yugoslavia

DATA SOURCES

We searched meeting records from UNICEF regional health officers and directors, reports and meeting records from the WHO East Mediterranean Regional Office and the WHO—World Health Organization European Office, letters exchanged between UNICEF and Yugoslavian public health directors and field officers, UNICEF and WHO financial reports related to research into tinea capitis, and control reports prepared by UNICEF delegates detailing campaign costs. We also searched documents from the UN–UNICEF archives in New York City, WHO archives in Geneva, the Institute of Public Health of Serbia, Belgrade city archives, and Israeli state archives in Jerusalem. Two leading newspapers from Yugoslavia in the 1950s, *Borba* and *Politika*, were searched for stories related to the tinea capitis elimination campaign or to policy declarations by the Yugoslavian government.

To identify people involved in the Yugoslavian tinea capitis elimination campaign of the 1950s, we placed advertisements in two Serbian newspapers (*Politika* and *Novi Pazar*; Figure 6.2) and made media appearances to disseminate information about the research to the public and to encourage individuals who were irradiated in the campaign to contact us. One hundred eighty-six people contacted our team and were interviewed. The interviews included a set of questions designed to gather information about demographic details, year and location of treatment, specific treatment details, personal medical history, and any personal comments. Thirteen of the individuals who responded to our advertisements lived in

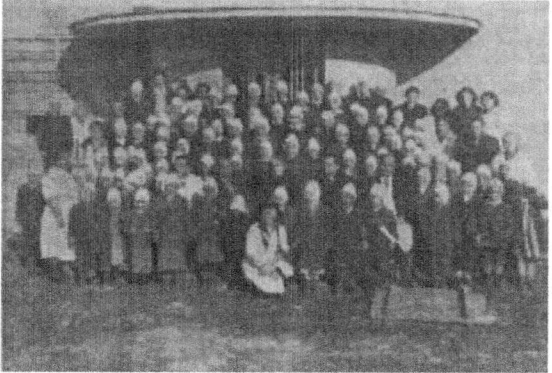

Figure 6.2 Our newspaper ad. Translation: "If you are one of the 50,000 children who had been treated for ringworm in the period 1951–1960 by x-ray–induced hair removal and Lime cap ointment, we would like to get in touch with you. We are trying to refresh memories on this important episode of public health in our country. Please contact us using the details provided."

Belgrade and were thus able to provide additional, videotaped, in-depth interviews after providing written informed consent. The interviews focused on personal aspects of the treatment and its consequences, as well as on the diagnosis, treatment, health outcomes associated with the irradiation, and information regarding the social context in which the campaign was done. We also interviewed 15 physicians, now in their 80s and 90s, who took part in the campaign. The interviews focused on their personal and professional experiences.

We searched previous Yugoslavian scientific reports and publications on tinea capitis. We searched Medline, and electronic databases at the libraries at the Serbian Medical Association and the Serbian Institute of Public Health using the following search terms: *mikoze*, mycosis, tinea capitis, and UNICEF campaign. We also searched for relevant papers in the National Library of Serbia and found 151.

Before World War II, tinea capitis was sporadic in Yugoslavia and was treated by the then-current standard of care, which included ionizing radiation. However, because ionizing radiation was not widely available, the therapeutic regimens that were used to treat tinea capitis generally included manual epilation before the application of fungicides, such as copper compounds, copper oleate, or ointments containing salicylanilide preparations to the scalp. In 1946, after World War II, the disease became widespread. In 1949, at a Zagreb conference that included all Yugoslavian health authorities, the government officially declared tinea capitis to be a major public health problem and applied to UNICEF for help in eliminating the disease. In 1950, a full-scale campaign to treat tinea capitis was launched with UNICEF assistance.[14] Both Yugoslavian and UNICEF reports describe a widespread operation during the 1950s to eliminate tinea capitis with treatment that included ionizing radiation. The number of individuals screened (878,659) and the number treated (49,389) in Serbia were among the highest ever reported in a public health campaign in Europe and North America.[15] The campaign was headed by the Serbian Institute of Public Health, and treatment was free of charge.[16] Ignjatovic[17] provides a detailed description of the campaign's organization and its course of action between 1950 and 1957. Tinea capitis was diagnosed in

36,379 children, 29,667 of whom received treatment. There are no records for the 6,712 children diagnosed with tinea capitis who were not treated by the year 1957. We assume that some of them were not treated at all because they were younger than 4 years old. In addition, many patients (19,722) who were not part of the UNICEF campaign received treatment for tinea capitis through referrals from family doctors. Thus, altogether about 50,000 individuals were treated, mostly children aged 5 to 15 years.[18]

Because these figures do not include the last 2 years of the campaign, 1958 to 1960, our estimation of the number of individuals involved is conservative. According to UNICEF and WHO reports of the Joint Committee on Health Policy, 24 mycological centers were established throughout Yugoslavia. Each was equipped with an x-ray machine, first-aid facilities, equipment for manual epilation, and a hospital ward with an average of 30 beds where children could stay during treatment.[19] Staff included 17 doctors (dermatologists or physicians who had completed courses in mycology and x-ray therapy), 120 junior medical personnel or senior medical students, and 120 auxiliary medical personnel or second-year medical students.[20]

At least four of the doctors we interviewed were senior physicians in the campaign and had clear memories of the events. Each reported that the treatment followed the medical doctrine of the time and expressed their personal belief that the campaign was of great national public health importance. According to UNICEF financial reports, the cost of the equipment and supplies provided to the campaign was US$151,741 (the equivalent of $1.1 million in 2009). Equipment provided by UNICEF included 20 x-ray machines, four of which were mobile (set up in ambulances), and 12 vans to transport children and staff. Between 1950 and 19, the Yugoslavian government contributed 35 million dinars (the equivalent of $2.7 million in 2009).[21]

Before the campaign, the length of hospital stays for a patient receiving treatment for tinea capitis was as long as 2 months; during the campaign it was reduced to about 7 days. This reduction in hospitalization time made it possible to treat many patients and was one of the main factors that made the campaign possible.[22]

After a diagnosis of tinea capitis was made at screening sites, groups of children with the infection were taken to regional hospitals, where the hospital mycology staff confirmed the diagnosis and created an individual record for each patient. The treatment included x-ray–induced hair removal (Figure 6.3) followed by application of a zinc ointment. All children who received treatment were quarantined during hospitalization.

The irradiation treatment protocol followed the standard practices of the time and was identical to the Kienböck–Adamson method.[23] The scalp was divided into five regions, one or two of which were irradiated each day. Before irradiation, thick scabs were removed manually and any infected areas were treated to prevent interference with x-ray penetration into the skin and to ensure successful epilation. The radiation dose was determined by a physician radiologist from the hospital and the procedure was done by radiology technicians. We were not able to obtain

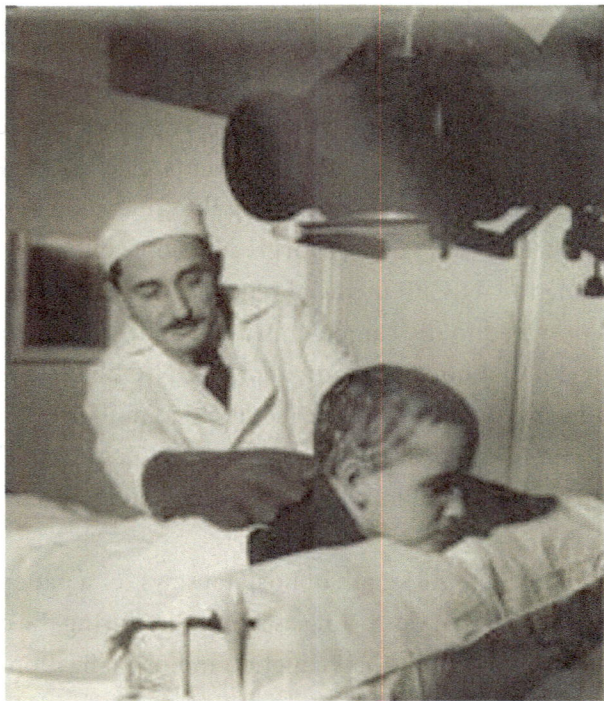

Figure 6.3 A young patient receiving a dose of radiation

original Serbian documents from the period that explicitly specified the radiation dose given to patients. However, Cikaric[24] describes irradiation treatment in Serbia during the 1950s and reports that for the treatment of various nonmalignant disorders (both infectious and degenerative), including tinea capitis, the maximum dose given was 400 roentgens (equivalent to $1,032 \times 10^{-4}$ C/kg). A dose of 400 roentgens is similar to the dose given during the Israeli tinea capitis campaign, and also to the dose recommended by the Kienböck–Adamson technique, which was thought safe for inducing temporary alopecia. Zinc ointment was applied 1 to 2 days after irradiation. The ointment was made with gelatin (30 g), glycerin (50 g), zinc oxide (30 g), and distilled water (90 g). A container of this mixture was placed in warm water. When the mixture had melted, it was applied directly to the scalp and to a few pieces of gauze that were used to cover the entire scalp. The gauze was then secured to the scalp with loose bandages. The gauze and ointment hardened into a thick plaster-like consistency and was known as the zinc hat. The zinc hat had a dual purpose: to contain the infection and to epilate any newly grown hairs when the hardened hat was removed. After application of the zinc hat the patients were discharged from hospital and returned home, where further treatment was provided.[24] In Serbia, the zinc hat was removed at a clinic close to the patient's home. The hat was removed after 21 days, at which point any remaining hair was manually epilated (Figure 6.4) and topical ointments to treat tinea capitis were applied to the scalp. Treatment after removal of the hat was given at the patient's home and included thorough daily washing of the scalp with soap and warm water, followed by topical application of diluted tincture of iodine (20 g of tincture plus 80 g of alcohol) and 10% salicylic acid cream. Patients and their parents were provided with the necessary soaps and ointments free of charge and received training to enable them to continue the treatment at home. The treatment usually lasted for 7 weeks, although for some mild cases the treatment was shorter.[25]

The 13 individuals who took part in the in-depth interviews shared sentiments of being forgotten, surprise at seeing our advertisements, and feelings of relief that something was finally being done for them.

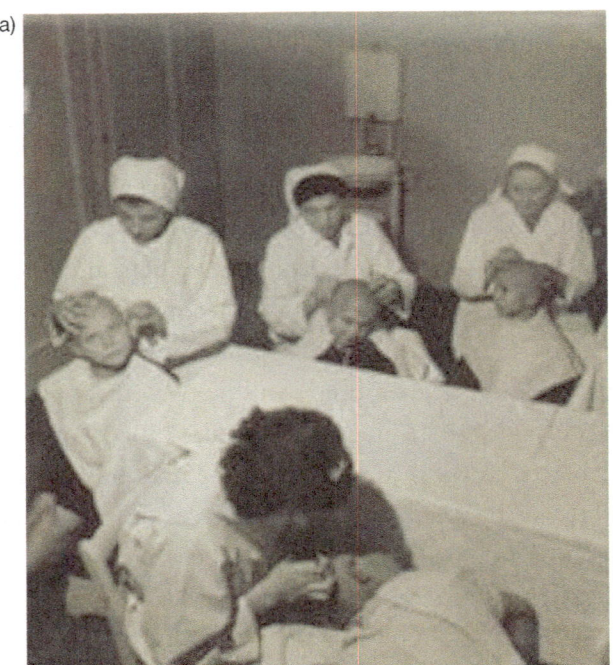

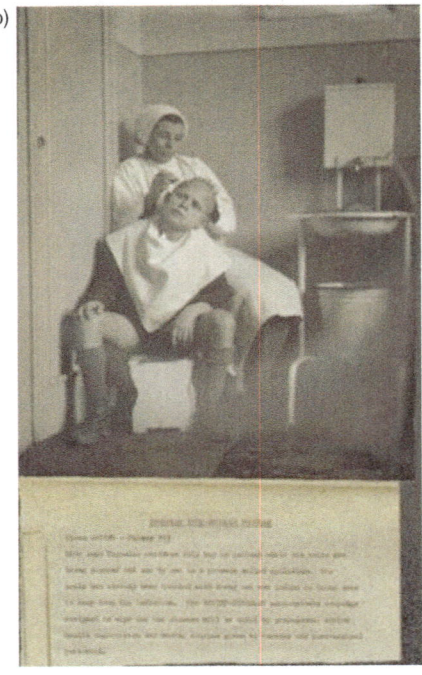

Figure 6.4 Manual epilation of remaining hair after x-ray treatment

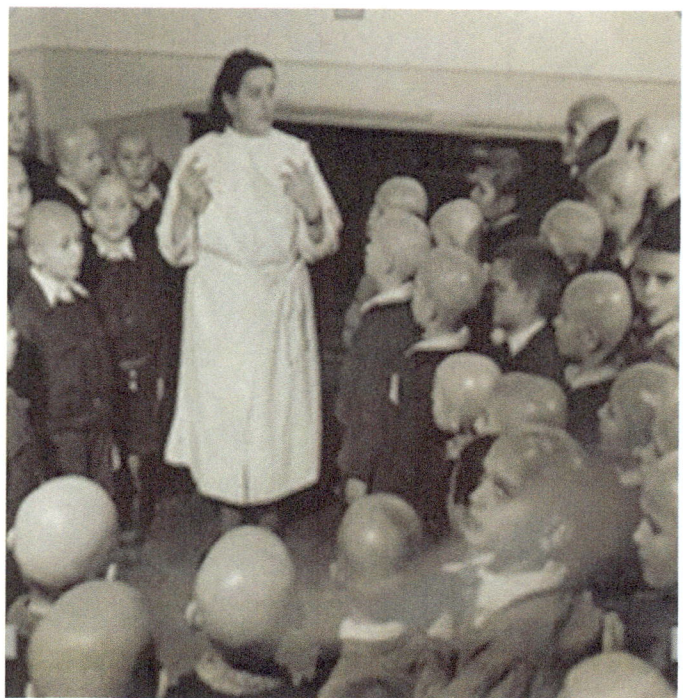

Figure 6.5 Children after epilation and irradiation completed

The interviewed individuals retained vivid memories of events despite the fact that half a century had passed since their treatment. Most of the interviewees felt traumatized by their treatment because they had been separated from their families. Around 30% expressed explicit concern about the possible consequences of the x-ray treatment on their current health status. Roughly two thirds of all patients in Serbia who received treatment for tinea capitis as part of the Yugoslavian campaign were treated at the Mycosis Hospital in Belgrade. Records at the Historical Archives of Belgrade City identify all patients who received treatment at the hospital during this period. These records provide an opportunity to study these patients and to assess their health as a result of the x-ray treatment they received.

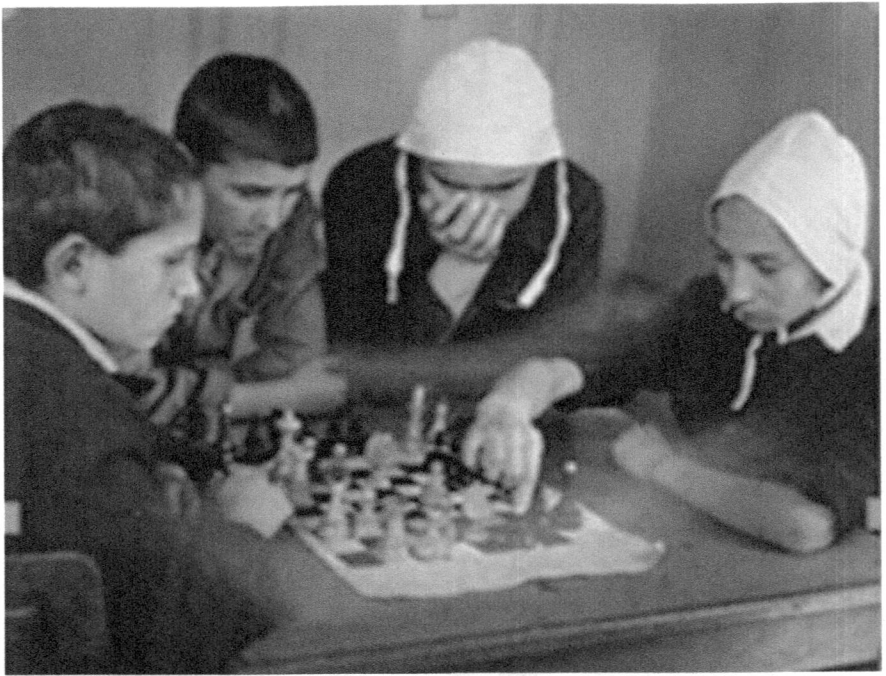

Figure 6.6 Children with the zinc hat

DISCUSSION

Among the factors that made the 1950s tinea capitis elimination campaign in Yugoslavia possible were its regional organization, the use of local health care personnel, the reduction of the hospitalization period (from 2 to 3 months to about 7 days, similar to the hospitalization period in Israel, where in-hospital treatment lasted 3 to 5 days for many patients), and the reduction of the length of time that children were separated from their families. Treatment was compulsory, and treating children in the absence of their parents, with full compliance to the medical authorities, was common practice at that time.[26] These practices might now seem severe, but given the historical context, labeling them as authoritarian would be unjust. We should, however, question how this major public health campaign has been erased from the collective memory of the contemporary medical community in Serbia. One possible explanation is that stigmatization of tinea capitis as the "poor people's disease" resulted in feelings of shame for the patients, who subsequently kept silent about their experience. Then, as the medical personnel involved moved on to other specialties, the memory of the campaign faded into history. In Israel, a history of tinea capitis remains a stigma for some of the treated population, as indicated by the incomplete participation in the compensation program.[27]

Research into the Israeli tinea capitis elimination campaign revealed some important clinical implications that must also be taken into consideration in Serbia. Irradiation therapy is associated with deleterious late health outcomes, such as an increased risk for cancer in the irradiated area.[28] Because of the similarities between the Israeli and Yugoslavian campaigns (i.e., the large number of patients, the age range of patients, the length and dates of the campaign, and the irradiation protocol), similar health consequences should be expected in both populations. There is a latency period of over 30 years between irradiation and the appearance of solid tumors of the brain.[29] If we assume that patients treated for tinea capitis in the Yugoslavian campaign were 5 to 15 years of age in 1950 to 1957 (the period for which Ignjatovic's report[17] provides detailed accounts), the patients would in 2010 be 58 to 75 years of age. The population census of Serbia indicated that in 2007, 22.5% of the population (about 1.7 million people) were 55 to 74 years of age.[30] The individuals who received radiation therapy during the tinea capitis campaign would constitute about 3.0% of the current population in this age range, which is, coincidentally, the time of life when sporadic and radiation-induced cancer is most prevalent. The Israeli cohort study by Modan et al.[3] estimated the relative risk associated with exposure to radiation for malignant brain tumors to be 57.3 and for malignant thyroid tumors to be 2.76. In 2007 in Serbia, the incidence of brain tumors was 21.77 per 100,000 people and the incidence of thyroid tumors was 8.16 per 100,000 people aged 55 to 74.[28,29] We used these data to estimate the incidence of both brain and thyroid tumors in the Serbian population in 2007[31] if the campaign to eliminate tinea capitis had not taken place. We calculated age-specific crude incidence rates of 20.21 and 7.75 per 100,000 people for malignant brain (ICD-10 diagnosis

C71) and thyroid (ICD 10-0-3 diagnosis C73.9) tumors respectively. We can therefore postulate that in 2007, if the campaign to eliminate tinea capitis in Yugoslavia had not taken place, there would be 7.17% fewer malignant brain tumors and 5.02% fewer thyroid tumors reported in Serbia (i.e., 32 of 506 recorded cases of malignant brain and thyroid disease would not have occurred). In Israel, discussions about the need for early detection and other preventive strategies for the irradiated population are ongoing. Physicians should be aware of particular subsets of a population who might be at increased risk for radiation-associated late health effects so that any disease can be detected early and treated promptly.

CONCLUSIONS

In this historical review we emphasize the need for medical communities to keep records of infectious diseases that seem to have been eradicated or that are no longer a serious issue because of advances in medicine. Evaluation of previous elimination campaigns can provide important lessons for those now planning similar campaigns and can reveal any unintended consequences of such efforts that might necessitate urgent action or increased awareness for specific diseases in subsets of the population.

These findings about the UNICEF-assisted campaign to eliminate tinea capitis in Yugoslavia, which involved the irradiation of about 50,000 children, should be incorporated into the working knowledge of the medical community in Serbia and in other countries that used a radiation-based technique. Physicians should have increased vigilance for symptoms of relevant diseases, mainly cancer, among the elderly people in these countries. The information presented here changes the context and improves our understanding of the Israeli campaign to eliminate tinea capitis by showing that it was not an isolated event. The findings also raise important questions regarding the retrospective responsibility of the medical profession for the adverse effects of a treatment once thought to be standard. Whether or not to inform the irradiated population of their possible increased risk for certain diseases should be discussed, as should the possibility of financial compensation or any other legal implications for those individuals involved. Medical communities in countries where irradiation-based tinea capitis campaigns took place should be made aware of the Serbian and Israeli experience so that necessary considerations are incorporated into the routine diagnosis, treatment, and follow-up of patients who might have been treated during such campaigns. As health care professionals, we have a moral obligation to revisit this episode in Serbian medical history to ensure that any unintended and undesirable consequences of our past actions be accounted for and mitigated.

ACKNOWLEDGMENTS

We thank the late Stephen J. Kunitz (University of Rochester School of Medicine), Shimon M. Glick (Ben Gurion University School of Medicine), Avi Israeli (Hebrew University), and Boaz Lev (Israel Ministry of Health) for their helpful suggestions. We also thank the Gertner Institute for Epidemiology and Health Policy Research for supporting this project.

NOTES

1. This study was published first in *Lancet Infect Dis.* 2010;10(8):571–576. Courtesy of the Lancet ID.
2. Kraut AM. *Silent Travelers: Germs, Genes and the Immigrant Menace.* Baltimore and London: Johns Hopkins University Press; 1994.
3. Raguet M. Prophylaxie des teignes scolaires au Maroc. *Maroc Medical.* 1956;35:377.
4. Raymond Jacques Adrien Sabouraud (1868–1938), a French physician, specialized in dermatology and mycology; see also Chapter 3.
5. See also Chapter 2.
6. Warner A, Modan B, Davidoff D. Doses to brain, skull and thyroid, following x-ray therapy for tinea capitis. *Phys Med Biol.* 1968;13:247–258; Modan B, Baidatz D, Mart H, Steinitz R, Levin SG. Radiation-induced head and neck tumors. *Lancet.* 1974;1:277–279.
7. Crawford GM, Luikart RH II, Tilley RF. Roentgen therapy in acne. *N Engl J Med.* 1951;245:726–728; Kaplan II. The treatment of female sterility with x-rays to the ovaries and the pituitary; with special reference to congenital anomalies of the offspring. *Can Med Assoc J.* 1957;76:43–64.

8. Warner et al.; Modan et al.; Sadetzki S, Chetrit A, Freedman L, Stovall M, Modan B, Novikov I. Long-term follow-up for brain tumor development following childhood exposure to ionizing radiation for tinea capitis. *Radiat Res.* 2005;163:424–432.
9. Modan et al.
10. Sadetzki et al.
11. Sadetzki S, Modan B. Epidemiology as a basis for legislation: How far should epidemiology go? *Lancet.* 1999;353:2238–2239; Siegel-Itzkovich J. Israel compensates for ringworm treatment. *BMJ.* 1995;310:350–351; Modan B. Israel compensation law for ringworm treatment. In: Cohen-Almagor R, ed. *Moral Dilemmas in Medicine.* Jerusalem: Van Leer Jerusalem Institute; 2002:388–411.
12. Israel State Archives Jerusalem, 2083/3; 4299–5/gimel, 189–9 gime; Shvarts S, Drori V, Stoler-Liss S. The international activity and health support in Palestine/Israel after WW2 and the Israel war of independence and the state first years. In: Debons D, ed. *Katyn and Switzerland: Experts and Medical Expertise in Humanitarian Crisis.* Geneva: University of Geneva; 2008:319–328.
13. Ilercil B. UNICEF program assistance to European countries. UNICEF Archives, CF/HST/MON/1989-003; 1–59; Tooby FW. Yugoslavia reports. UNICEF Archives, Long Island City, New York, USA: S-0535-0236, A483, F/NYH/PD, CF/NYH/05.
14. Yugoslav programme for antimycotic campaign. UNICEF archives, JC3/UNICEF-WHO/21, CF/NYH/PD, CF/NYH/05; People's Republic of Serbia. Ordinance of compulsory separation and treatment of persons suffering ringworm—Official Government Report Series. Sluzbeni glasnik NRS 1950; 8; Ignjatovic B. *Mycotic Diseases in Serbia (Tinea Capitis): Modern Campaign on Their Eradication. Antimycotic Campaign in Serbia.* Belgrade: Library of the Institute of Hygiene of the People's Republic of Serbia; 1959:1–91; Grin EI, Ozegovic L. Critical survey of mycological research and literature in Yugoslavia up to 1957. *Mycopathologia.* 1958;9:341–364.
15. Albert RE, Omran AR. Follow-up study of patients treated by x-ray epilation for tinea capitis. *Arch Environ Health.* 1968;17:899–918.
16. People's Republic of Serbia, Ordinance of compulsory separation; Ignjatovic; Grin and Ozegovic.
17. Ignjatovic.
18. Ibid.
19. Yugoslav programme; Ignjatovic.
20. Ibid.
21. Yugoslav programme; Stojanovic B. Exchange rate regimes of Dinar 1945–1990: An assessment of appropriateness and efficiency. Second conference on the southeastern European monetary history network (SEEMHN), 13 April 2007, 198–243.
22. Yugoslav programme; Ignjatovic.
23. Warner et al.; Adamson HG. A simplified method of x-ray application for the cure of ringworm of the scalp. *Lancet.* 1909;173:1378–1380; Steffen C. Dermatopathology in historical perspective: The man behind the eponym: Horatio George Adamson and Adamson's fringe. *Am J Dermatopathol.* 2001;23:485–488; Albert and Omran.
24. Ignjatovic.
25. Ibid.

26. Ibid.; Grin and Ozegovic.
27. Siegel-Itzkovich; Modan.
28. Warner et al.; Modan et al.; Sadetzki et al.; Sadetzki and Modan.
29. Sadetzki et al.; Sadetzki S, Chetrit A, Lubina A, Stovall M, Novikov I. Risk of thyroid cancer following childhood exposure to ionizing radiation for tinea capitis. *J Clin Endocrin Metab.* 2006;91:4798–4804.
30. Panev G. Population structures. In: *Population and Households of Serbia According to the 2002 Census.* Belgrade: Serbian Institute of Statistics, Institute for Social Sciences—Center for Demographic Research, Serbian Society of Demographers; 2006:107–249; Republic of Serbia, Serbian Institute of Statistics. Demographic projections according to gender, age and type of settlement, 2007.
31. Ibid.

7

The ringworm campaign in Portugal, 1940–1970

Historical review and present evaluation of x-ray–epilated individuals

PAULA BOAVENTURA, DINA PEREIRA,
PAULA SOARES, AND JOSÉ TEIXEIRA-GOMES

INTRODUCTION

Ringworm (tinea capitis) is a fungal disease that reached epidemic proportions in Portugal in the 1950s and 1960s, similarly to other countries. The rapid spread of the disease was so serious that the public health authorities had to take drastic measures to tackle the problem. Consequently, systematic screening of primary school children was undertaken throughout the country. Mobile teams were set up to go to primary schools and inspect children's heads, looking for the lesions of ringworm. The treatment mostly used was the topical application of an iodine tincture and a sulfur salt ointment. As there was no oral antifungal treatment available at that time, radiation-induced epilation was used as an efficient method to improve ringworm treatment and promote its eradication. With what was considered a relatively low dosage, epilation was quickly obtained over a period of a few weeks. Parents were instructed to remove the dead hair from their children's scalps, and the remaining infected follicles were removed by public health staff with tweezers. Thousands of children were irradiated in this manner, with a median dose of 325 to 400 roentgens (R). After complete epilation was achieved, the topical treatment was more easily applied.

At the Dispensário Central de Higiene Social in Porto (DCHSP), 5,356 individuals (mostly infants—80% were aged between 3 and 10 years old) were irradiated in this manner; we managed to follow up 1,375 of them. About 12% had pathology that could be related to the radiation they underwent as children, namely thyroid carcinoma, basal cell carcinoma, and meningioma. In this chapter we will divide our discussion into four main parts: diagnosis and disease evolution, epidemiology, treatment, and possible late effects from the treatment.

DIAGNOSIS AND DISEASE EVOLUTION

Ringworm was a highly contagious mycosis with a long evolution that infected children's scalps[1] and could lead to epidemic infections in schools and orphanages. It did not affect the child's general health status or even cause considerable cutaneous damage in most cases, but it did interfere with the child's welfare because it was so contagious.[2] Adult infection was considered unusual.[1]

On clinical observation, attention was paid to the scalp, the shape and distribution of the lesions, hair and hair stumps, and the presence or absence of inflammatory patterns.[3] During this observation, material for laboratory analysis was collected (short-tailed hair and adherent scales, scales from glabrous skin, nail fragments). There was also an attempt to identify the source of infection in order to eliminate it. Sometimes this observation was difficult due to the poor hygiene of the scalp (e.g., excessive physiologic desquamation caused by lack of washing, presence of parasites, secondary infection with serosity and crusts).[4] Another problem was the common use by the little girls of braided hair anointed with oils or Vaseline.

The infection could be due to several fungi: *Trichophyton violaceum* was the most common agent,[5] responsible for 60% of the cases; *T. tonsurans* (14%); *Microsporum canis* (10%); and *T. schoenleinii* (15%).[6] These numbers reflect the values from several publications presenting work performed between 1950 and 1958, with a total of 5,172 cases.[6] Neves,[7] in a 1960 mycologic study, detected 283 cases of ringworm and noticed that the incidence of *T. violaceum* seemed to diminish (41.0%) and that of *M. canis* seemed to increase (35.0%). He also mentioned two cases of *T. megninii* and one case of *T. mentagrophytes*.

The clinical expressions and evolution of these infections led to the classification of the disease into two main types: tonsure tinea and non-tonsure tinea.[8] Tonsure tinea caused hair breakage, but in non-tonsure tinea the hair did not normally break.[9] Tonsure tinea was then subdivided into trichophytic tinea and microsporic tinea. Trichophytic tinea was caused by several *Trichophyton* species, and microsporic tinea was caused mainly by *M. canis* and *M. felineum*.[10-12] Non-tonsure tinea (favus tinea) was caused by *T. schoenleinii*.

The trichophytic tineas presented variable patterns, depending on the host's sensitivity and the parasite species[1] (Figure 7.1A–C). Spots were produced with partial alopecia, with healthy hair (normal size) among the broken damaged hair (almost attached to the skin). The trichophytic tineas, due to their long adaptation to the human species, were more prone to induce a chronic status in the host, characterized by an absence of a visible reaction from the host.[2] The microsporic tineas were less well tolerated, and the skin showed a tendency to try to eliminate them through an inflammatory process that represented a natural mechanism of cure.[2] Both types of tinea disappeared before puberty, due to the global changes in the body, without causing visible traces in the scalp. The mechanism of cure was not fully understood but was probably due to alterations in the scalp's chemical composition due to the action of the sex glands.[1]

In microsporic tinea, a small, slightly erythematous spot would appear, and it would start to desquamate into small pityriasic scales (Figure 7.1D).

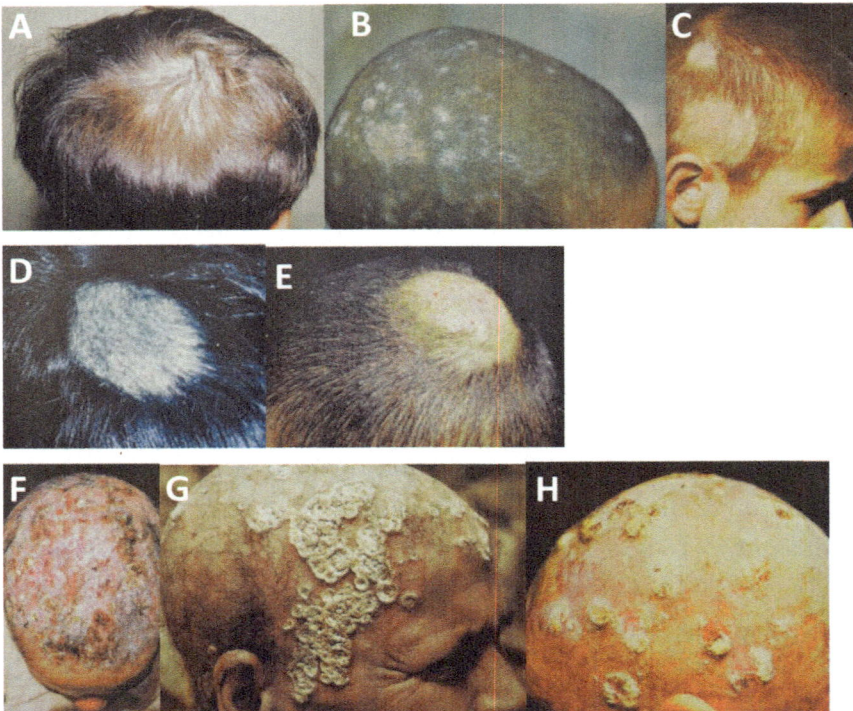

Figure 7.1 (A, B, C) Trichophytic tinea. (D, E) Microsporic tinea. (F, G) Favus tinea. Pictures gently provided by Prof. Aureliano da Fonseca.

The parasitized hair had a very characteristic pattern, cut a few centimeters above the skin, appearing to be covered by a whitish sheath that resulted from the mycelia agglomerating around the hair.[1] Commonly there was only one large spot; if there were many, there was almost always one that was larger than the others. The scales could be absent if the child's head had been washed recently, so it could be mistaken for alopecia areata. To distinguish the diseases, it was sufficient to observe the top of the hairs at the follicle exit. Spontaneous cure could occur due to the plaque transforming into a kerion[8] (Figure 7.1E).

Favus tinea had the appearance of small subepidermal yellow spots in which a milky liquid formed. Once dried, it turned into a yellow crust, with its convex part exposed, from which one or more hairs would emerge[1] (Figure 7.1F–H). These crusts were firmly adherent to the scalp;

once detached, they would leave a small humid depression, bright and hemorrhagic, that would emit an unpleasant mousy smell. The hair in the affected areas would lose its brightness. Following the natural course of the infection, the continuous pressure of the crust would frequently lead to atrophy of the hair follicle. The infection would cover the entire scalp and, once all the follicles had been destroyed, spontaneous cure would occur through the transformation of the scalp into scar tissue of definitive alopecia. It caused severe and irreversible tegument alterations and was usually observed in advanced stages of the disease, in children and adults whose life conditions were difficult.[2] Though the diagnosis was usually easy to make, sometimes favus tinea could be confused with seborrheic dermatitis or psoriasis.[1] It was also more likely to recur.[13] This was considered the worst form of ringworm disease, followed by trichophytic tinea, which was a more benign form than the microsporic tinea; luckily favus had the lowest incidence of the three modalities due to its weak contagiousness.[8]

The presence of the fungus had to be microscopically demonstrated in order to establish a diagnosis, to eventually predict the prognosis, and to choose the therapeutic approach, as the direct examination of the parasitized hair could not allow the identification of the fungus species, only its genus.[1] An auxiliary and very useful method for tinea diagnosis was the Wood light. It emitted UV rays that crossed a glass containing barium and sodium with a 9% nickel oxide silicate filter that allowed the radiation between the violet wavelength and the ultraviolet wavelength (3650 angstroms) to pass and produce fluorescence of the skin and of the parasitized hair.[1] This fluorescence varied with the fungus species. In microsporic tinea, greenish or violet striae appeared; in trichophytic tinea, the fluorescence was bluish or greenish; in the favus tinea, the fluorescence was gray-bluish or yellowish. This light could also be used to determine the extent of the lesions and to assess the cure during and after the treatment.[1]

The incidence of the three modalities of ringworm varied from region to region and from country to country. Fonseca conducted an epidemiologic study of the disease in northern Portugal, where 2,105 cases were studied,[1] and found that 63.3% of the cases were trichophytic tinea, 23.4% favus tinea, and 13.3% microsporic tinea. There was almost no difference between males and females, with only a slightly increase toward more females infected. The majority of the trichophytic tinea cases occurred in school-aged children (59.1% for children from 6 to 10 years old), but microsporic tinea was more prevalent until 5 years of age. Other authors agreed that microsporia was more frequent in early childhood and trichophytia in school-age children.[6,14,15] The increased prevalence of microsporia in the early childhood was attributed to the fact that usually the youngest children played more with animals (namely cats), and this infection was due to zoophilic agents.[10] In short, it was observed that microsporic tinea would appear only in early childhood; trichophytic tinea would occur in early childhood and late childhood, predominating in the first years of this second period; and favus tinea was particularly prevalent in individuals older than 12 years.[4]

Tonsure tinea was described as rare in adults, as opposite to non-tonsure tinea (favus tinea), but Fonseca et al. found 93 cases through the clinical examination of the mothers and older sisters of the children infected with trichophytic tinea.[16] It was exceptionally found in adult males. This situation was clinically relevant, as only eight women accepted the treatment due to the need to have their hair cut. Thus, the majority would constitute a disease reservoir. The reasons for the tonsure tinea appearance after puberty were not clear. The best-accepted explanation was that the disease was acquired in childhood and, for some reason, puberty did not involve the common alteration of the scalp oils, preventing spontaneous cure.

EPIDEMIOLOGY

The etiologic characterization of ringworm in Portugal began in 1922 with the work of Froilano de Melo et al.[17,18] After that, numerous studies were performed in the northern, central, and southern parts of Portugal. They lasted for different periods of time, but as a whole covered more than three decades.

Ringworm existed all over Portugal as an endemic disease of childhood.[6] It was more common in populations with fewer economic resources, especially those ones living near the coast, but also in rural areas[2,10] (Figure 7.2).

The majority of the piscatorial and rural populations had no concern about the disease, unlike the situation in the industrial and urban centers.[2] Fonseca[19] reported that the disease came from the coast to the rural and urban centers, transported by children who went to the beach in the summer. In fact, he detected the fungus in the pillows of the beach huts. To support this idea, he observed that the disease was unknown in the areas where the children did not go to the sea. Moreover, the prevalence

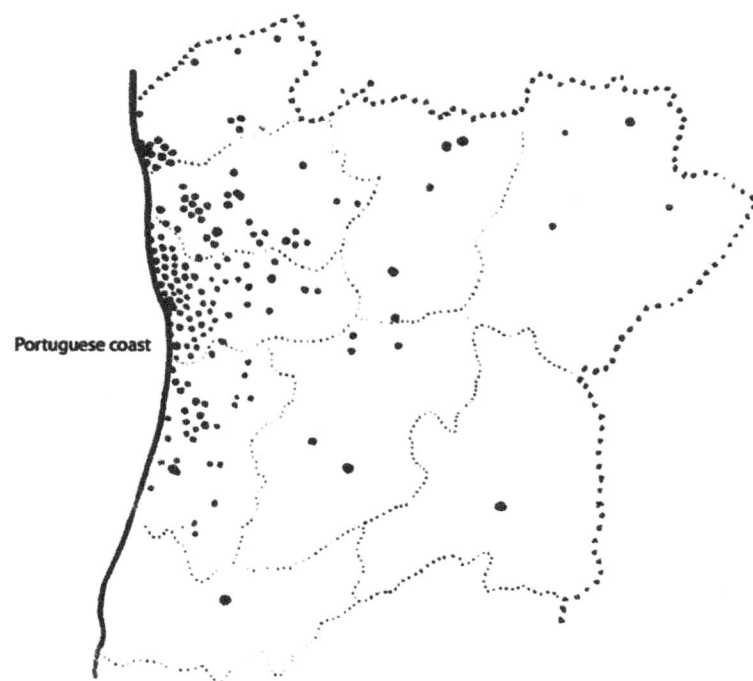

Figure 7.2 Ringworm distribution in northern Portugal
Adapted from Fonseca et al.[10]

of ringworm increased in those areas where going to the beach became more common, supported by the creation of beach holiday camps for children living in the countryside. Nevertheless, there were still some isolated foci of the disease that the author could not explain. The disease was then disseminated by the migration of the populations from the rural to the urban areas.[2,19] This migration sometimes led to the situation of families living in inadequate socioeconomic conditions, in groupings known as *ilhas* (literally "islands"), where families lived in one room and shared a bathroom. Sometimes there was not even a bathroom, and bathing took place in the living space using a basin. There was no piped water, so it had to be taken to the room in buckets to be warmed; thus, the same water was used to bathe several children.

It was common knowledge that, after the contagion, the fungi required certain conditions for its fixation and development, namely long curled hair and infrequent hair washing.[19] In winter, with the fear of contracting colds and other diseases, people used to wash their children's heads less frequently, especially if bathing conditions were deficient. That could allow the fungi to become established during the winter, and in spring, with an environment of oil, humidity, and heat, they would begin to grow. This explains why, in addition to the coastal areas, a high incidence of ringworm was observed near the fluvial areas.[19] To prevent the disease, Fonseca highly recommended hair washing twice a week or even daily in cases where the disease was already established. The disease was more easily spread among families, with the older children contaminating the younger ones, and the disease was common in children under 3 years of age.[19] For that reason, the second piece of advice proposed by Fonseca to prevent disease spread was to observe the individuals who lived with affected ones. In another article,[20] the author suggested that the children most prone to contagion were 4- to 8-year-olds.

Although the disease was more common in public schools, especially those in poorer socioeconomic areas, it was also present in private schools.[21] It usually presented with a more discrete pattern and was more difficult to recognize. Moreover, many parents refused to cut their children's hair, so these patients became ringworm-disseminating agents, especially to younger siblings and younger acquaintances.

It is impossible to estimate the number of cases in Portugal during that period or during the period in which the disease was more actively diagnosed and treated. Esteves stated in 1953[2] that there were no statistical data, or a global survey, that would allow an accurate evaluation of the spread and distribution of the disease. The author emphasized, as did others, that the cases were numerous among poorer groups, especially in the coastal areas. Costa Maia gave an estimate for 1950 in northern Portugal, based on investigations by Fonseca[11] and himself.[17] According to him, 60,000 to 70,000 cases would be expected in the school-age population (6 to 14 years old). He made this estimate by applying the incidence values obtained for ringworm disease (32%) to the number of school-age children in northern Portugal (Minho, Douro Litoral, and Trás-os-Montes) who were registered in the national census of 1950. Nevertheless, Costa Maia acknowledged that this estimate was rough and did not include preschool children or those who did not attend school (mostly 6- or 7-year-olds and those over 11 years old). In 1956, Fonseca presented a much lower estimate of 10,000 children, based on surveys performed in 13 municipalities in northern Portugal that showed percentages of the disease between 0.4% and 12.6%.[22] He observed 76,427 school-aged children. The higher prevalence was found in the municipalities of Póvoa de Varzim and Vila do Conde (12.6% and 10.0%, respectively[20]), which were mainly piscatorial regions. Almost all the children had poor hygiene habits due to poverty and family negligence. The same author found a prevalence of 2.1% in school-aged children in Porto in 1955.[21] He emphasized that ringworm also existed in children who did not attend school, who represented about 2.5 times the number of those who did attend school.

Nevertheless, the number of infected children all over the country exceeded the 10,000 to 60,000 mentioned for northern Portugal. This emphasizes the importance that ringworm infection represented for public health. Ringworm was found all over Portugal, although fewer cases were found in Alentejo.[2] It was also found in the Azores[23] and Madeira,[24] as well as in Mozambique[25,26] and Angola,[27] which at that time were Portuguese colonies.

With such high estimates of infected individuals, there were no doubts that the disease should be fought. The duration and extent of the disease were exacerbated in environments where parents were indifferent to the disease in their children.[2] Such indifference could be explained by rudimentary social obligations and was maintained by the common observation that, in most cases, the disease would disappear with age. Other factors responsible for the maintenance of this endemic disease were the long persistence of some lesions in adults' scalps and its localization in the nails, with favorable conditions for the fungus to live almost indefinitely.[2] Thus, eradication of the disease essentially required eliminating parasite reservoirs. This, in turn, required improving the cultural and economic standards of rural populations. Fonseca[11] referred to the need for an educational program on the disease, mainly for teachers and other educators, that should be complemented by a social work program, with social assistants and auxiliaries who could visit the families, teaching them how to correctly handle the disease and inquiring about and discovering possible hidden ringworm foci.

In northern Portugal, the favus tinea seemed to be more frequent, with favus lesions extending over the entire scalp and causing large areas of scar alopecia.[10] There the problem was even more acute, as this kind of infection had a longer duration and more serious sequelae.[17] In the dermatologic services of Lisbon, the annual registries showed a prevalence that normally did not surpass 5%.[10] The 23.4% prevalence found by Fonseca in 1953 in northern Portugal was attributed to the low social standards of part of the population in the north.

TREATMENT

Given the high frequency of ringworm in Portugal and the public health problem it represented, it was important to better understand and fight the disease. Several centers in Portugal dedicated themselves to regularly study and treat the disease. As the main areas of disease spread were the coastal and rural ones, where the means for adequate treatment were not always available, Brigadas Móveis de Profilaxia da Tinha (Mobile Teams for Tinea Prophylaxis) were organized to assist these populations and to carry out a plan to fight the disease that was established by the Direcção-Geral de Saúde (General Health Department). One of these teams was assigned to the northern part of the country and integrated in the DCHSP.[4] It started functioning in the municipality of Viana do Castelo in May 1954. Its necessity had been previously mentioned by Fonseca in 1953.[28] Fonseca even proposed creating two kinds of teams for the regions that had a high number of children, one for inspection and the other for observation and treatment (equipped with an x-ray apparatus). However, only one type of team was organized. It comprised a physician, a social assistant, a nurse, and an auxiliary and was equipped with appropriate x-ray equipment.[4,22] From May 1954 to February 1955, this team inspected 8,147 children; however, many children were not observed due to family refusal.[4] In 1956 there were several of these teams, distributed all over the country, but in northern Portugal there were only two.[22]

In Porto, the efforts of the DCHSP to fight the disease are shown in Table 7.1, which details the number of patients diagnosed in that institution in three consecutive periods.[29] The first x-ray epilations performed in Porto took place in 1930 in a private clinic (Fonseca, personal communication, 2011). Fonseca became acquainted with the disease in 1944, in soldiers' relatives at the Military Hospital of Porto; this led him to Vila do Conde, Póvoa de Varzim, and other endemic foci. Due to the high number

Table 7.1 NUMBER OF PATIENTS WITH TINEA, DCHSP, 1948–1962

Period	Number of patients
1948–52	2,105
1953–57	3,958
1958–62	3,508
Total	9,561

From reference 29.

of infected children he found, he took great pains to obtain the proper equipment to perform x-ray epilation. The first apparatus was installed in the DCHSP, and Fonseca traveled to the Hôpital Saint-Louis in Paris, the best dermatologic center in Europe at that time, to learn the technique. Much of what was achieved was due to the personal dedication of several physicians, even the mycologic studies, as there was little official support from the government.

In Lisbon, in the Hospital Curry Cabral (infectious diseases service), a clinical consultation dedicated to ringworm was implemented.[3] It was held on days when there were more patients and families scheduled so that the patients could get to know each other. This strategy facilitated the patients' adaptation to the exams and treatments and provided an opportunity to educate family members. Inpatient treatment was limited to patients living outside Lisbon who did not have the means to travel to Lisbon periodically. Decisions about the type of treatment given were based on the type of tinea, patient's age, presence or absence of inflammatory signs, lesion extension, previous treatments, particular conditions (e.g., economic situation, family or caregiver capacity to perform the treatments), and presence of onychomycoses. After considering these factors, patients were divided into those who could be cured with topical treatment only; those who needed x-ray epilation; and those with other tinea localizations (glabrous skin, nails), which represented chronic parasitic sources that could lead to scalp relapses.

The ringworm treatment consisted of two main procedures: (1) scalp disinfection with medication active against the microbial agent and (2) epilation with x-ray application to disinfect the scalp to an adequate extent and depth.[3] Due to profound penetration of mycelia into the hair follicle, it was difficult for any fungicidal to enter to the necessary depth and even inside the hair in order to produce adequate disinfection.[1]

The disinfection was performed with a liquid (iodine tincture) and an ointment (with sulfur salts). The liquid was applied in the morning and at night to the entire scalp, not only the affected areas. At night, after the liquid had dried, the ointment was applied. Every morning the scalp had to be washed vigorously with hot water and soap. The head had to be

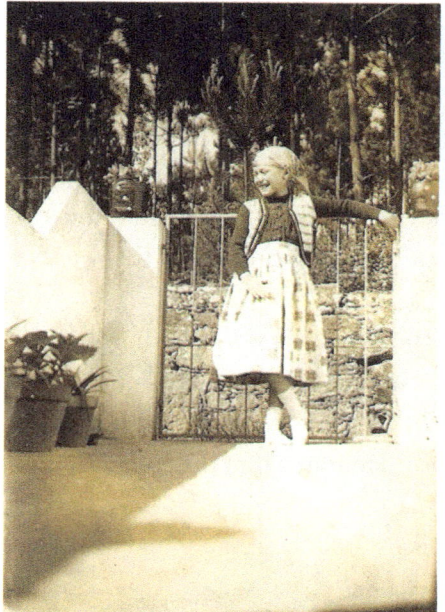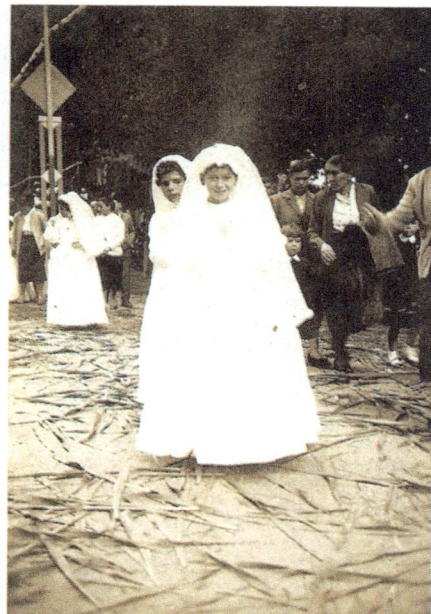

Figure 7.3 (A) Young girl with a scarf on her head after undergoing x-ray epilation treatment. (B) The same girl at her First Communion ceremony with false curled hair in the front of her face (she was still bald at the event).

protected all the time with a cap or a scarf of white cloth, which had to be replaced every 2 days[3,22] (Figure 7.3). The scarves had to be disinfected by boiling.[3] When the hair began to fall out, commonly 15 days after the x-ray irradiation, it was very important to remove the infected hairs with tweezers, avoiding hair breakage. Normally this operation was performed by the nurses or other health care personnel.[3,13] If the infected hairs broke off, the root could no longer be removed and the parasites would remain.[22] The hair usually began to regrow 5 to 6 weeks after it fell out.[3,13,22]

Epilation was performed with a Picker X-Ray Corp. apparatus using the Kienböck–Adamson method, which allowed the irradiation of the entire scalp in a short period of time. Only five fields were used, with a dose of approximately 300 to 400 R per field.[4,13,30,31] The five fields were in the frontal, vertex, occipital, and parietal regions and were determined by marking five points 11 to 13 cm apart from each other (depending on the size of the head).[30] The head was set in successive positions so the vertical rays from one field would be perpendicular to the vertical rays from the other fields.[13] The irradiation of the fields set in an anteroposterior orientation was performed in ventral decubitus, as shown in Figure 7.4. The ears were pulled to the front and kept still against the face with adhesive tape, after which they were protected with an appropriate lead cast. It was recommended that the face should also be protected.[13] Other authors did not refer to these protections, so it is not possible to know if this was the standard procedure.

According to Fonseca and Lisboa,[4] the five fields were irradiated in the same session, without a filter, with a focus–skin distance of 17 cm, 80 Kw, 6 mA that would apply a dose of 320 R per minute. These conditions are identical to those presented by Brandão.[13] He stated that the epilation dose

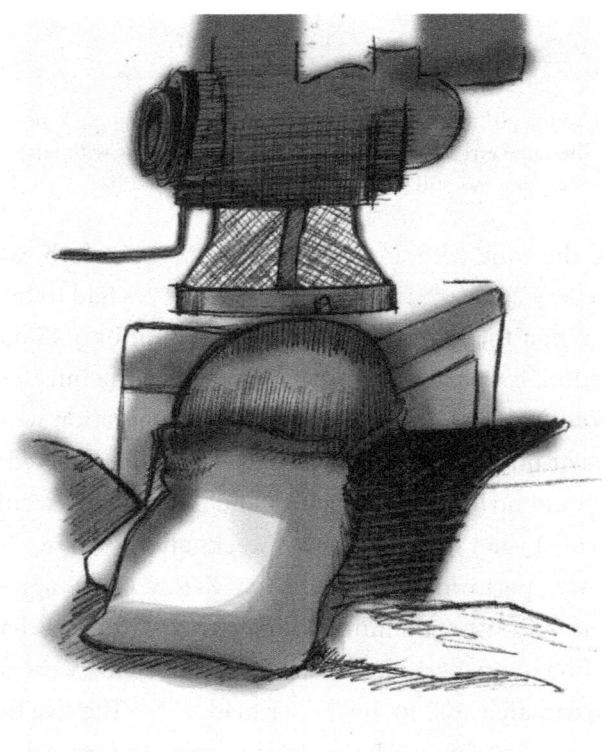

Figure 7.4 Diagram of the irradiation procedure
Based on a picture from reference 13.

depended on four main factors: the patient's age, the tinea diagnosis, the patient's constitutional type, and the cranial dimensions. For children 3 to 6 years old, the dose used was 300 to 330 R per field; for those 6 to 10 years old, it was about 350 R; and in adults, it was 400 R. If the diagnosis was favus, the dose would be slightly increased, due to the need for complete and uniform epilation, as well as delayed regrowth of the hair. Constitutional type was also an important factor, as lighter individuals were known to be more sensitive to radiation than darker ones. In exceptional cases of macrocephaly and microcephaly and other cranial malformations (Figure 7.5), it was sometimes necessary to modify not only the dose but also the classical five-field technique.

X-ray epilation according to the Kienböck–Adamson technique was referred to by other authors as an important weapon against scalp ringworm, provided it was carried out meticulously in every detail and administered by an operator with suitable training and experience in x-ray therapy of the skin.[32]

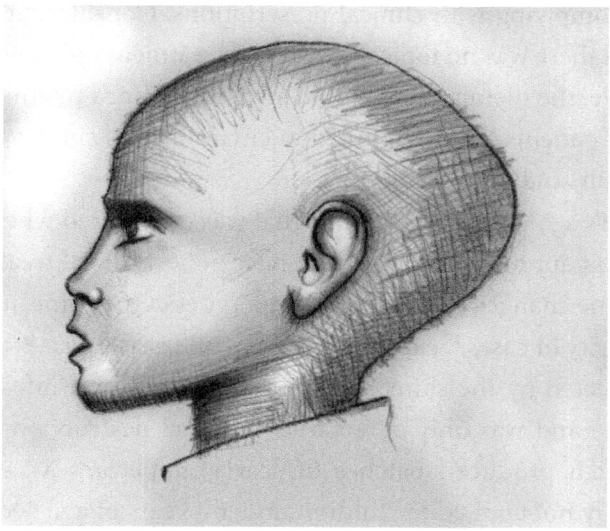

Figure 7.5 Example of a cranial malformation: scaphoid cranium
Based on a picture from reference 13.

By using ion-meters, operators discovered that the quantity of radiation received was not uniform: Areas located between the center of the fields received a dose that was 30% to 50% higher than the dose that was supposed to be applied (390 to 450 R). Nevertheless, this was still considered to be less than the dose that would induce permanent epilation (600 R), and the procedure was considered theoretically to be without risk.

For cases of favus tinea, the use of x-ray epilation was considered mandatory.[11,13,19] For trichophytic tinea, patients with mild disease (localized and with recent evolution) could be treated with salicylanilide cream, but those with extensive trichophytic tinea were sent for x-ray epilation.[11] The treatment with salicylanilide was considered much less effective than x-ray epilation (14.2% vs. 57.2%) in the evaluation by Fonseca and Lisboa in the municipality of Viana do Castelo.[4] The authors found a higher percentage of treatment rejection in the patients assigned to the salicylanilide treatment compared to those assigned to the x-ray epilation treatment. Because of the sympathy that families had for the treatment with "the apparatus," as they called it, but at the same time, having some fear that the children might go bald due to the epilation, they were relatively more careful in complying with clinical prescriptions. Considering this difference, and as there was no topical antifungal treatment more effective than salicylanilide, the therapeutic method advised for tinea treatment in large numbers of patients and in population environments similar to the ones found in their study was x-ray epilation.

The child's age was another factor that was considered when choosing the treatment approach. For children near puberty, local treatment, plus the endocrine changes that the body undergoes at that time, led to a cure in the majority of cases,[13] except for those with favus tinea. *T. schoenleinii* was not affected by the skin's immune capacities; thus, infection lasted past puberty and was only cured with the total destruction of the hair follicle, which produced patches of scarry alopecia.[19] X-ray epilation was generally not applied to children under 3 years of age because it was believed that the x-rays could interfere with the nervous centers and the ossification process of the cranium.[13] Nevertheless, Brandão states that this danger did not really seem to exist; rather, the real argument for not using this procedure was the difficulty keeping these children still. All patients in whom 3 months of topical treatment did not work were also irradiated.[13]

Some effects from the irradiation treatment have been described as accidents. The immediate ones (mainly nausea, vomiting, loss of appetite, and fever)[8,13] were attributed to a variety of causes, such as nervous excitement before and after the treatment, excessive ingestion of food before or after the treatment, and use of very high voltages.[13] Fonseca stated that no patient had problems with the x-ray application, besides rare headaches or nausea a few hours after the irradiation.[9,11] Some possible more severe late effects were mentioned; the most frequent was radiodermatitis, frequently resulting in definitive epilation, accompanied by skin lesions of variable severity.[8,13] These accidents were considered to be almost nonexistent if the correct technique was applied[8] and were reported to result from the administration of exaggerated doses or from superimposition of the fields, which could occur due to improper head fixation.[13] Definitive epilation could also result from anatomic defects in the head.[30] For instance, a very prominent occipital swelling, if not situated in the center of the occipital field, could diminish the focus–skin distance, causing a more persistent epilation that could become permanent. As all of these side effects were considered rare, the technique continued to be used, as it was considered by most authors as the only effective one.[8]

The criterion adopted for the cure was the absence of short-tailed hair and scales 3 to 4 months after the hair regrowth.[4,13] Penela and Esteves[30] stated that it was common for the hair to grow stronger in the scalp regions previously affected by the disease, so they advised the use of these areas for sample collection for the final exams performed to evaluate the cure.

If the disease recurred, a new x-ray epilation treatment was mandatory in the case of favus tinea; in other cases, it depended on the lesion's extension. In any case, the second epilation treatment was not to be performed less than 6 months after the first treatment to avoid the risk of causing radiodermatitis, which could lead to alopecia.[13] Esteves et al.[33] found a great difference in the cure rate with each method: 75% to 95% after x-ray epilation versus 34% with local treatment. They emphasized that x-ray epilation proved to be successful but had to be complemented with very careful manual removal of all infected hairs.

The hospitalization regimen, as noted above, was used only when there were no facilities for the ambulatory treatment or when disease was more severe (e.g., extended refractory lesions with localizations in glabrous skin and nails). One of the more significant difficulties involved in applying this regimen was the long time needed until the cure (about 5 months in the Hospital Curry Cabral).[3] Moreover, contagious individuals had to be isolated from those who were only under surveillance for treatment follow-up; proximity to contagious patients would increase their danger of reinfection.

With the appearance of griseofulvin, which began to be used in Portugal in 1960, the cure for ringworm became easy and took only a few weeks.[34] One of the first reports on the use of this new antimycotic agent was the one performed by Esteves and Neves in 1959,[35] so the department of dermatology of the Hospital Curry Cabral in Lisbon was among the first centers in the world to administer griseofulvin.[27] The authors said that finding new treatment methods for tinea had been one of the goals of their work over the last 13 years, so they decided to experiment with this new antimycotic. They used it in 14 cases of tonsure tinea caused by *T. violaceum*, *T. tonsurans*, and *M. canis*, with a dose of 1 g/day in patients aged 2 or more years and 0.5 g in those younger. All the cases were cured clinically and mycologically (direct examination and culture) after 3 to 5 weeks of treatment. The same dose of griseofulvin apparently cured four children with favus after 5 weeks of treatment and 2 weeks of observation. As far as we know, that was the first report on the action of griseofulvin in favus tinea in the world. It was clear that the fungus did not invade the portion of hair that grew during treatment,[35] and this confirmed Gentles' hypothesis[36] that griseofulvin renders keratin refractory to the parasite.[36] The efficacy of the drug was not so clear in five adults with chronic and extensive forms of tinea. There were no records of symptoms of intolerance to the drug in the 23 patients treated, nor any changes in the routine laboratory exams performed before and after treatment.[35] In the subsequent work that involved a total of 91 children, cure was obtained in 71, and the authors said that the failure rate obtained was higher than that reported by others.[27] A considerable simplification of the treatment of ringworm and reduction of the associated cost was achieved by the use of weekly doses of 12.5 mg/kg of fine-particle griseofulvin.[37]

In the last period of the DCHSP ringworm consultation reported by Fonseca and Macedo,[29] between 1958 and 1963, the treatment was, whenever possible, griseofulvin. Nevertheless, x-ray epilation was still used when there was no drug available or the patients could not afford it, which occurred in 55% of the cases. In a survey performed between 1955 and 1972 in the primary schools of Porto, Fonseca et al.[38] found an 84% reduction in the disease, which could mean that it was being eliminated. Nevertheless, comparing the data obtained from the inquiries in the schools with the ones from the dermatologic services of Porto, they concluded that although ringworm was disappearing from the city, it remained present in the country, mainly in the rural areas, where a disease reservoir was being maintained.

Griseofulvin is still used for effective ringworm treatment, alone or together with other drugs.[39-41] However, the infection is still evident and is increasing in undeveloped and even in highly developed countries.[42-44] Some reports have been published in Portugal[45,46] finding a relatively high incidence of *T. schoenleinii* as a second ringworm agent.[45]

POSSIBLE LATE EFFECTS FROM TREATMENT

X-ray epilation was widely used in many countries to treat ringworm, and follow-up studies of these irradiated individuals have been performed. The largest might be the one from Israel, with 10,000 individuals.[47-51] These follow-up studies have shown a two- to 10-fold increased risk for head and neck neoplasia, namely for basal cell carcinoma (BCC),[48,49,52,53] meningioma,[50,54,55] and thyroid carcinoma.[51,56] The thyroid is highly sensitive to radiation, especially when exposure occurs at a younger age.[51,57-59] An association between radiation exposure and parathyroid hyperplasia has also been described[60-63] in small cohorts other than the Israeli one.

The latency period between radiation exposure and diagnosis of neoplasia can be as long as 20 to 40 years for non-melanoma skin cancer[64–66] and for meningioma.[67–69]

We had access to the registries of the individuals who underwent x-ray epilation in the DCHSP between 1950 and 1963. This registration included 5,356 individuals, with name, address, age, treatment date, tinea diagnosis, and dose received. The majority of the individuals (70%) were 6 to 15 years old, reflecting the inspections done at schools at that time.

We started to locate and contact the individuals in March 2006. The DCHSP registry did not include date of birth, making it more difficult to locate the individuals and to ensure we reached the right person (we only could be sure when we got feedback from our contact). Moreover, people change addresses quite often, women can change their name when they marry, and some lack of accuracy in the initial registry data was detected.

We used several approaches, all of them time-consuming and sometimes redundant. We began using the Portugal Telecom (PT) online database, which allowed us to find about 15% of the supposed present addresses. After that, we used several databases from the national health system, even though we did not obtain the present address of around a third of the cohort. We also used the media—newspapers, radio, and television—in 2007, 2010, and 2011 (Figure 7.6).

We contacted the cohort members by sending a letter briefly describing the childhood therapeutic intervention they had undergone, proposing a free clinical observation, and asking them to contact us through a free telephone line. A second letter was sent whenever no answer was obtained to the first one.

The breakdown of cohort members into participants and non-participants is presented in Figure 7.7. This breakdown is being continuously updated, as clinical observations are ongoing; these figures reflect the latest update.

Two hundred thirty-eight individuals refused to participate: 76 lived far away, had incompatible schedule hours, or had difficulty traveling; 44 were ill; 20 considered themselves healthy; and the remainder refused to participate for unexplained reasons, did not receive the letter, or missed

A CARTA ENVIADA ÀS VÍTIMAS

O teor da carta enviada pelo Ipatimup: "Sabemos que há cerca de 50 anos foi tratado no Dispensário de Higiene Social, R. Anibal Cunha (à Carvalhosa), por causa de uma doença de pele da cabeça que obrigou à irradicação do couro cabeludo para fazer cair o cabelo e permitir a aplicação da tintura. A irradiação a que foi submetido nessa altura pode ter efeitos prejudiciais à sua saúde. Por essa razão, gostaríamos de o poder observar (Hospital Pedro Hispano - consulta externa - secratariado A) para ficarmos seguros que o tratamento não lhe causou danos. para isso, pedimos-lhe que os contacte através do telefone gratuito nº 800 20 73 70, 3ªs, 4ªs e 5ªs das 9 às 12 horas. Fora desse horário por favor deixe o seu nome, morada e nº de telefone, que oportunamente o contactaremos"

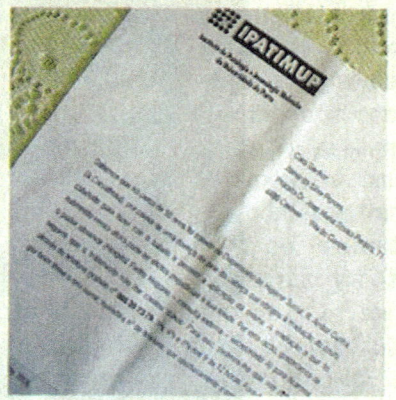

Figure 7.6 A newspaper item drawing attention to the letter that is being sent to patients by the research team, briefly describing the childhood therapeutic intervention they have experienced and proposing a free clinical observation, with a free telephone line for contact

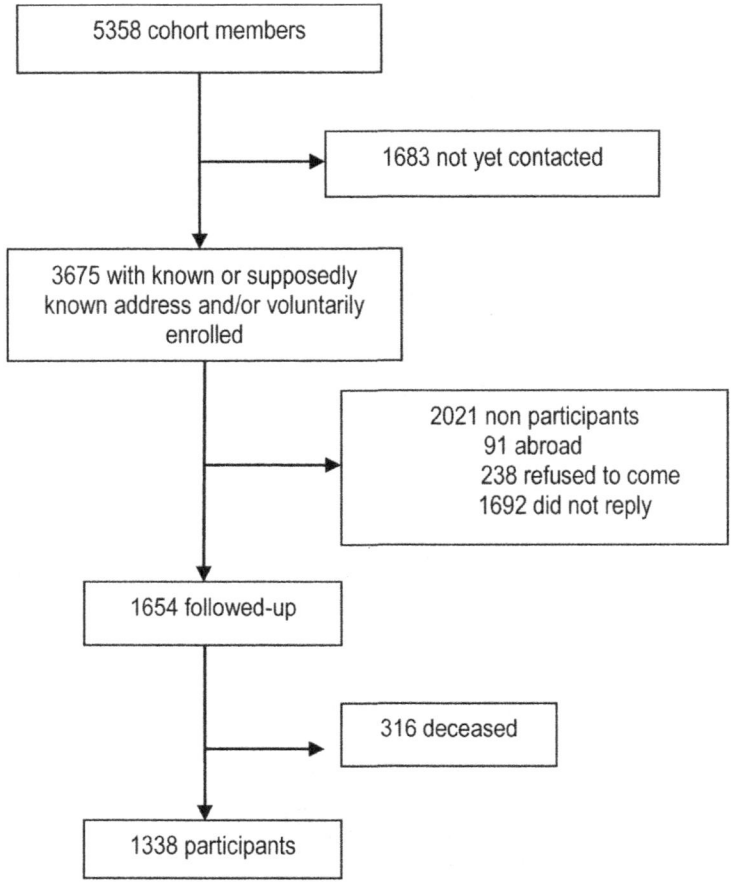

Figure 7.7 Breakdown of contacted individuals, participants, and non-participants from the DCHSP cohort

the appointment. Some individuals who refused to be observed had pathology possibly related to the radiation treatment: seven with brain tumors (four meningiomas), six with cerebrovascular accidents (an association between ringworm irradiation treatment and carotid sclerosis has recently been proposed[70]), six with BCC, and six who had undergone thyroidectomy (one for carcinoma). Several individuals who participated in the clinical observation told us that they were happy and/or surprised with our contact, as it made them feel they had not been forgotten, even though so many years had passed since their treatment. They expressed feelings of relief for finally being able to talk freely about the disease.

The clinical observation was always performed by the same clinician (Teixeira-Gomes), using a defined protocol that included careful observation of the head and neck areas in order to detect suspicious skin lesions and a clinical history. We suggested a cervical ultrasound to everyone who had not a previous history of total thyroidectomy, and a serum calcium measurement. A fine-needle aspiration biopsy (FNAB) was suggested for those with clinical thyroid nodules smaller than 15 mm with suspicious scan characteristics, and to all individuals with nodules larger than 15 mm. We suggested that those with a suspicious skin lesion undergo excision. The participants were asked to send us the reports from these exams/surgeries.

During the clinical observation, the participants were asked to provide a sample of blood and oral mucosal cells (under informed consent) for future genetic studies. In patients who had undergone head or neck surgery, we tried to recover the paraffin-embedded material to extract DNA.

Besides observing these individuals from the DCHSP cohort, we also observed more 280 individuals who did not belong to the cohort, as they were irradiated in other facilities, in Porto or in other regions of Portugal. They contacted us to schedule a clinical appointment upon hearing about our investigation in the media. The clinical results obtained during their observation were not included in the present report as there is no record of the radiation dose they received.

The main features of participants and cohort members were published after we had observed 1,287 individuals (Table 7.2).[71] The participants tended to be those who were younger when they received radiation. This may be due to the long delay between the irradiation and the actual contact—in some cases more than 50 years. Individuals who were older at the time of irradiation may have died, are more frequently ill, or are simply less likely to come for a clinical observation after such a long delay since irradiation. We also observed more women than men. A possible explanation is that women may be more likely to come for a clinical observation as they are more concerned about their health than men.[72]

Table 7.2 REGISTRY VARIABLES OF THE RINGWORM IRRADIATED COHORT IN THE 1950–1963 STUDY (N = 5,358), FROM THE DCHSP, AND PARTICIPANTS IN THE PRESENT STUDY (N = 1,287)

	Cohort member n (%)	Participants n (%)
Sex		
Female	2,804 (52.3)	767 (59.6)
Male	2,554 (47.7)	520 (40.4)
Type of infection		
Favus tinea	1,164 (21.7)	215 (16.7)
Microsporic/Tricophytic tinea	4,191 (78.2)	1,072 (83.3)
Not known	3 (0.1)	0 (0)
Age at irradiation		
≤5 years	1,352 (25.2)	419 (32.6)
>5 and ≤15 years	3,765 (70.3)	850 (66.0)
>15 years	185 (3.4)	18 (1.4)
Not known	56 (1.1)	0 (0)
Irradiation dose		
325–475 R	5,024 (93.8)	1,206 (93.7)
≥630 R	318 (5.9)	74 (5.8)
Not known	16 (0.3)	7 (0.5)
Thyroid pathology	—	33 (2.6)
Thyroid carcinoma	—	18 (1.4)
Follicular adenoma	—	462 (35.9)
Thyroid nodules		
All subjects	5,358 (100.0)	1,287 (100)

In the clinical observation, we talked to the patients about their ringworm experience and their childhood living conditions. We also talked on the phone to some x-ray–epilated individuals who contacted us to tell their stories. In total, we did 100 interviews and asked the irradiated individuals if they felt that the irradiation treatment had changed anything in their lives. We found that most of these individuals came from families with four to 11 children, living in houses with two or three rooms, without an indoor bathroom and no piped water. The bath was a weekly event, sometimes twice a week. These conditions explained the difficulty in eradicating the disease, as they did not favor the application of the important hygiene measures the treatment required.

From these testimonials, we learned that individual perceptions of the disease and its treatment vary widely. One factor that is expected to influence the individual's reaction to the situation is the age at the time of diagnosis. The temporary complete alopecia and use of a head covering required by treatment would draw attention at school, but this degree of exposure was not experienced by younger children who did not attend school. For those irradiated while attending school, 25 out of 70 (36%) said that the treatment affected their lives; the corresponding figures for younger children were six out of 30 (20%). The most common complaint was the stigma of being ignored by the other children and even teachers, and of being called "bald head." Another common complaint was about the topical treatment, the iodine tincture ardency, and the use of the tweezers for short-tailed hair removal. Some people had more dramatic complaints: five said they had to interrupt their studies due to the disease, five said they were distressed for life, two said they had learning disabilities, and three said they had difficulty coping with the stress situation. Some studies have addressed the problem of mental health disturbances in the irradiated individuals, but this line of investigation was not pursued.[73,74] In the present interviews we had the feeling that the distress described was more closely related to the difficulty coping with the situation.

In contrast, three women recalled the treatment period as a good time, because their mother made them wigs with their own hair after it was cut, or allowed them to wear many different hats.

A curious aspect mentioned by several patients (11 out of 100 [11%]) was a change in the hair pattern when it grew back. They stated that straight hair grew back curly and/or white hair appeared. We did not find any reference in the literature to this occurrence. Alopecia or thinning hair was another situation described, especially by the women. We evaluated the presence of alopecia or thinning hair in every woman we clinically observed[75] and showed that the risk for alopecia in these irradiated women was much higher (an eight-fold increased risk) in the individuals with favus tinea. Of course, alopecia could also be a consequence of the irradiation treatment, as described by others,[76,77] with a four-fold increased risk whenever a dose of 630 R or more was received (Table 7.3). We also confirmed that the risk of developing alopecia was higher in women who had received higher doses.

We published our data concerning the prevalence of thyroid pathology in the clinically observed individuals.[71] In Table 7.2, we present these data as well as the comparison between the DCHSP cohort members and the clinically observed individuals already mentioned. At the observation 18 individuals had been previously diagnosed with thyroid carcinoma, and we diagnosed 15 more cases. In total, we found a 2.6% prevalence of thyroid carcinoma, which is similar to the 2.1% found by Imaizumi et al.[78] in a survey study of Hiroshima and Nagasaki atomic bomb survivors using a similar protocol (thyroid ultrasonography). If we exclude from our study the prospective diagnosis, the prevalence decreases to 1.4%, similar to the

Table 7.3 ASSOCIATION BETWEEN TINEA DIAGNOSIS, IRRADIATION DOSE, AND AGE OF RINGWORM DETECTION AND ALOPECIA PREVALENCE

		Alopecia prevalence	
	%	RR (95% CI)	RR* (95% CI)
Tinea diagnosis			
Other	3.0	1	1
Tinea favosa	28.0	9.49 (5.36–17.79)	7.92 (4.49–13.99)
Irradiation dose			
<630 R	5.2	1	1
≥630 R	28.6	5.50 (2.96–10.22)	3.93 (2.61–5.91)
Age at time of irradiation			
≤4 years	3.6	1	1
5–9 years	5.3	1.48 (0.57–3.84)	1.33 (0.54–3.27)
≥10 years	13.9	3.87 (1.46–10.24)	2.29 (0.93–5.68)

* Adjusted for the other variables. RR, relative risk; CI, confidence interval.

Adapted from reference 75.

0.95% referred to by Sadetzki et al.[51] in retrospective studies. Our data are also in accordance with the higher risk for thyroid tumors referred to by Shvarts et al.[79]

Eleven participants presented with meningiomas (0.87%), all previously diagnosed; six had been irradiated at age 5 years or earlier (1.6%) and the other five had been irradiated after 5 years of age (0.7%). Three of these 11 cases presented with relapses. Ron et al.[80] showed an increased risk of meningioma of 9.5 times in the irradiated Israeli cohort. As the estimated prevalence for meningioma in the United States in non-irradiated individuals is 0.098%,[55] the prevalence found in the present study fits with Ron et al.'s[80] data. As noted, six of the 11 meningioma patients were irradiated earlier in life; a larger sample would be necessary to confirm an eventual increased prevalence of meningioma in younger irradiated individuals, as referred to by others.[68] Based on the fact that the irradiation treatment may confer a low risk for meningioma development, but one that persists for life, a cerebral nuclear magnetic resonance (NMR) study for screening all the irradiated individuals has been suggested by other authors.[81] Other head and neck neoplasias observed in our cohort were two parotid carcinomas (0.16%), two neurinomas (0.16%), and two hypophysis tumors (0.16%). The cerebral NMR screening would also be important for detecting these other head and neck tumors.

We also asked for calcium measurements in participants, and we detected hypercalcemia in 54 individuals. We asked them to obtain a second calcium evaluation; when this second value was high or borderline, measurement of serum parathyroid hormone and calcium levels in 24-hour urine was suggested to diagnose or rule out primary hyperparathyroidism (PHPT). The results from this study allowed us to diagnose and treat (so far) five cases of PHPT in individuals who were not aware of their problem. PHPT frequency has been related to childhood irradiation treatments, although the data are scarce.[63,82-84]

We found a high BCC prevalence in the irradiated individuals we have been observing, with figures similar to those described in other ringworm-irradiated cohorts. This tumor, although it has a low mortality, carries considerable morbidity,[85] and we concur with Meibodi et al.[86] that it is very important to create awareness in these irradiated individuals and encourage them to seek medical attention for any suspicious lesions (namely dermatologic ones).

CONCLUDING REMARKS

The ringworm epidemic in Portugal represented a remarkable situation both in terms of life events for those affected and in terms of disease epidemiology and health care strategies adopted. There was no oral treatment until 1958, and when it finally appeared, it was not available to all the infected individuals. Thus, the physicians had to revert to the scalp x-ray epilation method, in use in several other counties, in order to treat and prevent the spread of this highly contagious disease. The data we have obtained so far[71,75] on the possible late effects of ringworm epilation treatment support and underscore the arguments presented by Shvarts et al.[79] that physicians should be aware of particular subsets of the population who might be at risk for radiation-associated late health effects. Close follow-up of these higher-risk irradiated cohorts is justified so that head and neck lesions can be identified and treated.

ACKNOWLEDGMENTS

This work was supported by a grant from Calouste Gulbenkian Foundation (ref. 76636) and FCT (project: PIC/IC/83154/2007) and further funding from the Portuguese Foundation for Science and Technology (FCT), by a grant to P.B. (SFRH/BPD/34276/2007). IPATIMUP is an Associate Laboratory of the Portuguese Ministry of Science, Technology and Higher Education and is partially supported by the FCT. The work was conducted with the support of the Public Health Department of ARS-Norte. We are especially grateful to Prof. Aureliano da Fonseca for the photographs of tinea capitis patients, for the information that he kindly provided, and for reading the manuscript. We thank Prof. Sobrinho Simões for the valuable suggestions. Gratitude is also due to all the individuals who agreed to participate in this study as well as to all the physicians who provided us with clinical information. The authors thank Ana Reis for proofreading. Prize ACS-MERCK SERONO in Cancer Epidemiology, 2010.

REFERENCES

1. Fonseca, A. Patologia e tratamento das tinhas. *Sep O Médico* 30 (1951).
2. Esteves, J. A tinha como flagelo médico-social da criança. *O Médico* 1, 23–27 (1953).
3. Esteves, J. Organização e métodos na clínica e estudo da tinha. *Sep O Médico* 110, 500–503 (1953).
4. Fonseca, A., Lisboa, M. A tinha do couro cabeludo no concelho de Viana do Castelo: estudo epidemiológico e tratamento *Sep O Médico* 201–202 (1955).
5. Philpot, C. Geographical distribution of the dermatophytes: a review. *J Hyg Camb* 80, 301–313 (1978).
6. Neves, H., Carmo-Sousa, L. Medical and veterinary mycology in Portugal for 1949–1959. *Mycopathologia* 13(2), 135–152 (1960).
7. Neves, H. Mycological study of 519 cases of ringworm infections in Portugal. Significance of multiple localizations. Tinea as a single infection. *Mycopathologia* 13 (1960).
8. Leitão, A. Tratamento actual da tinha. *Jornal do Médico* 861 (1960).
9. Fonseca, A. Alguns aspectos médico-sanitários da tinha do couro cabeludo. *O Médico*, 109 ().
10. Fonseca, A. Aspecto epidemiológico da tinha no Norte de Portugal. *O Médico* 4, 833–837 (1953).
11. Fonseca, A., Osswald, W., Macedo, C. A tinha no couro cabeludo no concelho da Póvoa de Varzim: Inquérito eoidemiológico, tratamento e resultados. *O Médico* 1, 837–842 (1953).
12. Neves, H., Figueiredo, M.M. Imlicações etiológicas e epidemiológicas colhidas da análise de 2582 casos de tinha. *O Médico* 440 ().
13. Brandão, N. A roentgenterapia das tinhas do couro cabeludo (aspectos técnicos e problemas). *O Médico* 1, 857–864 (1953).
14. Esteves, J., Fonseca, A., Antunes, M.M. Aspectos epidemiológicos da Tinha em Portugal: Distribuição dos casos em função da idade, sexo e tipo de parasitismo. *Portugal Médico* 39 (1955).
15. Cabrita, J. Human mycoses in Portugal (1960–1973). *Mycopathologia et Mycologia applicata* 54, 347–360 (1974).
16. Fonseca, A., Osswald, W., Macedo, C. Importância e epidemiologia da Tinha Tonsurante após a puberdade. *Separata de Trabalhos da Sociedade Portuguesa de Dermatologia e Venereologia* 18(2), 85–93 (1960).

17. Costa-Maia, J. *Alguns aspectos de epidemologia, profilaxia e combate da Tinea Capitis*. Tese de Doutoramento, 1953.
18. Esteves, J. Algumas características etiológicas da endemia portuguesa de tinha. *O Médico* 831–832 (1953).
19. Fonseca, A. A tinha do couro cabeludo: Factores epidemiológicos e tratamento. Estado actual da luta contra a tinha. *O Médico* 25, 183–184 (1962).
20. Fonseca, A. Estudo epidemiológico da tinha do couro cabeludo no norte de Portugal (inquérito e factores epidemiológicos). *Actas Dermo-Sifiliográficas Fevereiro* 285–391 (1955).
21. Fonseca, A., Macedo, C. Alguns aspectos epidemiológicos da tinha do couro cabeludo na cidade do Porto. *Sep O Médico* 306, 1–10 (1957).
22. Fonseca, A. Alguns aspectos médico-sanitários da tinha do couro cabeludo. *O Médico* 109–115 (1956).
23. Salta, A.J., Antunes, M.M. Frequência e agentes etiológicos das tinhas de S. Miguel e Sta Maria (Açores). *Sep O Médico* 114, 925 (1953).
24. Sampaio, N. Sobre as Tinhas da ilha da Madeira. *Actas do II Congresso Luso-Espanhol de Dermatologia, Lisboa* 263 (1950).
25. Neves, H., Ramos, S.F., Figueiredo, M.M. Causative agents of ringworm in Lourenço Marques (Mozambique). *Derm Trop* 2, 153 (1960).
26. Van Uden, N., Neves, H. Contribuição para o estudo da flora dermatofítica de Moçambique. *An Inst Med Trop* 18, 263 (1961).
27. Neves, H. The unitary concept of ringworm. *Mycopathol Mycol Appl* 30, 1–18 (1966).
28. Fonseca, A. Esboço de organização de luta contra a tinha do couro cabeludo no norte de Portugal. *O Médico* 1 (1953).
29. Fonseca, A., Macedo, C. A Consulta da Tinha no Couro Cabeludo no "Dispensário Central de Higiene Social do Porto" no Quinquénio 1958–1963. *Sep O Médico* 690, 500–503 (1964).
30. Penella, S., Roda, J. Tratamento das Tinhas (Serviço N° 3 do Hospital do Desterro). *Amatus Lusitanus* (1943).
31. Fonseca, A., Osswald, W., Macedo, C. A acção do Dispensário Central de Higiene Social do Porto na luta contra a tinha: quinquénio de 1953–1957: Alguns aspectos epidemiológicos, tratamentos e resultados. *Sep O Médico* 403, 379–383 (1959).
32. Crossland, P. Therapy of tinea capitis: the value of x-ray epilation. *Calif Med* 54, 351–353 (1956).
33. Esteves, J., Brandão, F.N., Neves, H., Custódio, J.S. Ensaio de integração, funcional de serviço hospitalar em actividade dermatomicológica (1945–1958). *Bol Clin Hosp Civ Lisboa* 23, 307 (1959).
34. Fonseca, A. A tinha do couro cabeludo no século XVIII. *Sep Jornal do Médico* 122, 374 (1987).
35. Esteves, J., Neves, H. A griseofluvina no tratamento da tinha do coiro cabeludo e de outras localizações desta doença: primeiras observações. *Sep Jornal do Médico* 39, 341–344 (1959).
36. Gentles, J.C. Experimental ringworm in guinea pigs. Oral treatment with griseofulvin. *Nature* 182 (1958).

37. Neves, H., Cabral, A.J.L., Nunes, F., Caldeira, J.B. Progresso no tratamento da tinha do coiro cabeludo com doses semanais de griseofulvina. *F P O Médico* 24, 557 (1962).
38. Fonseca, A., Osswald, W., Macedo, C. A tinha do couro cabeludo nas crianças das escolas primárias da cidade do Porto no ano de 1972. *Jornal do Médico*, 161 (1972).
39. Hallgren, J., Petrini, B., Wahlgren, C.F. Increasing tinea capitis prevalence in Stockholm reflects immigration. *Med Mycol* 42, 505–509 (2004).
40. Khaled, A., Nbarek, L.B., Kharfi, M., Zeglaoui, F., et al. Tinea capitis favosa due to *Trichophyton schoenleinii*. *Acta Dermatovenerol Alp Panonica Adriat* 16, 34–36 (2007).
41. Ginter-Hanselmayer, G., Seebacher, C. Treatment of tinea capitis: a critical appraisal. *J Dtsch Dermatol Ges* 9, 109–114 (2011).
42. Chen, B.K., Friedlander, S.F. Tinea capitis update: a continuing conflict with an old adversary. *Curr Opin Pediatr* 13, 331–335 (2001).
43. Ginter-Hanselmayer, G., Stary, A., Messeritsch-Fanta, C. Current situation of tinea capitis in southeastern Austria. *Clin Dermatol* 20, 183–186 (2002).
44. Hackett, B.C., O'Connell, K., Cafferkey, M., O'Donnell, B.F., Keane, F.M. Tinea capitis in a paediatric population. *Ir Med J* 99, 294–295 (2006).
45. Lopes, V., et al. [Three years incidence of dermatophytes in a hospital in Porto (Portugal).] *Rev Iberoam Micol* 19, 201–203 (2002).
46. Valdigem, G.L., et al. A twenty-year survey of dermatophytoses in Braga, Portugal. *Int J Dermatol* 45, 822–827 (2006).
47. Ron, E., Modan, B. Benign and malignant thyroid neoplasms after childhood irradiation for tinea capitis. *J Natl Cancer Inst* 65, 7–11 (1980).
48. Ron, E., et al. Radiation-induced skin carcinomas of the head and neck. *Radiat Res* 125, 318–325 (1991).
49. Shore, R.E., et al. Skin cancer after x-ray treatment for scalp ringworm. *Radiat Res* 157, 410–418 (2002).
50. Sadetzki, S., et al. Long-term follow-up for brain tumor development after childhood exposure to ionizing radiation for tinea capitis. *Radiat Res* 163, 424–432 (2005).
51. Sadetzki, S., Chetrit, A., Lubina, A., Stovall, M., Novikov, I. Risk of thyroid cancer after childhood exposure to ionizing radiation for tinea capitis. *J Clin Endocrinol Metab* 91, 4798–4804 (2006).
52. Karagas, M.R., et al. Risk of basal cell and squamous cell skin cancers after ionizing radiation therapy. For the Skin Cancer Prevention Study Group. *J Natl Cancer Inst* 88, 1848–1853 (1996).
53. Gallagher, R.P., et al. Chemical exposures, medical history, and risk of squamous and basal cell carcinoma of the skin. *Cancer Epidemiol Biomarkers Prev* 5, 419–424 (1996).
54. Hubert, D., Bertin, M. [Radiation-induced tumors of the nervous system in man.] *Bull Cancer* 80, 971–983 (1993).
55. Claus, E.B., et al. Epidemiology of intracranial meningioma. *Neurosurgery* 57, 1088–1095 (2005).

56. Lubin, J.H., Schafer, D.W., Ron, E., Stovall, M., Carroll, R.J. A reanalysis of thyroid neoplasms in the Israeli tinea capitis study accounting for dose uncertainties. *Radiat Res* 161, 359–368 (2004).
57. Ron, E., et al. Thyroid neoplasia following low-dose radiation in childhood. *Radiat Res* 120, 516–531 (1989).
58. Wakeford, R. The cancer epidemiology of radiation. *Oncogene* 23, 6404–6428 (2004).
59. Sadetzki, S., Mandelzweig, L. Childhood exposure to external ionising radiation and solid cancer risk. *Br J Cancer* 100, 1021–1025 (2009).
60. Tamura, K., Shimaoka, K., Spaulding, S., Shedd, D. Association between primary hyperparathyroidism and previous irradiation. *J Surg Oncol* 19, 193–196 (1982).
61. Menis, E.D., Roiter, I., Legovini, P., Bassi, N., Conte, N. [Acute hyperparathyroidism associated with follicular carcinoma in the thyroid: possible role of juvenile cervical irradiation. Description of a case.] *Minerva Endocrinol* 22, 19–22 (1997).
62. Hedman, I., Tisell, L.E. Associated hyperparathyroidism and nonmedullary thyroid carcinoma: the etiologic role of radiation. *Surgery* 95, 392–397 (1984).
63. Stephen, A.E., Chen, K.T., Milas, M., Siperstein, A.E. The coming of age of radiation-induced hyperparathyroidism: evolving patterns of thyroid and parathyroid disease after head and neck irradiation. *Surgery* 136, 1143–1153 (2004).
64. Maalej, M., et al. Radio-induced malignancies of the scalp about 98 patients with 150 lesions and literature review. *Cancer Radiother* 8, 81–87 (2004).
65. Mseddi, M., et al. [Basal cell carcinoma of the scalp after radiation therapy for tinea capitis: 33 patients.] *Cancer Radiother* 8, 270–273 (2004).
66. Saladi, R.N., Persaud, A.N. The causes of skin cancer: a comprehensive review. *Drugs Today (Barc)* 41, 37–53 (2005).
67. Pollak, L., Walach, N., Gur, R., Schiffer, J. Meningiomas after radiotherapy for tinea capitis: still no history. *Tumori* 84, 65–68 (1998).
68. Sadetzki, S., Flint-Richter, P., Ben-Tal, T., Nass, D. Radiation-induced meningioma: a descriptive study of 253 cases. *J Neurosurg* 97, 1078–1082 (2002).
69. Gosztonyi, G., Slowik, F., Pasztor, E. Intracranial meningiomas developing at long intervals following low-dose X-ray irradiation of the head. *J Neurooncol* 70, 59–65 (2004).
70. Shai, E., et al. Carotid atherosclerotic disease following childhood scalp irradiation. *Atherosclerosis* 204, 556–560 (2009).
71. Boaventura, P., Soares, P., Pereira, D., Teixeira-Gomes, J., Sobrinho-Simoes, M. Head and neck lesions in a cohort irradiated in childhood for tinea capitis treatment. *Lancet Infect Dis* 11, 163–164 (2011).
72. Vintém, J.M., Guerreiro, M.D., Carvalho, H. Desigualdades de género e sociais na saúde e doença em Portugal: Uma análise do Módulo "Saúde" do European Social Survey, 2004 *VI Congresso Português de Sociologia, 25–28 Junho de 2008* 325 (2008).
73. Omran, A.R., et al. Follow-up study of patients treated by X-ray epilation for tinea capitis: psychiatric and psychometric evaluation. *Am J Public Health* 68, 561–567 (1978).

74. Ron, E., Modan, B., Floro, S., Harkedar, I., Gurewitz, R. Mental function following scalp irradiation during childhood. *Am J Epidemiol* 116, 149–160 (1982).
75. Boaventura, P., Bastos, J., Pereira, D., Soares, P., Teixeira-Gomes, J.M. Alopecia in women submitted to childhood X-ray epilation for tinea capitis treatment. *Br J Dermatol* 163, 643–644 (2010).
76. Modan, B., et al. Factors affecting the development of skin cancer after scalp irradiation. *Radiat Res* 135, 125–128 (1993).
77. Lawenda, B.D., et al. Permanent alopecia after cranial irradiation: dose-response relationship. *Int J Radiat Oncol Biol Phys* 60, 879–887 (2004).
78. Imaizumi, M., et al. Radiation dose-response relationships for thyroid nodules and autoimmune thyroid diseases in Hiroshima and Nagasaki atomic bomb survivors 55–58 years after radiation exposure. *JAMA* 295, 1011–1022 (2006).
79. Shvarts, S., Sevo, G., Tasic, M., Shani, M., Sadetzki, S. The tinea capitis campaign in Serbia in the 1950s. *Lancet Infect Dis* 10, 571–576 (2010).
80. Ron, E., et al. Tumors of the brain and nervous system after radiotherapy in childhood. *N Engl J Med* 319, 1033–1039 (1988).
81. Boljesikova, E., Chorvath, M. Radiation-induced meningiomas. *Neoplasma* 48, 442–444 (2001).
82. Bouallouche, A., Vermeulen, C., Cathelineau, G. [Hyperparathyroidism following cervical irradiation. A case and review of the literature.] *Sem Hop* 59, 129–132 (1983).
83. Cohen, J., Gierlowski, T.C., Schneider, A.B. A prospective study of hyperparathyroidism in individuals exposed to radiation in childhood. *JAMA* 264, 581–584 (1990).
84. Ippolito, G., Palazzo, F.F., Sebag, F., Henry, J.F. Long-term follow-up after parathyroidectomy for radiation-induced hyperparathyroidism. *Surgery* 142, 819–822 (2007).
85. Johnson, M.L., Johnson, K.G., Engel, A. Prevalence, morbidity, and cost of dermatologic diseases. *J Am Acad Dermatol* 11, 930–936 (1984).
86. Meibodi, N.T., Maleki, M., Javidi, Z., Nahidi, Y. Clinicopathological evaluation of radiation-induced basal cell carcinoma. *Indian J Dermatol* 53, 137–139 (2008).

8

"Deadly Medicine"

Michael Reese Hospital's Pandora's box and the campaign to warn the public of the late health effects of ionizing radiation in the United States

ITAI BAVLI AND SHIFRA SHVARTS

USE OF X-RAYS FOR BENIGN DISEASES

The practice of using x-rays for the medical treatment of benign diseases began in the 1920s, peaked in the 1940s and 1950s, and then gradually became less frequent by the 1960s.[1] Radiation therapy was considered to be good medical practice and a very effective treatment for benign illnesses, such as cervical adenitis, hemangiomas of the head and neck, tinea capitis (ringworm), birthmarks, infertility, pertussis, hypertrophy of the tonsils and adenoids, deafness, enlargement of the thymus gland (which was incorrectly believed to cause crib death), acne, and more.[2] The immediate results were often promising. For example, acne scarring was reduced, some forms of deafness improved,[3] and radiation treatment was very effective in eliminating ringworm (Figure 8.5).[4]

Head and neck radiation was a common practice worldwide. In the United States, more than 2 million people are estimated to have been treated with radiation for benign conditions (Figure 8.7),[5] and hundreds of thousands of people were treated with radiation therapy for ringworm of the scalp (and other benign ailments) in other parts of the world, including Syria, Egypt, Morocco, Tunisia, Canada, Latin America, and Europe.[6] In Yugoslavia (see Chapter 6), a United Nations Children's Fund (UNICEF)-assisted campaign to eliminate tinea capitis resulted in treating approximately 50,000 children with radiation.[7] In Portugal (see Chapter 7), health authorities treated approximately 30,000 children with radiation for scalp ringworm,[8] and tens of thousands in France underwent similar treatments.[9] In Israel, approximately 31,000 children with ringworm were treated with radiation.[10]

X-ray treatment gradually came to an end during the 1960s after other effective treatments had been developed (e.g., griseofulvin for ringworm)[11] and studies were starting to suggest that benign and malignant tumors of the thyroid gland (as well as leukemia) were being detected 5 or more years after the exposure in individuals who had received radiation treatment during childhood or who had been exposed to atomic bomb radiation or fallout.[12]

LONG-TERM ADVERSE EFFECTS OF RADIATION TREATMENT

Among the many risk factors for cancer, exposure to ionizing radiation is one of the most studied and measured epidemiologically. The primary reason is the exposure of large populations to radiation from the explosion of the atomic bombs over Hiroshima and Nagasaki. These two events constituted one-time high external exposures to ionizing radiation (i.e., the entire dosage was absorbed by the entire body in a single incident). The information gathered over a lengthy period many years (20 to 30) after the event made it possible to elucidate in-depth correlations between the estimated dosages among various groups within the exposed population and the development of numerous types of cancers at a greater frequency than expected in similar populations that had not been exposed to radiation. The data showed a higher prevalence of some kinds of cancers among those exposed to high dosages, but it was not possible to distinguish any higher prevalence among those exposed to lower dosages against the backdrop of high *natural* rates.[13]

The absence of definitive evidence of the effect of low-dose radiation on the human body has led to many controversies regarding the threshold below which radiation was considered safe and the maximum protection dose a person can be exposed to in a given year.[14] During the 1950s and 1960s, evidence was insufficient to reach firm conclusions about the hazards that low doses present.[15]

One of the first studies to show a link between therapeutic radiation to the head and neck following treatment for ringworm and brain tumors was published in 1968 by Albert and Omran[16] from New York University. The study was an extension of earlier work by Albert et al.[17] on subjects who had undergone radiation treatment in the United States that demonstrated a greater prevalence of brain tumors among people who had been exposed to radiation to treat ringworm of the scalp as children. Following that study, numerous epidemiologic articles were published on the link between childhood head and neck radiation and late health effects. The most influential study was published in 1973 by DeGroot and Paloyan from the University of Chicago, who found that children treated with radiation tended to develop thyroid cancer and other ailments as adults.[18] They concluded and warned that there were still many individuals in the United States who had been treated with radiation as children but had not received follow-up medical care, and that an effort must be made to alert the public and physicians.[19]

Less than a year later, another pioneering study was published by Modan et al.[20] on 10,834 children who had been treated with radiation for ringworm of the scalp in Israel. They showed that those who had been exposed to radiation were at significantly greater risk of developing both malignant and benign brain, thyroid, and parotid gland tumors. Thereafter, scientific research on x-ray therapy increased and reports on the causality between the treatment and cancer, and other adverse effects, were widely published.

MICHAEL REESE HOSPITAL'S CAMPAIGN TO LOCATE FORMER RADIATION PATIENTS

A few months after DeGroot and Paloyan's publication in 1973,[21] a worker at Michael Reese Hospital in Chicago (Figure 8.1) found a box containing a registry of 5,266 former patients who had been treated with radiation for benign diseases. The hospital had to make a decision about what to do with the registry and whether to contact the people and inform them that they are at greater risk of developing cancer. Although the x-ray therapy given at the time was considered effective and safe, the hospital feared that many patients would sue for damages.[22] After much deliberation, and recognizing that radiation-associated thyroid carcinoma is an urgent problem, hospital officials decided to contact the patients and arrange for follow-up medical examinations.[23]

Ivan Dee, the director of public relations at the hospital, described the situation to the *Chicago Tribune*: "There was a great dispute among

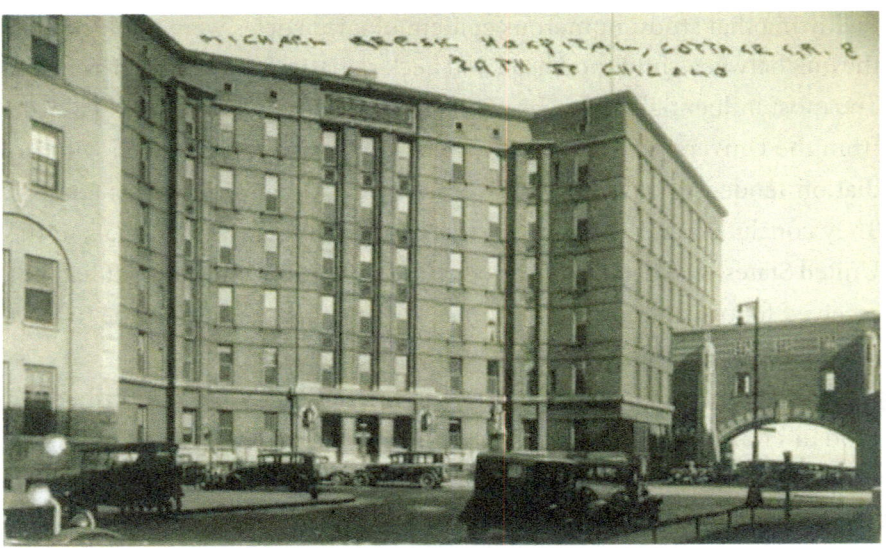

Figure 8.1 Michael Reese Hospital, 2929 South Ellis Avenue, Chicago, IL (1881–2008). The date of the image is estimated to be the 1920s or 1930s.
Chicago History Post Cards. In: Kaplan, Jacob. Michael Reese Hospital: http://forgotten chicago.com/features/michael-reese-hospital/.

the medical staff as to whether we should recall these patients and warn them of the danger . . . Many [at the hospital] were afraid that the recall would make the hospital appear negligent and open it up for malpractice suits . . . The decision to go ahead was made on responsible ethical grounds . . . We had a duty to our former patients to call them back for checkups."[24]

Efforts to contact former patients who were considered part of the population at risk began in December 1973, and in January 1974 the hospital began to examine those who had been contacted. To facilitate the program, letters were sent and phone calls made to all patients who may have undergone x-ray treatment and were at higher risk of developing thyroid cancer.[25]

Rachel Warshaw-Dadon, who underwent irradiation treatment at the hospital as a child, described the way the hospital contacted her:

> I was born in Chicago in 1949. My father was a professor of nuclear physics and my mother a chemist. In 1952, I suffered repeated bouts of tonsillitis; I was given radiation therapy at Michael Reese Hospital. Though my parents should have known the danger of the radiation treatment, they did not, and agreed that I receive the treatment, based on the scientific knowledge at that time. In about 1973, when I was living in Boston, I received an urgent notice from Michael Reese Hospital: "Attention, you might have thyroid cancer and we are responsible for it. We ask your forgiveness." The letter directed me to go to the nearest reputable hospital to be tested for untoward results of the radiation therapy, with the expectation that I might have thyroid cancer. I went to Harvard Medical School and underwent several examinations. Michael Reese paid the expenses.[26]

In the interview with her, Mrs. Warshaw-Dadon emphasized that although her parents were scientists (both had worked on the Manhattan Project), they decided to send her for radiation treatment. She mentioned that her parents should have guessed that radiation therapy would have adverse effects but based their decision on the knowledge they had at that time (1952) based on a medical procedure that was considered effective and safe.

Media coverage

In early 1974, the hospital's attempts to track down former patients for medical examinations started to appear in the media, especially the newspapers.[27] As a result, many additional former patients, or those who believed they underwent the treatment, began to contact the hospital for appointments and more information.[28] The hospital officials realized that there were many more patients who were unaware of the late health effects of radiation and that a follow-up program was needed. Thus, efforts to contact former patients were renewed in July 1974.[29] Medical malpractice suits that were filed against the hospital were dismissed (Figure 8.2). The courts accepted the hospital's defense that, at the time, treating children with radiation was standard and was considered an effective procedure, meaning that no malpractice was involved.[30]

Locating former patients was a complex task, as most had moved, many did not remember or did not know that they or their relatives underwent radiation treatment in childhood, and records were not always available.[31] Despite these difficulties, the hospital made extensive efforts to locate its patients, often making many phone calls before giving up.[32]

The hospital's campaign and the media coverage it attracted led other hospitals throughout Illinois, where the treatment was prevalent, to launch similar campaigns. For example, in March 1974, Northwestern Memorial Hospital in Chicago announced that it was trying to locate former patients who had been treated with radiation at the hospital more than 20 years prior.[33] In February 1975, an attempt was made to contact former patients at Evanston Hospital and a "recall clinic" was established to examine former patients.[34] At this stage, national news channels started to cover the situation in Illinois. Programs describing the problem emphasized the positive role of the media coverage that prompted more health institutions to search for their former patients. Media reports advised those who knew

X-ray malpractice suit dismissed here
James Pearre
Chicago Tribune (1963 Current file); Dec 14, 1976;
ProQuest Historical Newspapers Chicago Tribune (1849 - 1987)

X-ray malpractice suit dismissed here

By James Pearre

THE FIRST of 40 malpractice suits filed against Michael Reese Hospital by persons who received neck X-ray treatments there 15 to 35 years ago has been dismissed by a Circuit Court Judge.

The X-ray treatments, which subsequently were found to increase the risk of thyroid cancer, were "standard procedure" in the 1940s and '50s, Judge David Canel ruled. Canel cited medical reports stating that X-ray irradiation of the face and neck once was considered a safe and effective method of treating severe acne and chronic swelling of the tonsils, adenoids, and thymus gland.

In 1973, after researchers discovered an increased incidence of thyroid cancer among persons who had received irradiation treatment, Reese began efforts to locate 5,000 former patients, inform them of the risk, and urge them to have thyroid examinations.

DOZENS OF OTHER hospitals subsequently began similar recall programs, but administrators of the hospitals have expressed fears that they, like Reese, would be sued by some of the patients, a Reese spokesman said.

Joan Matlaw, a Michael Reese staff attorney, said 40 patients have sued Reese in connection with the treatments in the last two years. She called the Canel ruling "very encouraging."

Canel's ruling, issued Thursday, involved a suit filed against Reese by Dr. Harold Shinsky, a Michigan dentist, who received neck X-ray treatments at Reese in 1949, when he was a child. Shinsky developed a malignant thyroid tumor, which was surgically removed about 1970. He sued Reese in 1974.

Besides failing to prove negligence, Canel said, Shinsky exceeded the statute of limitations for malpractice suits by suing more than two years after he knew or should have known about the alleged negligence.

IT HAS BEEN estimated that as many as 70,000 persons may have received the neck X-rays treatments at Chicago hospitals from the 1940s through the early '60s.

About 3,000 of the 5,000 Reese patients have been contacted thus far, and 1,000 have been given free thyroid examinations at the hospital, a spokesman said.

Approximately eight our of every 100 of the recalled patients examined at Reese since January, 1974, were found to have developed thyroid cancer.

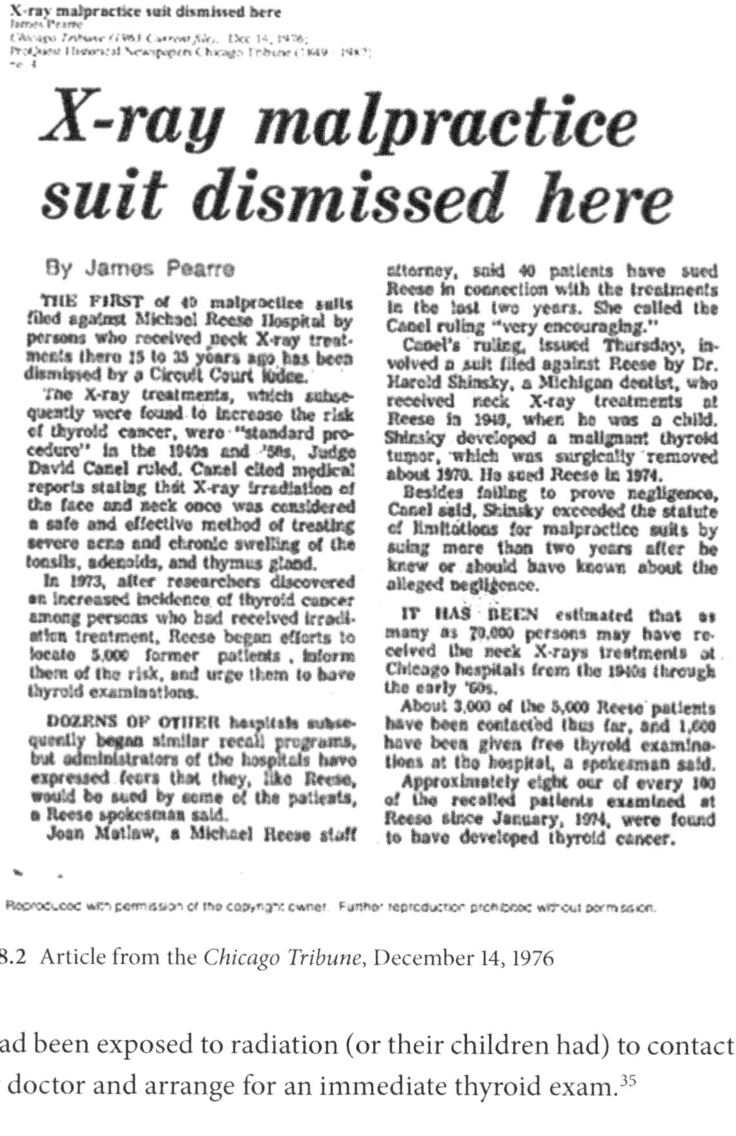

Figure 8.2 Article from the *Chicago Tribune*, December 14, 1976

they had been exposed to radiation (or their children had) to contact their family doctor and arrange for an immediate thyroid exam.[35]

Expanding the efforts to locate and examine radiation patients

Because hospitals ran into difficulties locating former patients, Illinois state health authorities (e.g., Illinois Hospital Association, Illinois State Medical Society, and allied groups) joined the efforts to alert the public of the late effects of radiation. They used the media (newspapers and television) to reach a greater audience (Figure 8.3). As a result, thousands of former patients started to contact medical centers and sought medical advice and examination across Illinois.[36]

Media coverage of Michael Reese Hospital's campaign prompted health institutions in other parts of the United States to start their own campaigns to locate and examine people who had received radiation to the head and neck, including a screening program in Milwaukee, Wisconsin. In 1974, the Medical College of Wisconsin began to examine people who had undergone radiation treatment at the center and located nearly 2,000 patients.[37]

Media coverage of the situation in Chicago also led medical centers in Detroit, Michigan, to search for their former patients who had undergone radiation treatment as children. A unique situation was created in Detroit when a television journalist from Detroit's Channel 4, Robert Vito, who himself had been treated with radiation at Michael Reese Hospital as a child, was contacted to come in for an appointment and a cancerous growth was detected on his thyroid gland. The reporter decided to single-handedly launch a campaign to locate patients at risk in the Detroit area. He began asking medical institutions one question: "When are you starting your recall program?"[38]

In February 1975, Vito began a series of reports on the radiation treatment he had received as a child and the cancer he got as a result. Six hours after the first report, his station was flooded with calls from 3,000 people asking for more information. A short time later, at least 16 hospitals in the Detroit area began contacting their former radiation patients.[39] Vito's reports and publication in the media of the late health effects of radiation treatment led to many screening campaigns in Detroit and other locations throughout Michigan.[40]

Media coverage (radio, TV, and newspapers) of the issue had led many alarmed individuals and physicians to contact the National Cancer Institute (NCI) and other national health institutions and ask for more information. In response to these requests, the NCI, together with the U.S. Food and Drug Administration (FDA) and other organizations,[41] held

X-ray treatment patients prove to be hard to locate

By Brenda Stone

ILLINOIS hospitals are having poor results in tracking down former patients who risk developing thyroid cancer because of X-ray treatments given 15 to 30 years ago.

At least 10 hospitals in the last year have sent letters to former patients, urging them to return to the hospital for examination or to seek medical advice from their current physicians.

However, the majority of such letters have been returned to the hospitals as "undeliverable," a spokesman for the Illinois Hospital Association said.

MEANWHILE, 20 Chicago hospitals and 27 others throughout the state have established thyroid screening programs to make tests readily available to persons who know or think they might have had the X-ray treatments as children.

The persons being sought are those who had X-ray treatments to the head and neck area during the late 1940s to early 1960s as therapy to shrink enlarged tonsils, adenoids, and thymus glands. In a few cases, the therapy was also used for severe acne.

In recent years a growing body of medical evidence indicates that those persons may have up to three times higher risk of thyroid cancer and other thyroid abnormalities than persons who did not receive the therapy.

AT MICHAEL Reese Medical Center, where a large-scale study of the problem has been under way since 1974, fewer than 10 per cent of nearly 5,000 patients have responded to personal letters, said Dr. Lawrence Frohman, a principal investigator in the study.

Frohman said the poor response is largely because most of the patients were children and the majority have moved several times or changed their names thru marriage since they were treated.

At the University of Illinois Hospital, 374 letters have been sent and 200 returned marked "unknown" or "incorrect address," a spokesman said. At Children's Memorial Hospital, 105 of 142 letters never reached their destinations.

BUT DESPITE the slim response to the letters, several thousand Chicago-area residents have sought medical advice and examination as a result of media reports and a public information campaign being headed by the Illinois Hospital Association, the Illinois State Medical Society, and allied groups.

Said Frohman, "Anyone who knows or thinks they might have had this type of X-ray therapy years ago should be examined.

"From what we've seen at Reese so far [among 1,950 patients examined], a person who was irradiated may have a one in four chance of having a thyroid abnormality and one in 12 chances of having a thyroid cancer.

"The odds are certainly in their favor, but the risks are too great to ignore," Frohman said. He cautioned, however, that persons at risk "should not panic" because if a thyroid cancer is found, it generally is slow-growing, usually does not spread, and is highly treatable, typically by surgery.

Where to go for thyroid tests

City	Hospital	Cost for Screening Former Patients	Others
Aurora	Copley Memorial	No charge	No charge
Berwyn	MacNeal Memorial	No charge	No charge
Blue Island	St. Francis	No charge	Estabd. fees
Chicago	Chicago Osteopathic	No charge	Estabd. fees
	Children's Memorial	No charge	Estabd. fees
	Cook County	To be determined	To be determined
	Grant	No charge	Estabd. fees
	Holy Cross	No charge	Estabd. fees
	Loretto	No charge	Estabd. fees
	Louis A. Weiss Memorial	No charge	Estabd. fees
	Mary Thompson	No charge	Estabd. fees
	Mercy	No charge	Estabd. fees
	Michael Reese	No charge	Estabd. fees
	Mt. Sinai	No charge	Estabd. fees
	Northwestern Memorial and Northwestern University Medical Clinics		
	Presbyterian-St. Luke's	No chrg. Program limited to former patients	
	St. Anne's	No charge	Estabd. fees
	St. Anthony	Not applic.	Estabd. fees
	St. Elizabeth's	No charge	Estabd. fees
	St. Joseph	No charge	Estabd. fees
	St. Mary of Nazareth	No charge	Estabd. fees
	University of Chicago Hospitals and Clinics	No charge	Estabd. fees
	University of Illinois		
Chicago Hts.	St. James	No charge	No charge
Elgin	St. Joseph	No charge	Estabd. fees
Elmhurst	Memorial of Du Page County	No charge	Estabd. fees
Evanston	Evanston	No charge	No charge
	St. Francis	No charge	Estabd. fees
Evergreen Pk.	Little Company of Mary	No chrg. Program limited to former patients	
Harvey	Ingalls Memorial	No charge	Estabd. fees
Maywood	Loyola University Medical Center	Estabd. fees	Estabd. fees
Melrose Park	Westlake Community	No charge	Estabd. fees
Oak Park	Oak Park	No charge	Estabd. fees
	West Suburban	No charge	Estabd. fees

Figure 8.3 The article describes efforts made by local hospitals throughout Illinois to locate former patients. Under the heading "Where to go for thyroid tests," the article provides information about the thyroid screening program throughout Illinois.

a medical conference on the late health effects of radiation to the head and neck in infancy and childhood on September 24 and 25, 1975. The goal of the conference was to improve communication with physicians regarding the late effects of radiation and to guide medical centers on how to respond to the situation. At the conference, local hospitals were recommended to locate and examine their former patients, and a national strategy for coping with the situation was drafted.[42]

By 1976, continuous media reports led health officials in western Pennsylvania to search for tens of thousands of individuals who were thought to have received radiation to the head and neck.[43] Similar to the efforts made by Chicago hospitals, they sent letters and made phone calls to all for whom records of childhood irradiation existed.[44] In the greater Pittsburgh area alone, medical authorities searched for a group of approximately 10,000 former patients who had been exposed to possibly cancer-causing radiation treatment during childhood.[45] In early 1977, medical centers in Connecticut began their own campaigns. Windham Community Memorial Hospital in Willimantic announced the beginning of a recall campaign to contact former patients in January 1977.[46] Similar to previous campaigns launched in other places, local and national media covered the story.[47]

In addition to media reports describing the efforts made by different medical centers to locate and examine former patients, personal stories about people who had undergone radiation treatment were published in the national news. The stories emphasized the tragedies and suffering of those who had undergone the treatment and were later diagnosed with cancer, and the sometimes complex relationship between parents and their children who underwent a treatment during childhood that put them at risk.[48]

In January 1977, the television show *60 Minutes* (Figure 8.8)[49] devoted a program to ways in which medical centers and health authorities across the United States were searching for former irradiated patients. The program investigated the actions that were being taken by medical centers and national health authorities across the United States to inform the concerned public about the late health effects of radiation. According to the program, in most medical centers, no effective campaign had been launched to warn and bring in former patients for medical examinations, and only a few hospitals had taken it upon themselves to alert the public and trace former patients.[50] Even though the national medical organizations involved (i.e., American Medical Association, American Hospital Association, and NCI) had encouraged all medical centers to start recall programs, only a few had done so. *60 Minutes* investigators called 20 of the largest hospitals in the United States and found that no recall program was launched.[51]

THE NATIONAL CAMPAIGN TO WARN THE PUBLIC

The NCI takes the lead

On July 13, 1977, the NCI launched a campaign about radiation-related thyroid cancer. The goals of the program were twofold. First, the NCI aimed to warn the medical community about the risk and to brief physicians about how to examine, diagnose, and treat thyroid tumors that had resulted from past radiation treatment. To this end, the NCI published "Information for Physicians: Irradiation-Related Thyroid Cancer," which could be ordered from the NCI's central office in Bethesda, Maryland, at no charge.

Second, they aimed to warn the public of the long-term risks of therapeutic radiation. Hundreds of thousands of pamphlets (Figure 8.4) were distributed in shopping centers across the United States, asking people who had undergone radiation treatment during childhood to go to their family doctor for a thyroid checkup: "Did you as a child or a young adult have X-ray treatments involving your head or neck? If so, it is important that you have an examination by your physician."[52] The pamphlets also included a list of diseases for which radiation treatment had been considered good medical practice: ringworm of the scalp, enlargement of the thymus gland, deafness due to lymphoid tissue around the Eustachian tubes, enlargement of the tonsils and adenoids, and acne.[53]

(a)

FOR FURTHER INFORMATION

Write to:
Office of Cancer Communications
Dept. T
National Cancer Institute
Bethesda, Maryland 20014

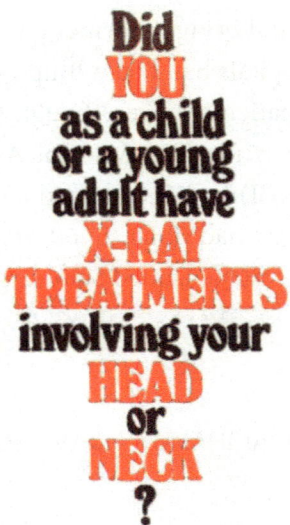

U.S. DEPARTMENT OF HEALTH,
EDUCATION, AND WELFARE
Public Health Service
National Institutes of Health
National Cancer Institute

DHEW Publication No. (NIH) 77-1706

(b)

WHY HIGH RISK?

THE THYROID GLAND at any time from 5 to 30 or more years after such X-ray exposure.

Fortunately, these tumors are usually slow-growing and benign (noncancerous). They remain confined to the neck for long periods, even when they are cancerous. When discovered early, they can be successfully removed.

A link recently has been recognized between tumors of the thyroid gland and X-ray treatments administered years before for various noncancerous conditions of the head, neck or upper chest.

For several decades beginning in the early 1920's, radiation therapy was considered good medical practice and effective treatment for conditions including:
- ringworm of the scalp
- enlargement of the thymus gland
- deafness due to lymphoid tissue around the Eustachian tubes
- enlargement of the tonsils and adenoids
- acne

WHAT IS THE THYROID?

It is a gland at the base of the throat. It affects your growth development and rate of metabolism.

Because short-term effects of the treatments appeared to be excellent, thousands of children and young adults in the United States received radiation for these conditions, particularly before antibiotics became available.

Unfortunately, the thyroid gland also frequently received some radiation during these treatments.

Figure 8.4 Original NCI pamphlet distributed in July 1977
Courtesy of the National Archives, USA.

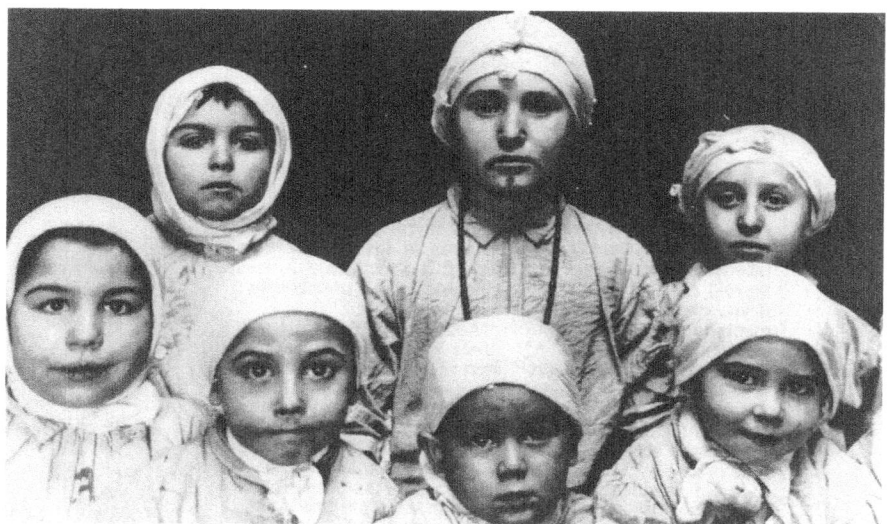

Figure 8.5 Children after ringworm treatment on Ellis Island
Courtesy of the National Park Service, Statue of Liberty, National Monument and Ellis Island.

In addition, notices were published in newspapers (Figure 8.6) and television presenters opened their programs with warnings; for example:

- The National Cancer Institute wants you to have your thyroid checked by a doctor if you ever had X-ray treatments.[54]
- WASHINGTON [UPI] – The government is stepping up its effort to alert an estimated 1 million Americans believed to have an increased risk of developing thyroid cancer because of exposure to head and neck radiation up to 40 years ago.[55]
- U.S. to intensify tumor alert on X-ray therapy long ago[56]
- U.S. issues warning on thyroid cancer[57]
- National Cancer Institute says X-rays used for treatment of illness in neck and head area could cause thyroid cancer[58]
- National Cancer Institute says many Americans may be at risk of thyroid cancer due to X-rays of neck and head[59]
- National Cancer Institute says X-ray treatments for illness in head and neck area may increase chances for thyroid cancer.[60]

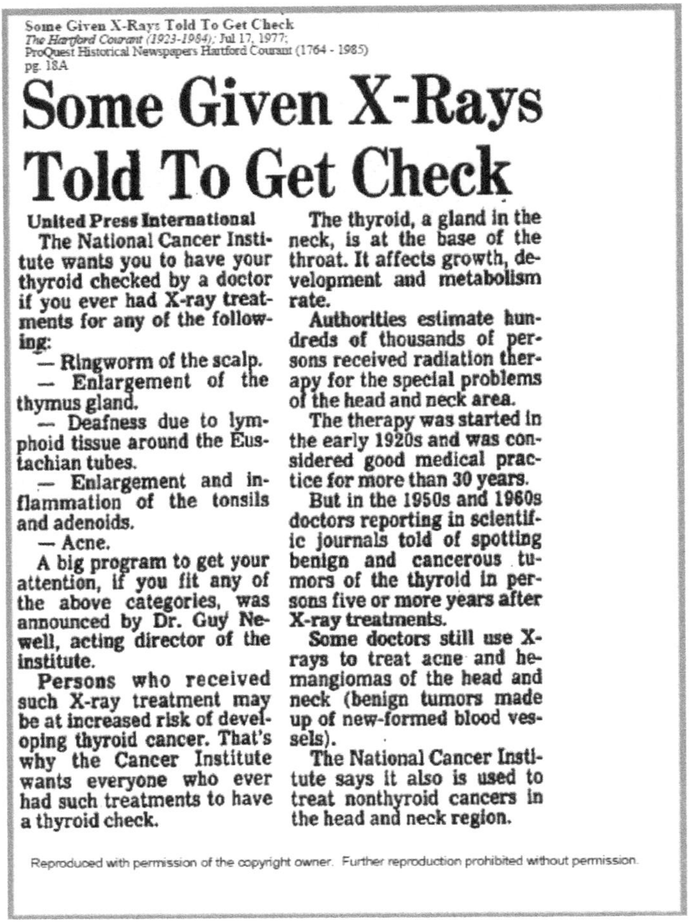

Some Given X-Rays Told To Get Check
The Hartford Courant (1923-1984); Jul 17, 1977;
ProQuest Historical Newspapers Hartford Courant (1764 - 1985)
pg. 18A

Some Given X-Rays Told To Get Check

United Press International

The National Cancer Institute wants you to have your thyroid checked by a doctor if you ever had X-ray treatments for any of the following:

— Ringworm of the scalp.
— Enlargement of the thymus gland.
— Deafness due to lymphoid tissue around the Eustachian tubes.
— Enlargement and inflammation of the tonsils and adenoids.
— Acne.

A big program to get your attention, if you fit any of the above categories, was announced by Dr. Guy Newell, acting director of the institute.

Persons who received such X-ray treatment may be at increased risk of developing thyroid cancer. That's why the Cancer Institute wants everyone who ever had such treatments to have a thyroid check.

The thyroid, a gland in the neck, is at the base of the throat. It affects growth, development and metabolism rate.

Authorities estimate hundreds of thousands of persons received radiation therapy for the special problems of the head and neck area.

The therapy was started in the early 1920s and was considered good medical practice for more than 30 years.

But in the 1950s and 1960s doctors reporting in scientific journals told of spotting benign and cancerous tumors of the thyroid in persons five or more years after X-ray treatments.

Some doctors still use X-rays to treat acne and hemangiomas of the head and neck (benign tumors made up of new-formed blood vessels).

The National Cancer Institute says it also is used to treat nonthyroid cancers in the head and neck region.

Figure 8.6 NCI's public warning as it appeared in an article from the *Hartford Courant*, July 17, 1977

The NCI's education campaign in the media to alert the public and physicians of the late effects of radiation prompted additional hospitals to call their former patients for medical examinations. In New Jersey, for example, the state tried to work with hospitals and warn former patients; as a result, testing programs were launched throughout the state, including free screening for people who thought they may have been treated as children or young adults with radiation for benign diseases.[61] The campaign

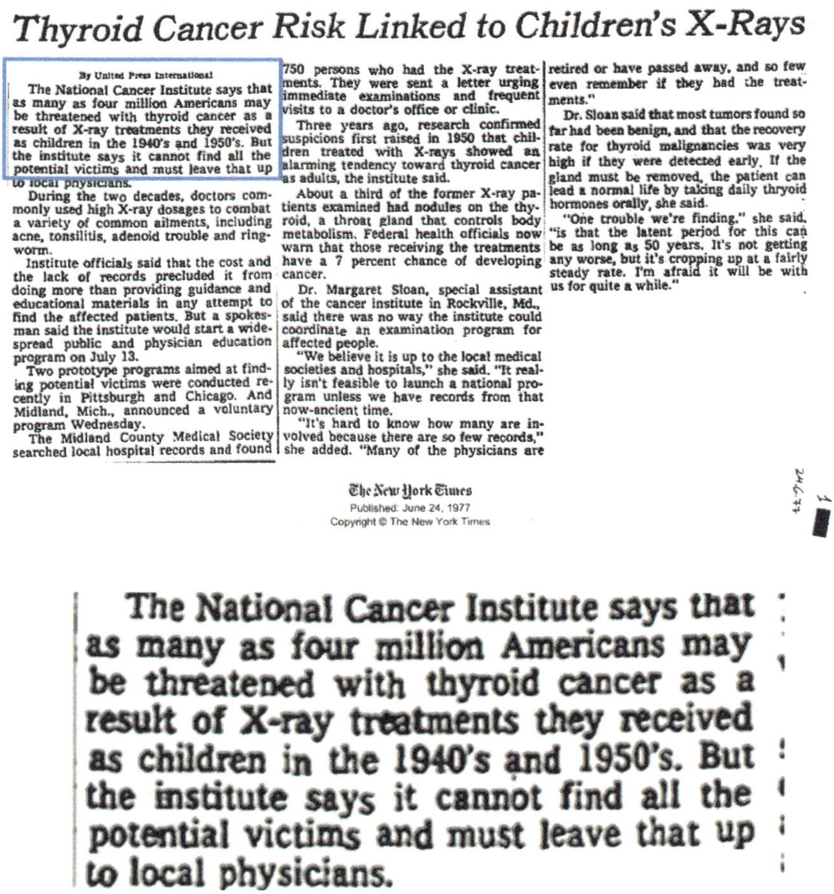

Thyroid Cancer Risk Linked to Children's X-Rays

By United Press International

The National Cancer Institute says that as many as four million Americans may be threatened with thyroid cancer as a result of X-ray treatments they received as children in the 1940's and 1950's. But the institute says it cannot find all the potential victims and must leave that up to local physicians.

During the two decades, doctors commonly used high X-ray dosages to combat a variety of common ailments, including acne, tonsilitis, adenoid trouble and ringworm.

Institute officials said that the cost and the lack of records precluded it from doing more than providing guidance and educational materials in any attempt to find the affected patients. But a spokesman said the institute would start a widespread public and physician education program on July 13.

Two prototype programs aimed at finding potential victims were conducted recently in Pittsburgh and Chicago. And Midland, Mich., announced a voluntary program Wednesday.

The Midland County Medical Society searched local hospital records and found 750 persons who had the X-ray treatments. They were sent a letter urging immediate examinations and frequent visits to a doctor's office or clinic.

Three years ago, research confirmed suspicions first raised in 1950 that children treated with X-rays showed an alarming tendency toward thyroid cancer as adults, the institute said.

About a third of the former X-ray patients examined had nodules on the thyroid, a throat gland that controls body metabolism. Federal health officials now warn that those receiving the treatments have a 7 percent chance of developing cancer.

Dr. Margaret Sloan, special assistant of the cancer institute in Rockville, Md., said there was no way the institute could coordinate an examination program for affected people.

"We believe it is up to the local medical societies and hospitals," she said. "It really isn't feasible to launch a national program unless we have records from that now-ancient time.

"It's hard to know how many are involved because there are so few records," she added. "Many of the physicians are retired or have passed away, and so few even remember if they had the treatments."

Dr. Sloan said that most tumors found so far had been benign, and that the recovery rate for thyroid malignancies was very high if they were detected early. If the gland must be removed, the patient can lead a normal life by taking daily thyroid hormones orally, she said.

"One trouble we're finding," she said, "is that the latent period for this can be as long as 50 years. It's not getting any worse, but it's cropping up at a fairly steady rate. I'm afraid it will be with us for quite a while."

The New York Times
Published: June 24, 1977
Copyright © The New York Times

> The National Cancer Institute says that as many as four million Americans may be threatened with thyroid cancer as a result of X-ray treatments they received as children in the 1940's and 1950's. But the institute says it cannot find all the potential victims and must leave that up to local physicians.

Figure 8.7 According to this June 24, 1977, article in the *New York Times*, "as many as four million Americans may be threatened with thyroid cancer as a result of X-ray treatments they received as children in the 1940's and 1950's."

helped raise public awareness of the issue, prompting many individuals to contact their closest medical centers, and made the late effects of radiation known not only to a limited group of researchers or private hospitals, but also the public. This was one of the first known campaigns in which national health authorities used the media to warn the public of the late effects of a standard treatment that had been widely accepted.

The FDA's response

Though the NCI took the lead and launched the public campaign, the FDA also responded to the first data linking the late effects to radiation. In June 1974, approximately 1 year after DeGroot and Paloyan's findings and approximately 4 months after the pioneering publication by Modan et al. on the link between childhood radiation for the treatment of ringworm and brain tumors, the FDA published a short article on the delayed effects of head and neck radiation[62] in the *FDA Drug Bulletin*, a journal whose goal was to improve communication between the FDA and practicing physicians.[63]

The *Drug Bulletin* quoted the studies in New York[64] and Israel[65] on neoplastic developments in persons who had received x-ray epilation for tinea capitis (ringworm). Casper Weinberger, Secretary of the U.S. Department of Health, Education, and Welfare (DHEW), noted that the purpose of the article was "to alert physicians to possible delayed effects of ionizing radiation in individuals treated with X-ray for ringworm of the scalp."[66]

In September 1977, a few months after the NCI warned the public and the medical community, the FDA's Bureau of Radiological Health published medical alerts for the professional community, summarizing the work of a committee established to investigate the health effects of ionizing radiation. Under the title "A Review of the Use of Ionizing Radiation for the Treatment of Benign Disease," the Bureau of Radiological Health made general recommendations for the medical profession regarding when and how to use radiation treatments and provided information on the late effects of radiation treatments. In both cases, the FDA communicated with physicians and not with the public.[67]

UNCERTAINTY, MEDIA REPORTS, AND THE NCI CAMPAIGN

The late health effects of radiation treatment appeared many years after the treatment was no longer administered; thus, ambiguity existed regarding whose role it was to assess and respond to the risks.[68]

The NCI acted as part of its responsibilities under the NCI Act of 1971. This was an era of transition (since the late 1960s and early 1970s) from focusing on detection and treatment of cancer (i.e., control) to focusing on efforts to prevent cancer (i.e., prevention). The agency shifted its focus from educating the public and physicians about cancer and improving knowledge about the disease to preventing the further development of cancer already established in the body and giving more attention to preventable factors, such as tobacco, asbestos, and radiation.[69] In a way, the NCI's campaign represented a combination of both eras: control and prevention. The campaign aimed not only to alert those who were at risk and treat them (early detection of thyroid cancer saved lives) but also to educate physicians and the public about the link between childhood radiation and thyroid cancer.[70]

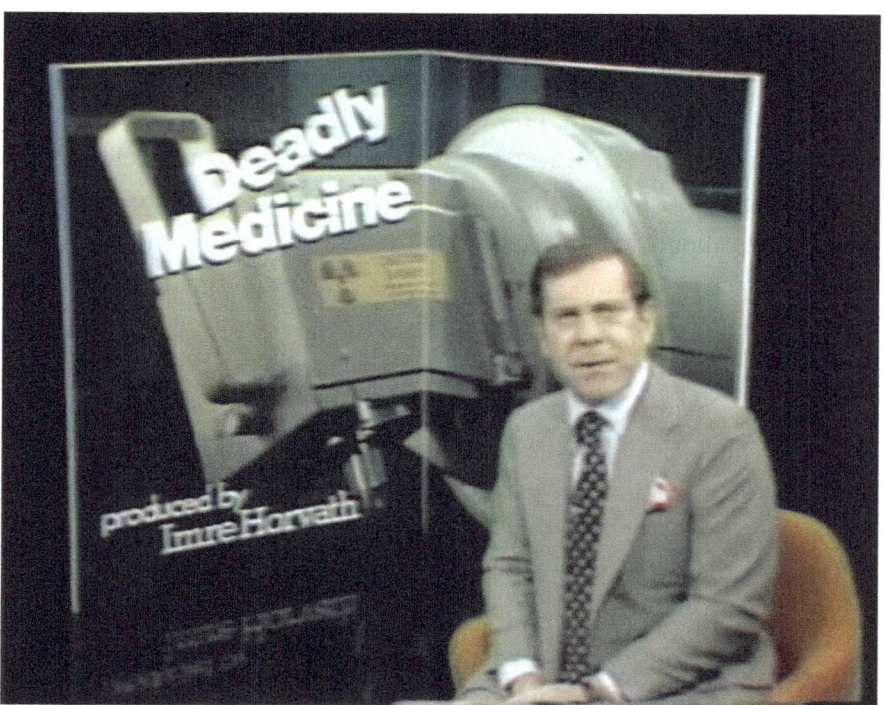

Figure 8.8 The *60 Minutes* broadcast in January 1977 that examined the late effects of radiation

Furthermore, the campaign was carried out during an era of uncertainty and controversies with regard to the effects of low-dose radiation. The controversy about radiation risk mostly centered around atomic bomb radiation, atomic fallout, and exposure to nuclear plants. Ambiguity existed regarding the lack of a threshold below which radiation was considered to be safe (i.e., tolerance dose) and the potential of any risk of radiation per year (i.e., maximum protection dose).[71]

In 1948, after the first data were collected from studies on atomic survivors, the US National Committee on Radiation Protection abandoned the concept of tolerance dose, realizing that even very low doses can be dangerous, replacing it with a maximum permissible dose standard.[72] During the 1950s, more controversy ensued when the Atomic Energy Commission attempted to persuade the public that atomic energy was safe and did not pose a danger below a certain rate of exposure.[73] This claim was criticized by critics of nuclear power and environmentalists who emphasized the danger of any exposure to radiation.[74]

The question of radiation safety moved beyond the strict scientific debate[75] and became more politically sensitive. Considerations, such as whether the benefit of nuclear testing or nuclear plants outweighed the risk they posed, structured the debate as the public became more involved and anxious about radiation risks.[76] In this context, when the treatment was no longer in use, more apparent links were established between the treatment and its late health effects.

Michael Reese Hospital's recall program and the snowball effect it had (i.e., the media attention it attracted) played an important role in informing the NCI of the severity and scope of the problem. However, it is difficult to ascertain how much influence media reports actually had on the NCI's decision.

The publicity of Michael Reese Hospital's campaign prompted several health institutions to follow suit, but most medical centers did not take action. One reason for their inaction was a fear of malpractice suits. As Michael Reese Hospital's Dee noted, "Some [hospitals] were quite reluctant to follow our lead because they were afraid that such a move would damage their reputation and cause legal problems."[77] According to Dee, the Michael Reese campaign was based on responsible ethical grounds. Malpractice suits were filed against Michael Reese Hospital after the hospital started the recall program but were dismissed by the courts because radiation therapy was considered at the time it was given to be a safe and effective treatment.[78]

Those who decided to follow Michael Reese Hospital's lead and start searching for and examining their former patients created more media attention and contributed to the snowball effect that led to a recognition of the link between tumors of the thyroid gland and radiation treatment during childhood. Although DeGroot and Paloyan's study showed a more apparent link between radiation to the head and neck area during childhood and thyroid cancer than previous studies, it is unlikely that one study alone could have prompted national health authorities to launch a nationwide campaign. At that time, little was known about the size of the population at risk and more data were required to determine the severity of the risk. As we have shown, media coverage played an important role in assisting national health authorities to obtain this information and to learn the scope of the problem, eventually realizing that the nation was facing a public health problem.

The relationship between the media and government is complex. Media reports can potentially inform governmental bodies about scandals, hazards, and other types of information. National health authorities care about media reports, which in some cases can affect their decisions.[79] Media reports can assist national health agencies in discovering new sources of health hazards. For example, in his book *The Cigarette Century*, Brandt describes how an investigative program ("Day One") revealed that the tobacco industry controlled the level of nicotine in the cigarettes it produced. The program prompted the FDA to try to act against the industry and to attempt to regulate nicotine under the agency's authority.[80] Media coverage can also assist health authorities in determining the state of knowledge and severity of different health topics. For example, a recent "Report to Congressional Requesters" from the General Accounting Office (GAO) argued that media reports of OxyContin misuse, addiction, and overdose deaths helped the FDA to learn the scope and severity of the danger of opioid use.⁸¹ As a result, the FDA added a black box warning to the drug and changed the information on the package insert.⁸²

Media coverage helped the NCI realize the severity and scope of the problem with childhood radiation in several ways. First, media reports of Michael Reese Hospital's recall campaign prompted other medical centers to follow suit. As a result, more people with a history of radiation were examined, more research was done, new scientific reports on radiation-induced thyroid cancer were published, and a more certain link was established. As mentioned in *HEW News* on July 13, 1977: "From the experience of recall programs at several medical centers, it is estimated that a quarter to a third of the individuals irradiated develop thyroid tumors. Perhaps a third of such tumors are cancerous."⁸³

Before local efforts were made to locate and examine former patients, there was insufficient evidence to determine how many individuals who had undergone radiation treatment were likely to develop thyroid tumors (cancerous and benign). It was the actions and new findings of various medical centers that helped the NCI realize that the nation was facing a public health issue.⁸⁴

In addition, recall programs by various medical centers resulting from the publicity of Michael Reese Hospital's campaign brought to the NCI's attention the fact that there was a large population at risk that was hard to locate; thus, effective recalls are mostly logistically impossible and an effort should be made to alert these people.⁸⁵ As no estimate was available for the number of irradiated people, media reports of recall programs helped the NCI realize that there was a very large population at risk.

Publicity also helped notify the NCI of the problem in a more direct way. Newspapers, radio, and television publications had alarmed physicians and individuals (or parents who were aware of the radiation history of their children). This led to many requests for information and advice directed to the NCI and the National Institute of Arthritis, Metabolism, and Digestive Disease by both physicians and individuals.⁸⁶ As a result, the NCI (and other organizations) held a medical conference on the late effects of radiation, where the recommendation to launch the campaign was discussed.

CONCLUSIONS AND IMPLICATIONS

The decision of Michael Reese Hospital to recall former patients, the media attention it attracted, and the snowball effect it had played an important role in assisting national health authorities in determining the hazards of radiation treatment of benign diseases and responding to them. The sequence of events presented here emphasizes the role of the media as a tool that can possibly assist national health authorities in learning of new health risks. If the media had not picked up the story, millions of Americans who had undergone radiation treatment during childhood might not have known the dangers, as early detection of thyroid cancer saves lives.

No other country has warned the public of the adverse effects of radiation treatment for benign diseases. Millions of people across the globe do not know that they are at an increased risk of developing cancer as a result of the treatment. We find this puzzling, especially because, since 1973, a large number of studies have been published linking the treatment and a variety of adverse effects. In Canada, for example, former patients were still looking for advice in 2001. Personal stories of people who had been exposed to childhood radiation for benign diseases and consequently been diagnosed with cancer were published in Canadian newspapers,[87] but no similar attempt was made to alert the public and contact these people (see the Appendix to this chapter).

This study raises ethical and legal questions, such as the obligation of health authorities to warn patients of the adverse effects of medical treatments, even if no malpractice was involved. It also raises the question of how effective the NCI's nationwide campaign was to warn the public. Further research that collects data on the number of people who were examined because of the campaign is likely to shed new light on this issue and to help write policy recommendation for similar instances.

Finally, the case study described here demonstrates that what is considered to be safe and effective by the medical community, can turn out to have deadly long-term adverse effects. From the historical analysis presented here, we learn that it is often hard to predict the potential for rare late health effects and, thus, promptly and transparently responding to new health risks is important. This study can also teach us how national health authorities share information with the public and physicians when a health problem is discovered.

APPENDIX

RADIATION TREATMENTS IN CANADA

An unknown number of Canadian children and young adults received radiation treatment to the head and neck for benign conditions (Figure 8.9). Many of these patients do not know or remember that they, or a relative, underwent the treatment. In 2001, former patients were still looking for advice. Personal stories of people who had been exposed to childhood radiation for benign diseases and consequently diagnosed with cancer were published in Canadian newspapers. One of these stories was that of Nancy Riva, who lost her two brothers and was diagnosed with cancer as a result of radiation treatment for inflamed thymus gland, which was believed to prevent crib death. Riva wanted to raise public awareness, encouraging people with a history of childhood radiation to have their thyroid checked.

Though evidence suggests that the treatment was prevalent in Canada, as in other parts of the world, little is known about the national health authorities' response at the federal and provincial levels to the discovery of the severe late effects. To the best of our knowledge, no attempt has been made to search for and alert these patients.

This is important because early detection of thyroid cancer and other ailments could have saved Canadians' lives. It is particularly interesting because the national campaign to warn the public in the United States was known in neighboring Canada. For example, on July 14, 1977, *The Globe and Mail* published an article titled, "U.S. increasing efforts to warn million potential cancer victims." The article detailed the adverse effects of the treatment and described the NCI's campaign to alert the public of the risk. Furthermore, in February 1978, Paul Walfish and Robert Volpé,

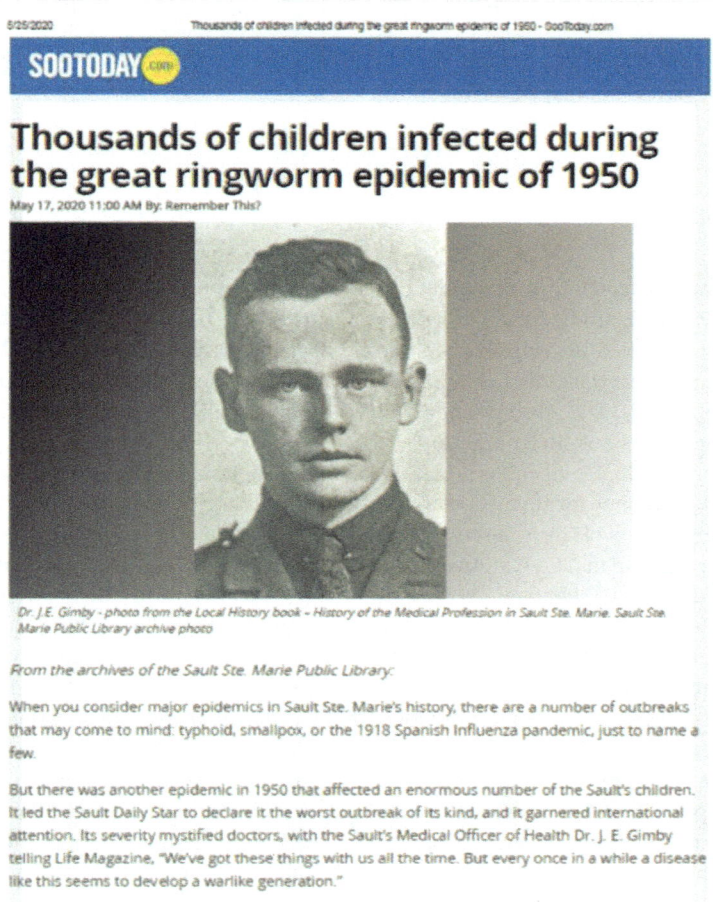

Figure 8.9 Radiation treatments in Canada
History of the Medical Profession: Sault Ste. Marie 1920's, Sault Ste. Marie Public Library Archives, North Branch, Ontario, Canada.

professors of medicine at the University of Toronto, published an article in *Annals of Internal Medicine*[88] discussing the long-term harms of radiation treatment in childhood and the national program to educate the public and physicians about these risks.

To date, no systematic attempt has been made to examine how many Canadians—and which populations—were given the treatment and are subsequently at increased risk of developing cancer. In addition, because there has been no known attempt to inform physicians of the late health effects of childhood radiation, health professionals are mostly unaware of the risk when seeing patients today.

NOTES

1. "Deadly Medicine" is the name of the *60 Minutes* program broadcast in January 1977 that examined the late effects of radiation. An early version of this study was published in Bavli, Itai, and Shifra Shvarts. Michael Reese Hospital and the campaign to warn the US Public of the long-term Health effects of ionizing radiation, 1973–1977. *Am J Public Health*. 2019;109(3):398–405 and in Hebrew in the Ringworm book, BGU pub. 2018.
2. Simpson CL, Hempelmann LH, Fuller LM. Neoplasia in children treated with x-rays in infancy for thymic enlargement. *Radiology*. 1955;64(6):840–845; Crossland PM. Therapy of tinea capitis: The value of x-ray epilation. *Calif Med*. 1956;84:351–353; Asherman YG. Curative irradiation of menstruation and fertility disorders [in Hebrew]. *Harefuah*. 1957;50(7):163–165; Siskind WM, Richtberg D. Tinea capitis in a city hospital: Treatment with x-ray. *NY State J Med*. 1958;58(12):2040; Cipollaro AC, Kallos A, Ruppe JP Jr. Measurement of gonadal radiations during treatment for tinea capitis. *NY State J Med*. 1959;59(1):3033–3040; Hocstaedt VB, Lager G. Curative irradiation of female and menstrual disorder: Setting directives [in Hebrew]. *Harefuah*. 1959;56(3):70; National Cancer Program, Special Communication: Irradiation-related thyroid cancer (August 20, 1976); Walfish PG, Volpé R. Irradiation-related thyroid cancer. *Ann Intern Med*. 1978;88(2):261–262; Shvarts S, Sevo G, Tasic M, Shani M, Sadetzki S. The tinea capitis campaign in Serbia in the 1950s. *Lancet Infect Dis*. 2010;10(8):571–576.
3. Rosenthal MS. *The Thyroid Cancer Book*. Canada: Your Health Press, a division of Sarahealth, Inc. in association with Trafford Publishing Trafford Publishing; 2002:26–27; Sadetzki S, Modan B. Epidemiology as a basis for legislation: How far should epidemiology go? *Lancet*. 1999;353(9171):2238–2239.
4. Maryanov AR. Treatment of tinea capitis with epilation by means of roentgen rays. *Maryland State Med J*. 1955;4(1):20–22; Crossland; Siskind and Richtberg; Cipollaro et al.; Shvarts et al.; Rosenthal, 26.
5. Rosenthal, 28; Thyroid cancer risk linked to children's x-rays. *New York Times*, June 24, 1977.
6. Rosenthal, 28.
7. Shvarts et al.
8. Gomes-Teixeira. Personal correspondence via e-mail, 2009.
9. Tilles G. *Teignes et teigneux: Histoire médicale et sociale*. Paris: Springer Verlag; 2009.
10. Bar-Oz A. The truth about the ringworm affair [in Hebrew]. *Harefuah*. 2016;155(10):637–641.

11. Katzanelbugen Y, Zandbank M. Griseofulvin: A new treatment for fungal diseases [in Hebrew]. *Harefuah.* 1959;57(3):59; Berlin H, Tajer A, and H Yair. Treatment with griseofulvin for ringworm and select cases of fungus on the skin and nails [in Hebrew]. *Harefuah.* 1960;60(4):115–116.
12. Duffy Jr BJ, Fitzgerald PJ. Cancer of the thyroid in children: A report of 28 cases. *J Clin Endocrin Metab.* 1950;10:1296–1308; Clark DE. Association of irradiation with cancer of the thyroid in children and adolescents. *JAMA.* 1955;10:1007–1009; Simpson et al.; Miller JM, Horn RC, Block MA. The increasing incidence of carcinoma of the thyroid in a surgical practice. *JAMA.* 1959;171:1176–1179; Saenger EL, Silverman FN, Sterling ThD, Turner ME. Neoplasia following therapeutic irradiation for benign conditions in childhood. *Radiology.* 1960;74:889–904; Riddley CM. Basal cell carcinoma following x-ray epilation of the scalp. *Br J Dermatol.* 1962;74:222–224; Socolow EL, Hashizume A, Neriishi S, Niitani R. Thyroid carcinoma in man after exposure to ionizing radiation: A summary of the findings in Hiroshima and Nagasaki. *N Engl J Med.* 1963;268:406–410; Conard RA, Rall JE, Sutow WW. Thyroid nodules as a late sequela of radioactive fallout in a Marshall Island population exposed in 1954. *N Engl J Med.* 1966;274:1391–1399; Conard RA, Dobyns BM, Sutow WW. Thyroid neoplasia as late effect of exposure to radioactive iodine in fallout. *JAMA.* 1970;214:316–324; National Cancer Institute. Information for physicians on irradiation-related thyroid cancer. *CA Cancer J Clin.* 1976;26(3):150–159.
13. Israeli, Miron. *Occupational Malignant Diseases and Compensation Schemes: A Report to the Rivlin Committee* [in Hebrew] Israel Committee of Nuclear Energy (2013).
14. Walker JS. *Permissible Dose: A History of Radiation Protection in the Twentieth Century.* Berkeley, CA: University of California Press; 2000; Proctor RN. *Cancer Wars: How Politics Shapes What We Know and Don't Know About Cancer.* New York, NY: Basic Books; 1996:159; Dry S. The population as patient. In Schlich T, Ulrich T, eds. *The Risks of Medical Innovation: Risk Perception and Assessment in Historical Context* (Vol. 21). New York, NY: Psychology Press; 2006:116–132; Holden C. Low-level radiation: A high-level concern. *Science.* 1979;204(4389):155–158.
15. Walker, 156.
16. Albert RE, Omran AR. Follow-up study of patients treated by x-ray epilation for tinea capitis. *Arch Environ Health.* 1968;17(6):899–918. The collection of data for the follow-up study began in 1962.
17. Albert RE, Omran AR, Brauer EE, et al. Follow-up study of patients treated by x-ray for tinea capitis. *Am J Public Health.* 1966;56:2114–2220.
18. DeGroot L, Paloyan E. Thyroid carcinoma and radiation: A Chicago endemic. *JAMA.* 1973;225(5):487–491.
19. Ibid., 491.
20. Modan B, Mart H, Baidatz D, Steinitz R, Levin SG. Radiation-induced head and neck tumours. *Lancet.* 1974;303(7852):277–279.
21. DeGroot and Paloyan.
22. See: Once a cure, now a threat. *Chicago Sun*, March 3, 2002.

23. Frohman LA, Schneider AB, Favus, MJ, et al. Thyroid carcinoma after head and neck irradiation: Evaluation of 1476 patients. In: DeGroot L, ed. *Radiation-Associated Thyroid Carcinoma*. New York: Grune & Stratton, Inc.; 1977:5.
24. Thyroid tests; no cover-up. *Chicago Tribune*, March 13, 1977.
25. Frohman et al., Thyroid carcinoma, 5–15; Frohman LA, Schneider AB, Favus, MJ, et al. Risk factors associated with the development of thyroid carcinoma and of nodular thyroid disease following head and neck irradiation. In: DeGroot L, ed. *Radiation-Associated Thyroid Carcinoma*. New York: Grune & Stratton, Inc.; 1977:231–240; X-ray malpractice suit dismissed here. *Chicago Tribune*, December 14, 1976.
26. Interview with Rachel Warshaw-Dadon, March 1, 2012. Mrs. Warshaw-Dadon provided us with written permission to quote her name in this interview.
27. Ex-patients hunted; cancer risk. *Chicago Tribune*, March 6, 1974.
28. Frohman et al., Thyroid carcinoma, 5.
29. Ibid.
30. Ibid., 5–15; *Greenberg J et al., Plaintiffs-Appellants, v. Michael Reese Hospital* (September 25, 1979); *William Lissner, v. Michael Reese Hospital* (April 12, 1989); X-ray malpractice suit dismissed.
31. U.S. Department of Health, Education, and Welfare. *HEW News*, July 13, 1977:8; National Cancer Institute, Information for physicians.
32. Seligmann J and Butler M, Dangerous legacy. *Newsweek*, April 14, 1975:82.
33. Stone B, Ex-patients hunted: 2d hospital seeks cancer-risk cases. *Chicago Tribune*, March 7, 1974:30.
34. Murphy ED, Scanlon EF, Swelstad JA, et al. A community hospital thyroid recall clinic for irradiated patients. In: DeGroot L, ed. *Radiation-Associated Thyroid Carcinoma*. New York: Grune & Stratton, Inc.; 1977:35–40.
35. *NBC Evening News*, February 14, 1975.
36. X-ray treatment patients prove to be hard to locate. *Chicago Tribune*, May 29, 1975.
37. Cerletty JM, Guansing AR, Engbring NH, et al. Radiation-associated thyroid carcinoma. In: DeGroot L, ed. *Radiation-Associated Thyroid Carcinoma*. New York: Grune & Stratton, Inc.; 1977:1–3; Cerletty JM. The organization, publicity, evaluation, cost and funding of a thyroid screening program. In: DeGroot L, ed. *Radiation-Associated Thyroid Carcinoma*. New York: Grune & Stratton, Inc.; 1977:261–269. Dr. James Cerletty from the Endocrine section of the Department of Medicine at the Medical College of Wisconsin described how news coverage of Michael Reese campaign affected the decision to start studying the issue: "Our study [the screening program] was capitulated into action by publication in the press and by radio of a news bulletin announcing the Michael Reese thyroid recall project" (p. 262).
38. Miller MJ. The metropolitan Detroit area "screening program." In: DeGroot L, ed. *Radiation-Associated Thyroid Carcinoma*. New York: Grune & Stratton, Inc.; 1977:281.
39. Dangerous legacy, *Newsweek*.
40. Ibid.

41. The National Institute of Arthritis, Metabolism and Digestive Diseases; the Bureau of Radiological Health of the FDA; the American College of Radiology; and the American Thyroid Association.
42. National Cancer Program, Special Communication.
43. An estimated 70,000 subjects in Chicago, 10,000 in Milwaukee, and 20,000 in Pittsburgh had undergone radiation treatment. Discussion of radiation and thyroid cancer screening programs: Summary of experience in current programs. Frohman LA, CarrollRG, Humburger J., et al., in: DeGroot L, ed. *Radiation-Associated Thyroid Carcinoma*. New York: Grune & Stratton, Inc., 1977:42–43.
44. Carroll R, Ellis LD, Moore D, et al. Organization of screening program for detection of thyroid cancer. In: DeGroot L, ed. *Radiation-Associated Thyroid Carcinoma*. New York: Grune & Stratton, Inc.; 1977:273.
45. Patients irradiated years ago sought because of cancer peril. *New York Times*, May 14, 1976.
46. Windham Hospital begins "recall" of x-ray patients." *Hartford Courant*, January 27, 1977.
47. Ibid.
48. For example, Brookeville woman, x-ray treated baby, develops tumor. *Washington Post*, August 12, 1976.
49. "Deadly Medicine," *60 Minutes*.
50. Ibid.
51. Ibid.
52. This was the sentence that appeared on the front page of the pamphlet. DHEW Publication No. [NIH] 77-1206, 1977.
53. Ibid.
54. Some given x-rays told to get check. *Hartford Courant*, July 17, 1977.
55. Tell cancer risk from old x-rays. *Chicago Tribune*, July 7, 1977.
56. U.S. to intensify tumor alert on x-ray therapy long ago. *Washington Post*, July 7, 1977.
57. U.S. issues warning on thyroid cancer. *Los Angeles Times*, July 7, 1977.
58. *CBS Evening News*, July 13, 1977.
59. *ABC Evening News*, July 13, 1977.
60. *NBC Evening News*, July 13, 1977.
61. Cancer check is urged for past x-ray care. *New York Times*, August 6, 1977.
62. FDA Drug Bulletin. Head and neck radiation: Problem of delayed effects. *Bulletin*, Food and Drug Administration, July 1974. Note that the bulletin concentrated on the delayed effects of radiation treatment for ringworm.
63. Schmidt AM "Letter: FDA Drug Bulletin," FDA Drug Bulletin. *Clin Toxicol.* 1974;7(5):551.
64. Albert and Omran.
65. Modan et al.
66. Epstein E. Letters to the editor. *Arch Dermatol.* 1975;111:925.
67. U.S. Department of Health, Education, and Welfare. *A Review of the Use of Ionizing Radiation for the Treatment of Benign Disease.* HEW publication (FDA) 78–8043, 1977. Although public warnings are not common FDA practice, there is at least

one known historical case. In 1956, the FDA launched a public campaign to warn the public about a fake cancer treatment offered by Harry Hoxsey's clinic. In April 1956, the FDA began distributing "public beware" posters to post offices across the United States, urging people not to go to the Hoxsey clinic and inviting them to write to the FDA for further information. Cantor D. Cancer, quackery, and the vernacular meanings of hope in 1950s America. *J Hist Med Allied Sci.* 2006;6:324–368.
68. It was not clear whose role it was—the NCI's or the FDA's—to assess new health risks and respond to them. The FDA, the regulator whose role it is to protect the public health, monitors safety issues with drugs and treatments and has clear procedures on how to respond to safety problems that surface after approval of a drug or a treatment. The NCI is a research institute that investigates cancer risks.
69. Cantor D. Introduction: Cancer control and prevention in the twentieth century. *Bull Hist Med.* 2007;81(1):3–4.
70. Devra Davis challenged the view that national health institutions, such as the NCI, and regulatory bodies, effectively worked to prevent cancer. She argued that hidden ties between the industry (such as chemical companies or big tobacco companies) and academic researchers and the government (among others) affected the way cancer risks were assessed. As a result, some of these risks were ignored, and actions aimed at protecting the public and preventing cancer took many years after the risks were already known (e.g., tobacco risks, workplace causes of cancer, chemicals). See D. Davis, *The Secret History of the War on Cancer* (New York, NY: Basic Books, 2007).
71. J. Samuel Walker, *Permissible Dose: A History of Radiation Protection in the Twentieth Century* (Berkeley, CA: University of California Press, 2000); Robert N. Proctor, *Cancer Wars: How Politics Shapes What We Know and Don't Know About Cancer* (New York, NY: Basic Books, 1996).
72. Walker, *Permissible Dose*; Proctor, *Cancer Wars*, 159; Sarah Dry, "The Population Is Patient."
73. The US Atomic Energy Commission was established in 1946. Its main role was to protect the public health and safety from the dangers of radiation produced by nuclear fission. See Walker, *Permissible Dose*, 14.
74. Walker, *Permissible Dose*; Proctor, *Cancer Wars*.
75. For a more detailed explanation of the various studies and methods used to measure the effect of low-dose radiation, see Proctor, *Cancer Wars*, chapter 7.
76. Walker, *Permissible Dose*, 156.
77. Thyroid tests, *Chicago Tribune*.
78. Lawrence et al., Thyroid carcinoma; Greenberg et al.; *William Lissner* lawsuit; X-ray malpractice suit dismissed here.
79. See: Carpenter D. *Reputation and Power: Organizational Image and Pharmaceutical Regulation at the FDA*. Princeton, NJ: Princeton University Press; 2010; Maor M. Organizational reputations and the observability of public warnings in 10 pharmaceutical markets. *Governance*. 2011;24(3):557–582; Maor M, Sulitzeanu-Kenan R. The effect of salient reputational threats on the pace of FDA enforcement. *Governance*. 2013;26(1):31–61.

80. Brandt AM. *The Cigarette Century: The Rise, Fall, and Deadly Persistence of the Product That Defined America*. New York, NY: Basic Books; 2007:358–361.
81. Government Accounting Office (GAO). GAO-04-011Report to Congressional Requesters: Prescription Drugs: OxyContin Abuse and Diversion and Efforts to Address the Problem (2003):9.
82. Ibid.
83. *HEW News*, 6.
84. Ibid.
85. National Cancer Institute, Information for physicians, 153.
86. Ibid., 151.
87. Irradiated at birth, now they're dying: How a procedure to prevent sudden infant death syndrome is being linked to cancer deaths. *Vancouver Sun*, February 9, 2001; Radiation therapy suspected in deaths: Treatment in 1940s for newborns questioned by woman whose two brothers died of cancer. *Time Colonist* (Victoria, British Columbia), February 9, 2001; Woman blames radiation for death of her brothers. *Prince George Citizen* (British Columbia), February 12, 2001; Regional report. *Windsor Star* (Ontario), February 12, 2001; Radiation used to help stop crib death linked to cancer. *Kamloops Daily News* (British Columbia), February 12, 2001; Radiation for SIDS blamed for cancer. *Calgary Herald*, February 12, 2001; Cancer risk sparks campaign: Irradiation of thymus glands at birth once standard practice. *Calgary Herald*, March 13, 2001.
88. Paul G. Walfsh, Robert Volpe. Irradiation-related thyroid cancer. *Ann. Intern. Med.* 1978;88(2):261–262.

9

Healing the children and the nation

The campaign to eradicate ringworm in Israel, 1925–1960

SHIFRA SHVARTS, AYA BAR OZ, ELI SHACHAR, SARI LEVI, SIGAL SAMCHI, AND ITAI BAVLI

INTRODUCTION

At the start of 1926, the head of the dermatology department of Hadassah Hospital in Jerusalem, Dr. Arieh Dostrovsky, announced with great exhilaration[1] that in April 1925 Hadassah had opened a therapeutic department within the x-ray institute, where specialized treatment for children with ringworm employing x-rays had been inaugurated: "With roentgen rays the disease is swiftly and completely cured. The whole cure takes a month. The cure in and of itself with an x-ray machine (irradiation) is sufficient, even a few minutes."[2]

Dr. Dostrovsky's declaration on the use of an x-ray machine for innovative treatment of ringworm patients marks, in essence, the beginning of the campaign to eradicate ringworm in Eretz-Israel,[3] which after the establishment of the State of Israel in 1948 came to be known as the "ringworm affair." This campaign, which began in 1925, ended in 1960 when the treatment for ringworm changed from x-rays to an oral antifungal medication.

The first section of this chapter examines plans to eradicate ringworm in the Jewish community of Eretz-Israel (henceforth, the Jewish community) during the British Mandate period (1917–1948), based on historical documents of the period. The second part covers the program for a "war on ringworm" in the first decade after independence in the State of Israel. Evidence will be presented that the medical protocol developed in Eretz-Israel during the British Mandate period for irradiation treatment of ringworm patients was based on the standard medical protocol that had been used in the Western world since 1910 and was not exclusive to Israel. In the first half of the 20th century, many campaigns were carried out, both in most European countries and in the United States, to eradicate ringworm using irradiation. Thus, the treatment of ringworm in Israel in the 1950s was not the product of negligence or paternalism; rather, it was carried out in accordance with the best method currently in medical practice in the Western medical community at the time. This fact stands in contrast to widespread public opinion in Israel that irradiation against ringworm of immigrant children in the 1950s was carried out by Israeli authorities irresponsibly, and even maliciously and deliberately to harm Jewish immigrants arriving in Israel from non-Western Muslim countries. This erroneous outlook drove the passage in 1994 of a compensation law for victims of irradiation for ringworm (the Ringworm Victims Compensation Law), a law that was not enacted anywhere else in the world.[4]

ERADICATION OF RINGWORM IN THE JEWISH COMMUNITY IN ERETZ-ISRAEL DURING THE BRITISH MANDATE PERIOD (1917–1948)

Scalp ringworm (tinea capitis) was very prevalent in the Jewish community in Israel during the period of Ottoman rule and was considered (along with trachoma) to be a core medical problem among children of the Jewish community. The British conquest of Palestine/Eretz-Israel[5] and the arrival in 1918 of the country of the American Zionist Medical Unit (AZMU), which grew to become the Hadassah Medical Federation,[6] represented a turning point in ringworm treatment. The Hadassah Zionist Women's Federation, founded in the United States in 1912, was the first and the most central player; Hadassah began to operate in the public health domain among the Jews of Eretz-Israel immediately after the British completed their takeover of the country from the Ottoman Turks.

Hadassah made improving the health of mothers and children its first objective, establishing a network of available and accessible health services for the public throughout the country, establishing hygiene departments in educational institutions, and formulating a plan to advance health and health education in accordance with progressive principles that the unit brought with them from the United States. In 1919, the unit conducted the first survey in the country to examine the prevalence of trachoma and ringworm (Figure 9.1). The survey, conducted in 20 Jewish educational

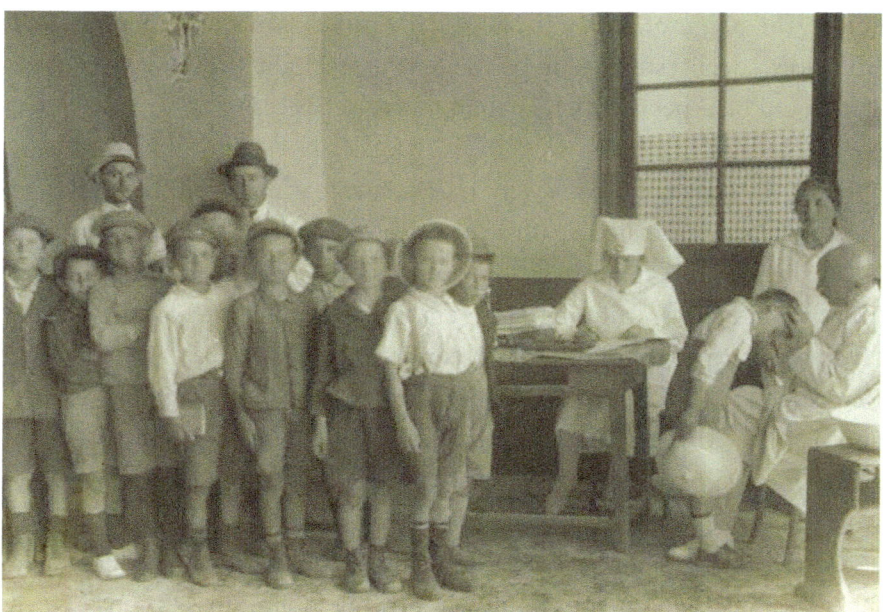

Figure 9.1 Checking children's heads for ringworm at the Jerusalem schools
The Donchin-Hadassah Collection.

institutions in Jerusalem, showed that 40% of the children in educational facilities in Jerusalem had ringworm, and the most prevalent kind was similar to the ringworm prevalent in Europe.[7]

Ringworm had already been known as a local disease in Eretz-Israel throughout the 19th century, but the worsening of living conditions and serious damage to the sanitation infrastructure, particularly during World War I, led to an epidemic. Hadassah focused on trachoma and ringworm not only due to the number of children affected but also to the social stigma associated with these diseases. Trachoma often led to grave vision defects and even to blindness and had a serious impact on the quality of life of children infected with it. While ringworm did not have as serious an effect on the health of children as trachoma did, it was perceived by the public as a disease of the poor and those with poor hygiene and thus carried a negative connotation that had a harsh impact on the affected children.

Since ringworm caused very noticeable bald spots, children with the disease were easy to identify, leading to ostracism by peers and social isolation. The plight of girls was particularly unforgiving, and they suffered from low social esteem due to the aesthetic blight the disease caused. This could be especially detrimental to their chances of finding marriage partners.

After the survey findings were in, Hadassah announced the launch of an eradication campaign against the disease, first in schools in Jerusalem by hair removal (manual epilation)[8] and application of an antifungal salve. The central agent in the ringworm eradication campaign was the School Hygiene Department of the Jewish community, headed by Dr. Mordechai Berachiahu.[9] This department viewed eradication of contagious diseases and hygiene education in educational facilities as a top priority, and assisted greatly in organizing and executing the campaign to eradicate ringworm in the schools and kindergartens.

Despite Hadassah's readiness to take action in all the educational facilities of the Jewish community, in practice not all institutions agreed to participate and allow their pupils to be examined.[10] All told, 3,573 children in 20 educational facilities were examined out of 17,000 children enrolled in Jewish educational institutions. Of these 3,573 examined, 976 (27%) across the country were found to have ringworm; 413 were cured after treatment, while 553 children (56%) remained infected. The children treated ranged in age between 3 and 18, and most were between ages 4 and 8. The highest percentage of affected children was registered in Jerusalem (63.3%) (Figures 9.2, 9.3, and 9.4).[11]

In Dostrovsky's estimation, because of the refusal of some schools to participate in the ringworm eradication campaign and the custom

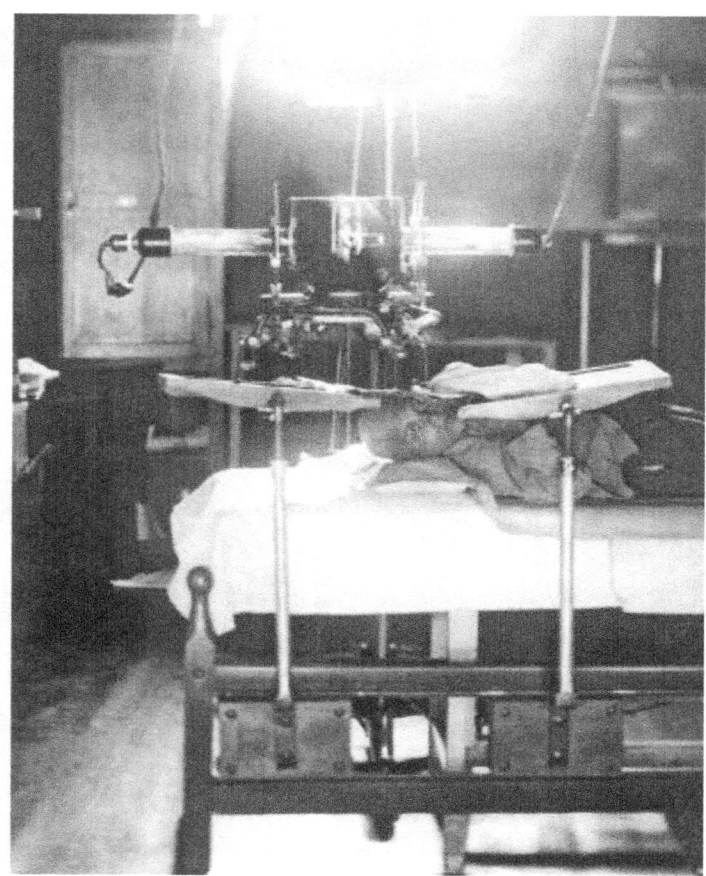

Figure 9.2 Irradiation treatment of a child with ringworm, Hadassah, 1920s
The Donchin-Hadassah Collection.

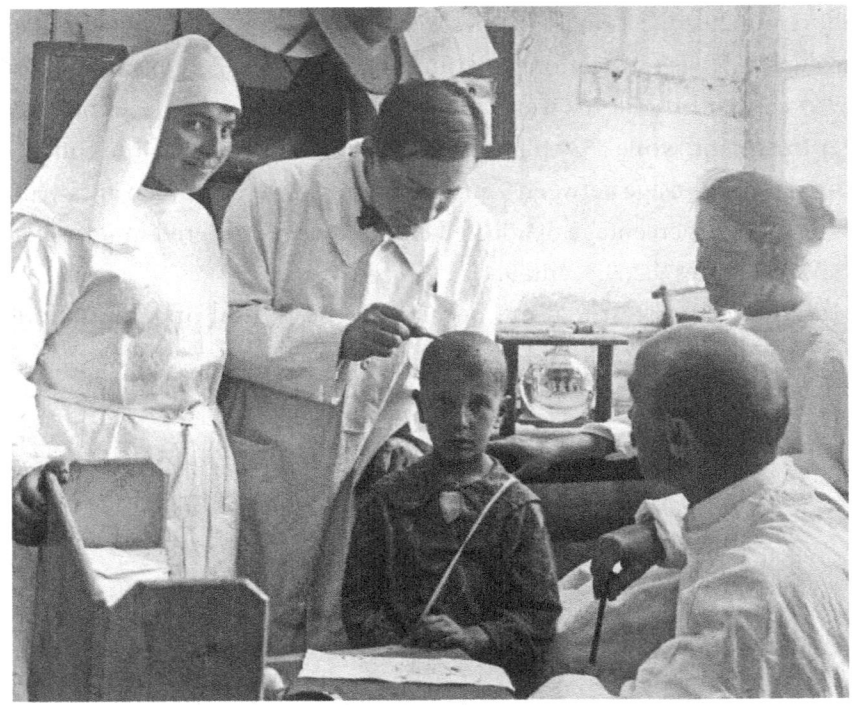

Figure 9.3 Checking child's head following irradiation treatment
The Donchin-Hadassah Collection.

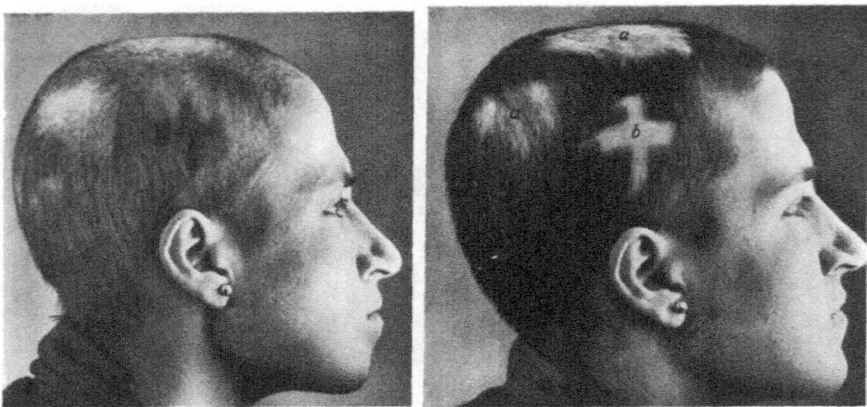

Figure 9.4 Ringworm
Prof. A. Drukmann collection, 1936. Hadassah Jerusalem Department of Radiology Archives.

of many families to send their children to different schools, many children who had been treated and cured became reinfected by family members or friends who went to schools that didn't participate in the program.[12]

In Tiberias it was reported that out of 677 pupils examined in the schools, 21% (most of them younger children) had ringworm.[13] Examination of children in the school system demonstrated that there was a considerable gap between various facilities in the rate of ringworm. Dostrovsky believed the differences stemmed from differences in the socioeconomic status of each student body. Thus, in the Tachkemoni School in Jerusalem, where parents came from relatively high socioeconomic strata, the percentage of children with ringworm was 23.7%, while in institutions where the pupils came from low socioeconomic strata and there were many orphans, the percentage of children with ringworm exceeded 60%. The situation was similar in kindergartens. The percentage of ringworm children in kindergartens with children from homes with good socioeconomic standing was 14.9%, compared to 41.3% in kindergartens whose enrollees were from poorer families.[14]

Dostrovsky's position that directly linked socioeconomic standing and disease and personal hygiene was shared by most of the physicians at the time and was cited many times in the daily papers in regard to ringworm as well as other diseases such as trachoma, tuberculosis, and lice.[15] This position was identical to the position of many doctors in Europe who viewed ringworm as a social disease that accompanied poverty and low socioeconomic status.

The campaign to eradicate ringworm was complex and required coordination among many health agents: doctors, nurses, and educational personnel.

The fact that the campaign was only partially successful due to difficulties with reinfection, and the inability to treat the disease effectively, led Hadassah's directorship to decide to treat ringworm with irradiation, which was considered the most advanced and effective treatment for the disease at the time.

X-ray treatment in Eretz-Israel

The first x-ray machine was brought to Eretz-Israel in 1905 by Dr. Armanak Afendi, an Ottoman Turk physician in Jerusalem,[16] but it is not known to what medical purpose it was applied. Hadassah began irradiation for ringworm in 1925 after purchasing an appropriate x-ray machine from the Siemens company. Irradiations for ringworm were first carried out in Jerusalem, and afterwards throughout the country.[17]

In addition to Hadassah's radiology institute, there were also private radiology institutes operating in Eretz-Israel where irradiation against ringworm and other dermatologic diseases such as acne and psoriasis was carried out. The radiologist Dr. Eliyahu noted explicitly in an ad published in a local newspaper that he was a participant in the campaign for "mass curing of chronic dermatological diseases, particularly diseases of the scalp of children and the elder person (ringworm)."[18]

In 1925, Dr. Dostrovsky, together with Dr. Avraham Drukmann (a radiologist graduate of medical school in Vienna who joined the Hadassah radiology department in 1925),[19] prepared plans for the campaign to eradicate ringworm, this time through irradiation. According to the plan, children who had been examined in the schools and kindergartens (those facilities that agreed to participate in the program) and were found to have ringworm were sent to the Hadassah Radiology Institute for a series of 5-day treatments. Following this, the subsequent complementary treatment was carried out by nurses from the School Hygiene Department. Irradiation treatment required several weeks and close follow-up, as well as grappling with deep apprehensions triggered among parents and children alike (particularly among girls) as a result of the total hair loss rendered by irradiation. The weak point of the treatment was the need to remove every hair left on the scalp after irradiation. To do so, at first *colifonium* (a sticky waxy substance made from the sap of coniferous plants) was spread on the entire scalp and used to remove from the roots any remaining hair, after which any remaining hairs were plucked out with tweezers.[20] Such treatment was very difficult for children but was designed to ensure that every single hair strand infected with ringworm would be removed, to prevent reinfection. This treatment was conducted by special nurses mobilized for this purpose.

Dostrovsky and Berachiahu feared primarily reinfection and the respread of the disease, and therefore they formulated clear directives to school administrators regarding this issue:

a. No pupil shall be accepted at school unless the child brings a license [certification] for such, a license written by a dermatologist who examined him (this examination is of course carried out free of cost).
b. All pupils who were not at school at the appointed time of the last examination by the doctor also need to bring a note from him, even though they are regular students.
c. For this purpose, it is necessary for every teacher to note in his class journal the students who have already been examined by the doctor. Every pupil who isn't marked in the class journal as checked needs to bring a note.[21]

Dostrovsky stressed that this directive was being carried out in all the schools in the Jewish community in the country, without exception.

In Dostrovsky's judgment, distancing pupils from school during the initial healing process was essential due to the difficulty of preventing reinfection before all the infected hair had fallen out. These directives were part of the conventional medical protocol worldwide. The period during which children were not allowed to return to school was even longer in France and the United States, and they were sent to special schools for ringworm children for the entire period until they were healed. Such extreme measures would not have been accepted by the Jewish community in Eretz-Israel in any case, and therefore to ensure eradication of the disease, it was imperative to suspend the pupils from school during the initial healing period.

In the years 1925 to 1928, 3,500 children were irradiated in Jerusalem at Hadassah's radiology department,[22] and during the first year of the campaign, another 343 children were irradiated at Hadassah Hospital in Tel Aviv.[23] In an intermediate survey published by Dostrovsky in late 1926, he stated that 600 children had been fully cured of ringworm, and added that in light of the success, he was optimistic about the possibility of successfully completing the campaign in all the participating schools.[24] At the same time, in some children the initial treatment series with irradiation did not cure their disease, and they were irradiated again. Dostrovsky and Drukmann conducted follow-up of approximately 2,300 ringworm children in Jerusalem who were treated with irradiation, and their research findings were similar to the data in scientific reports abroad: The children had few side effects, and the changes that took place in hair growth after irradiation (straight hair that became curly, more robust or thinner hair growth, and so forth) were also similar to manifestations reported in the medical literature.[25]

The unusually high rates of cure achieved with irradiation treatment, the relatively short period of treatment needed (compared to lengthy traditional treatment methods that sometimes lasted a year or more), and the low rates of cure by traditional methods reinforced Dostrovsky's insistence that all ringworm patients, without exception, be treated via irradiation.

Despite the close collaboration between the educational facilities and Hadassah in the ringworm eradication realm, and the optimism regarding the probability of success, several problems remained. The first was the failure of private schools to rigorously enforce directives to send children with ringworm home so they wouldn't spread their disease. The second problem was "by school girls who don't want under any circumstances to have their hair cut, as well as parents who were afraid of x-ray."[26] An additional difficulty emanated from the lack of a designated budget for irradiation; as a result, it was impossible to send 80 children (30 from Haifa, 30 from Tiberias, and 20 from Safed) for irradiation treatment.[27] Examination of children in the schools and identification of schoolchildren with contagious diseases such as ringworm was carried out in coordination with Mandatory health authorities.[28]

According to Dostrovsky and Berachiahu's reports, the campaign to treat children with ringworm with irradiation was very successful, and the disease almost disappeared from the public schools in Jerusalem. In Tel Aviv and Jaffa as well, where a portion of the schoolchildren were treated in the first stage of the campaign with chemical remedies, not irradiation, the percentage of ringworm children dropped from 19% to 9%, a very significant improvement.[29] Children in smaller clusters throughout the country were also sent for radiologic treatment in Jerusalem.

Thus, from 1928 to 1931, about 600 children were sent to Hadassah from the northern region—265 from Tiberias, 159 from Haifa, 139 from Acre, and 15 from the agricultural settlements.[30]

Ringworm among new immigrants

Following the eradication of ringworm in the schools, the initiators of the campaign (Dostrovsky and Berachiahu) subsequently faced the difficult challenge of preventing a renewed outbreak of the disease. It was clear to the two that the weak point was health supervision of new immigrant children, who continued to arrive in Eretz-Israel from Eastern Europe and Middle Eastern countries, primarily those coming from Yemen.[31] This issue has already been raised in 1925 at the beginning of the campaign for eradication of ringworm, and it remained on the public health agenda up until 1938. As Dostrovsky explained:

> One can't discount the assumption that in a known portion [of the cases], one can credit the spread of fungal disease among us on account of new immigration. Immigration is massive and, after all, most of the schoolchildren it has brought on its wings came from countries [where] the spread of ringworm is of epidemic proportions.[32]

He stated that there was a particular difficulty in educating and dealing with reservations of the parents of the new immigrants regarding the treatment method to be used, particularly the total hair loss as a result of irradiation.

With the increase in immigration in the late 1920s and early 1930s, the School Hygiene Department headed by Berachiahu declared that all the immigrants and their children would, upon arrival in the country, undergo systematic examination for early detection of contagious diseases, particularly trachoma and ringworm. Immigrants from Eastern Europe and their children were generally examined prior to their immigration (in their country of departure) and, if needed, they were treated there.[33] In other words, in the campaign for eradication of ringworm conducted by the Jewish health organization OZE (the Society for the Protection of Jewish Health) with funding from the Joint Distribution Committee, 26,700 children from Jewish communities in Eastern Europe were treated with irradiation between 1921 and 1938, the majority prior to immigration to the West (where severe cases of ringworm were grounds for barring entry) and a minority to Eretz-Israel (see Chapter 5).[34] Thus, most medical attention was now turned to immigrants from countries in the Middle East (mostly Yemen) where examinations were not conducted prior to immigration to Eretz-Israel.[35]

Upon arrival, the immigrant families were transferred to the Immigration Absorption Center. There they were examined, and anyone found to have a contagious disease (tuberculosis, trachoma, or ringworm) was sent for treatment. Berachiahu stated that since treatment for these diseases was lengthy, the immigrants were required to bring their children weekly to the Hadassah clinic, even after they had undergone the absorption process and been released from the Immigration Absorption Center, due to concern that children who had not completed treatment would enter kindergartens and schools and reinfect local ("veteran") children.[36] If parents refused to send their child with ringworm for irradiation treatment, the child was barred from school. Children who were treated by other (traditional or chemical) means by private doctors were not allowed to return to school unless they had a doctor's certification that they had received irradiation treatment, or had obtained special certification from Hadassah.[37]

The cost of irradiation was underwritten, usually jointly, by the School Hygiene Department and the patient's local (municipal) council.[38] If the local council refused to participate in underwriting treatment, the remaining sum charged by Hadassah was covered by the School Hygiene Department.[39]

Throughout the entire period of the British Mandate, medical responsibility for providing x-ray treatment for those with ringworm in the Jewish community in the country was placed exclusively in the hands of the dermatology and radiology departments of Hadassah, headed by Dostrovsky and Drukmann.[40] Hair samples for ringworm analysis were sent regularly to the Hadassah lab, and Hadassah was the final arbiter in cases of disagreement over whether to allow a child to return to school.[41] The medical protocol for treatment of ringworm in the country was uniform: irradiation employing the Kienböck–Adamson method, and weekly follow-up by a school nurse until hair regrowth commenced (see Chapter 2). Dostrovsky and Drukmann believed that treatment of ringworm with irradiation was the best and most effective method in existence at the time,[42] and this stance was the leading one by most dermatologists in Eretz-Israel.

Treatment at private clinics was also underwritten by the Jewish community's national leadership, the Jewish National Council (JNC), and Hadassah. For example, when children with ringworm were identified in Tiberias in 1942, Dr. Yehuda Bromberg, a member of the Hadassah management, gave permission to the health department of the JNC to underwrite irradiation treatments at the private clinic of Dr. Avraham Tuvia Sternberg in Tiberias.[43]

Dr. Ernst Feilchenfeld[44] cited that ringworm was also very prevalent among Arab residents, and that in 1934 he had treated some 100 Arab children with ringworm who came for irradiation treatment at his private clinic in Tel Aviv.[45] Dostrovsky himself noted that ringworm was prevalent among Arab schoolchildren in Jerusalem, and used as an example the Syrian (Schneller) orphanage in Jerusalem, where 25% of the 500 schoolchildren had ringworm.[46]

Irradiation for ringworm was very widespread in Eretz-Israel in the 1930s, not only due to the medical success of the treatment but also due to the influx to Eretz-Israel of many roentgenologists from central Europe after Hitler came to power. These doctors brought with them advanced x-ray machines and opened private radiology institutes in the main cities. According the records of the Israel Medical Federation, in 1938, 10 private radiology institutes operated in Jerusalem, in addition to the one at Hadassah Hospital; in Tel Aviv, 13 private radiology institutes operated parallel to the one at Hadassah Hospital in Tel Aviv and the General [*Clalit*] Sick Fund (GSF)'s Zamenhof Clinic[47] in Haifa five private institutes operated and in 1940 an additional institute was opened; in Tiberias one private institute served members of the GSF, as well, and the agricultural townships (*moshavot*) of Rishon le-Zion, Petach Tikvah, and Rechovot had one radiology institute in each. All these institutes were operated by experienced roentgenologists.[48]

The British Mandatory health authorities did not generally intervene in the operations of Jewish public health promotion organizations. The primary interest of the British was to prevent epidemics and mass morbidity, primarily malaria and typhus, and they did not deal with the health of mothers and children, issues that did not present any risk to their governing machinery. In the Health Order for the Public issued by the British in 1940, ringworm was not included on the list of contagious diseases that had to be reported to British Mandatory authorities.[49] This can be explained in light of the success of the campaign to eradicate ringworm, which had already decreased the number of infected children year after year to a very low level, and therefore there was no need to report the disease.[50] The director of Hadassah, Dr. Chaim Yaski, underscored in 1947 in his survey of the Hadassah University Hospital's dermatology department that ringworm had almost entirely disappeared in the Jewish community.[51]

Documents from the period from the end of the Second World War (1945) until establishment of the State of Israel (1948) show that all the children of immigrants who arrived during this period and were found to have ringworm were treated with irradiation in frameworks in operation at the same time—at Hadassah's hospitals in Jerusalem or in Tel Aviv and in the clinics of the GSF in Tel Aviv and Haifa. Afterwards, they were treated with follow-up and supervision of the School Hygiene Department headed by Berachiahu, and when deemed necessary, the children were sent for irradiation at private institutes.[52]

In a survey of the workings of the Immigrants Medical Service in the fiscal year 1946–47, the service during this period was the sole responsibility of Hadassah.[53] The administrative director of Hadassah, Haim Shalom Halevi, wrote that the primary health problem among immigrants was tuberculosis, followed by mental illness; ringworm was not mentioned at all in his survey.[54] One can assume that the success of the war on ringworm carried out by Hadassah during the Mandate period, and the reduction in the number of ringworm cases to a very low incidence rate, removed the disease from the agenda of the Jewish community in Eretz-Israel at the time, and it was considered no longer a relevant issue.

Summary

Treatment of ringworm with irradiation continued throughout the entire period of the British Mandate and up until the close of the first decade of statehood. The directives that Dostrovsky and Berachiahu formulated in the 1920s and that served them in the war on ringworm throughout the Mandate period were adopted by the Ministry of Health of the newly established State of Israel and were the foundation for eradicating the disease among immigrant children during mass immigration as well.[55] The success in eradicating the disease during the Mandate period was held up as a shining example of the operations of the State of Israel in this realm until 1960, when treatment of ringworm worldwide shifted to an oral antifungal medicine.

RINGWORM IN THE STATE OF ISRAEL

Where is the ringworm?

The establishment of the State of Israel in May 1948 and the mass immigration that followed placed the issue of immigrants' health onto the public agenda. The most burning health problems among immigrants, as they were classified by the Israeli government, were tuberculosis and typhus. Ringworm was not included among them and was not even raised in discussions in the government.

In its first year of operation, the Israeli Ministry of Health adopted the Mandatory health services ordinances as a basis for its operations and updated them ad hoc as needs arrived, when raised in discussion. One of the first actions of the Ministry was to update the 1940 Mandatory Public Health Ordinance that specified diseases of a potential epidemic nature that must be reported to Mandatory health authorities: plague, dysentery, trachoma, smallpox, typhus, malaria, leprosy, tuberculosis, poliomyelitis (infantile paralysis), syphilis, and contagious children's diseases (such as diphtheria, German measles, whooping cough, chickenpox, and meningitis).[56] Ringworm was not included. Also, the new Public Health Ordinance updated in 1949 did not include ringworm, and the diseases that were included were the same ones cited in the 1940 British ordinance.[57]

In February 1950, the Ministry of Health initiated an additional amendment to the Public Health Ordinance and even proposed a "war on venereal and social dermatological diseases,"[58] parallel to which expansion of the list of contagious disease that must be reported was sought. In the list of diseases cited in the Ordinance's Clause 11(a), various forms of ringworm were added. The edict was signed by Minster of Health, Haim-Moshe Shapira. It was stated explicitly that from now on, cases of ringworm must be reported to health authorities.[59] With this step, the Ministry transformed ringworm and its treatment into a disease for which the Ministry of Health was responsible and the responsibility of public health agencies in Israel (Hadassah, the Sick Funds). The primary reason for entering ringworm into the Public Health Ordinance was the fact that many children of the new immigrants who were arriving in the first waves of immigration after the state was established suffered from ringworm and trachoma on a wide scale that had to be addressed.

The documents that accompanied changes in the Public Health Ordinance reveal that all medical agents were required to report every ringworm patient; failure to do so was considered a criminal act and those found to have ringworm were required by law to receive treatment. It was stated that "The government administrator or the doctor is authorized to compel parents to accept medical treatment for their children who are sick with ringworm since this disease is contagious and presents a public health risk to the city, the village or the region since it is liable to spread among children mixing one with the other."[60]

At the same time, the ordinance did not stipulate who was authorized to treat ringworm; it only stated that treatment was compulsory. In practice, this directive transformed all the children who had been treated for ringworm in the State of Israel beginning in February 1950 into individuals who had been treated on orders from the state, whether treated privately or in public frameworks. Despite ringworm being added to the ordinance (and perhaps because of this), ringworm became a key subject that needed to be addressed or to be treated as a higher priority, like the other diseases cited in the order. However, examination of the Ministry's work plans for a "war on venereal disease and social dermatoses" reveals that treating ringworm was the last priority.[61]

In practice, treatment against ringworm was given according to what had already been prescribed by Hadassah's dermatology and radiology departments—that is, irradiation to trigger epilation, and afterwards complementary treatment (manual removal of all remaining hair, smearing the scalp with a salve, and wearing of a head cover) and monitoring until hair regrowth commenced.

The lack of public attention to ringworm in the first 2 years of statehood is further substantiated by the lack of media coverage. Newspaper coverage of mass immigration does not mention ringworm as a central health problem threatening the nascent state, as would be the case in later years.

Ringworm only received media coverage beginning in December 1950 in the context of the immigration of Yemenite Jews.[62] This point is important in understanding the development of public attitudes toward the disease, its treatment, and the ethnic linkages it came to carry afterward.

In late 1949, Hadassah conducted the first survey to examine the prevalence of ringworm in schools and kindergartens in Jerusalem and neighboring areas such as Ein Karem, an abandoned Arab village that had absorbed many homeless new immigrants. Dr. Felix Sagher, a Hadassah dermatologist[63] who oversaw examination of the children, reported that out of 70 children examined, 15 had ringworm and 10 were suspected to be infected with ringworm; among all the children in Ein Karem, 20% definitely had ringworm. In Jerusalem and its environs only children age 3 years and up were sent for irradiation treatment at Hadassah; those under 3 were treated with "a special medicine"[64] that was smeared on their scalps and the head was wrapped in a clean kerchief, without shaving the hair and without irradiation. According to Dr. Sagher, "The infected children cannot go to school for approximately two months and there is the need to isolate them in special classrooms in the school."[65]

In December 1949 the first meeting was convened to discuss Hadassah's proposal that it organize comprehensive treatment against ringworm among new immigrants, headed by the director of the Ministry of Health, Dr. Yosef Meir.[66] Dostrovsky represented Hadassah at the meeting and was accompanied by Drukmann, Mr. Haim Shalom Halevi (deputy director-general of Hadassah), Mrs. Bertha Landsman (member of the board of Hadassah), and Dr. Kalman Mann (medical deputy director-general of Hadassah). At the close of the meeting, it was decided that Hadassah—which had the most experience in organizing treatment against ringworm—would be responsible for this treatment on behalf of the State of Israel.

It was also decided that medical treatment would continue to use irradiation (as was customary in the medical community worldwide) according to the Kienböck–Adamson method. As for complementary treatment, proposals was made to treat the scalp with iodine or another solution in lieu of the painful epilation method (with tweezers and *colifonium*). However, Dr. Sagher made it clear that due to the type of ringworm prevalent in Israel, the only way to prevent reinfection was to carry out complete epilation after irradiation.

Similar discussion on the best treatment for eradicating ringworm was also published in the medical literature of the time. The articles dealt with treatment methods against the various ringworm fungi in Europe and the Mediterranean and addressed the question of which strains of ringworm fungi should be treated with *colifonium* to produce complete hair loss, in addition to irradiation-induced hair loss.[67]

The decision of the Ministry of Health to give Hadassah responsibility for handling the war on ringworm in Israel met with a positive response and was not challenged. Thus, the burden of handling ringworm treatment was shifted to Hadassah at a time when the Ministry of Health was close to collapsing under the burden of other health problems it was forced to deal with. The transfer of responsibility for treating ringworm received further affirmation a year later, in February 1952, when the Knesset decided to "endorse" this arrangement: "Among other operational realms for preventive medicine, one should mention the responsibility of the Ministry of Health for classifying and curing children infected with ringworm, in collaboration with the Ministry of Welfare, the Israel Defence Forces (IDF) and the Hadassah Medical Federation."[68]

In the coming months, Hadassah corresponded with local municipal authorities (mainly those that had a large population of immigrants) to formulate a unified plan of action to treat ringworm. Thus, Dr. Mann wrote to the mayor of the Tiberias municipality:

> We understand that you stand to appoint a doctor to your municipal clinic. In that in Tiberias ringworm is prevalent to a substantial extent and the city stands to absorb many families among Yemenite immigrants, many of whom are infected with this disease, it would be very desirable that the clinic doctor receive in-service training in curing ringworm. We would be pleased to enable the physician to receive the necessary in-service training at our dermatology clinic

in Jerusalem... The in-service training will take approximately 3 weeks.[69]

It was also agreed that Hadassah would send Dr. Sagher on regular visits to the city of Beer Sheva to oversee the complementary treatment against ringworm after irradiation had been carried out in the immigrant intake camp Shaar HaAliyah ("Immigration Gate") near Haifa.[70] In addition, Hadassah would establish a dermatology consultation clinic in Beer Sheva, and the clinic physician would also treat ringworm cases.

Hadassah's involvement was not limited solely to medical consultation or medical supervision of treatment against ringworm in Israel; it was also responsible for all aspects tied to ringworm—including treatment that new immigrants received abroad, primarily those who had immigrated from North Africa. Thus, Professor Drukmann wrote to Dr. Yosef Meir:

> In our ringworm cases that came from Morocco, I have seen cases that already received irradiation, and exhibit signs of *alopecia* and *atrophic dermatitis*[71] caused by too large a dosage of irradiation. These children will be permanent foci for reinfection, and throughout their entire lives will be afflicted in a cosmetic sense. In my opinion, [we] must not irradiate them again because the damaged skin from the irradiation is susceptible to *carcinomatosis*. This should be brought to the attention of the Joint[72] or other institutions engaged in this in Morocco. They need to stop the irradiations or do what needs to be done.
>
> P.S. I want to clarify that among us, over the last 20 years, there hasn't been the incidence of any cases of damage from irradiation for ringworm.[73]

Under the authority invested in Hadassah as the agent responsible for the national machinery for treating ringworm, Hadassah initiated the establishment of a children's hospital and adjacent therapeutic radiology

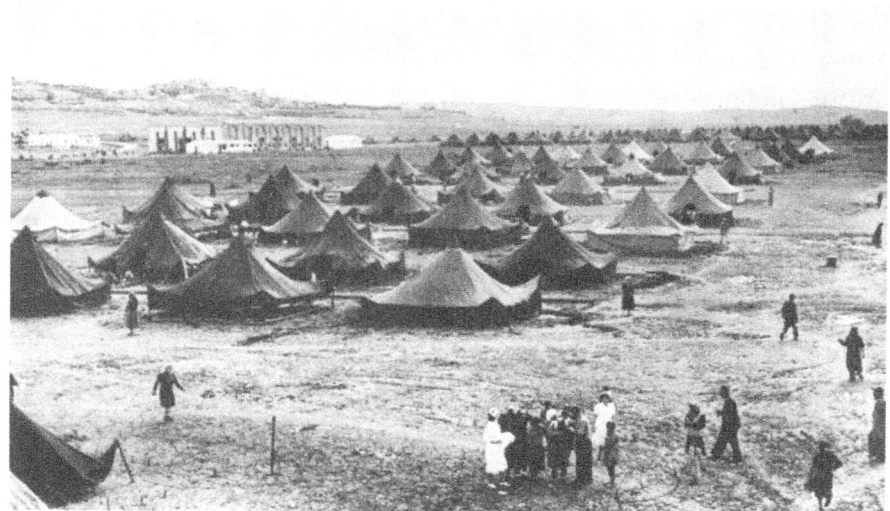

Figure 9.5 Immigrants' tent camp in the 1950s
Government Press Office website, 8 January 1949.

institute for ringworm in the Rosh HaAyin camp (a "tent city" not far from Petach Tikvah where many Yemenite immigrants were concentrated), and on June 22, 1950, Dostrovsky reported that the onsite treatment center had begun to operate (Figure 9.5). Dostrovsky said that 10% of the children in Rosh HaAyin had ringworm (at the time the camp held 12,000 immigrants, mostly from Yemen, including 3,000 children).[74]

The treatment station was operated by a doctor, a ringworm nurse, and a sanitation nurse, and the working plan encompassed examination and treatment of 30 children a week. The radiology institute operated for a year at Rosh HaAyin, and in 1951 it was closed after the "tent city" became the Rosh HaAyin *ma'abara* (transit camp).[75] According to various reports, during the period of its operation, the Rosh HaAyin facility treated between 400 and 1,000 children.[76] According to Drukmann, who oversaw the operation of the institute, ringworm treatment among the children at Rosh HaAyin was only partially successful due to organizational difficulties and numerous power outages.[77] On January 8, 1952, Hadassah announced that the radiology institute was being transferred from Rosh

HaAyin to the Schneller military camp in Jerusalem, which henceforth would serve as the national center for ringworm treatment. The former British military camp—which in the past had been an orphanage—was maintained (temporarily) by the IDF, but the medical team that worked there was Hadassah's. On January 9, 1951, the first 70 children arrived at the camp. Transforming a military camp into a youth camp was part of the non-military roles the IDF fulfilled (and continues to fulfill) parallel to its military functions—and in this particular case, it was part of a wider campaign undertaken by the IDF called *Korat Gag* (literally "a roof over one's head") designed to provide better living conditions for immigrant children in the transit camps (Figure 9.6).[78] Schneller was chosen because the camp had previously been an orphanage, and its physical plant made it possible to run social and educational activities for the children during their stay.[79] The children brought to Schneller were treated for ringworm in 5-week intervals, after which they were sent back home. Until it closed in 1953, the Schneller camp treated some 1,200 children.[80]

Parallel to organized treatment of children with ringworm in the Schneller camp—who were for the most part children from outside Jerusalem—Hadassah treated at its own radiology institute in Jerusalem some 1,000 children with ringworm who lived within Jerusalem, or in the Jerusalem Corridor. The patients were transported to the institutes daily, while complementary treatment after irradiation was provided at clinics staffed by Hadassah public health nurses.[81] When the Hadassah Hospital radiology institute was closed due to technical problems or because staff members were on vacation, or when the waiting list for treatment was very long, children were sent by health authorities to private physicians in Jerusalem who treated the cases under Hadassah supervision and Ministry of Health funding. Thus, for example, between 1949 and 1959, 696 children who were members of the GSF in Jerusalem were treated for ringworm by Dr. Avraham Izmojik, who treated the children under an agreement between the doctor and Hadassah.[82]

Even after the Schneller camp was closed (March 1, 1953), Jerusalem children continued to receive treatment against ringworm at the

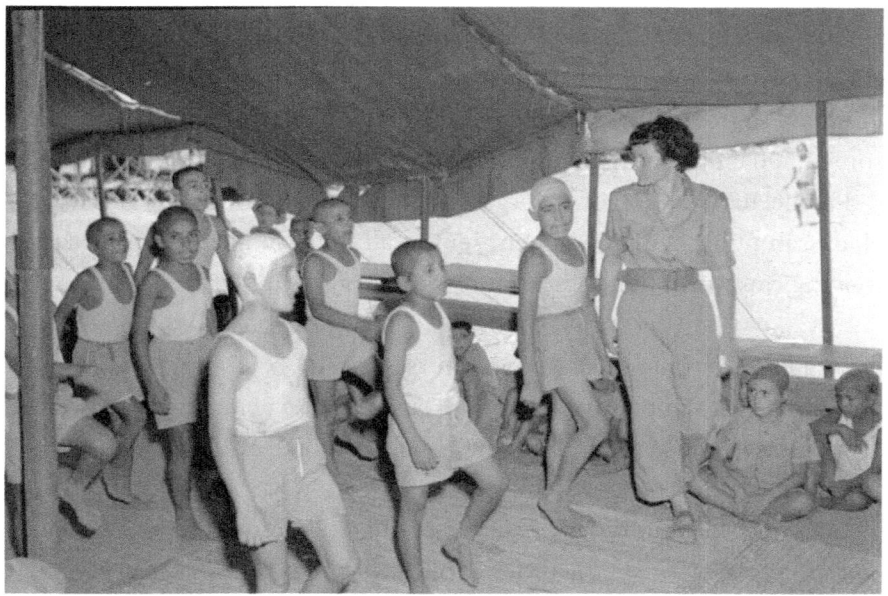

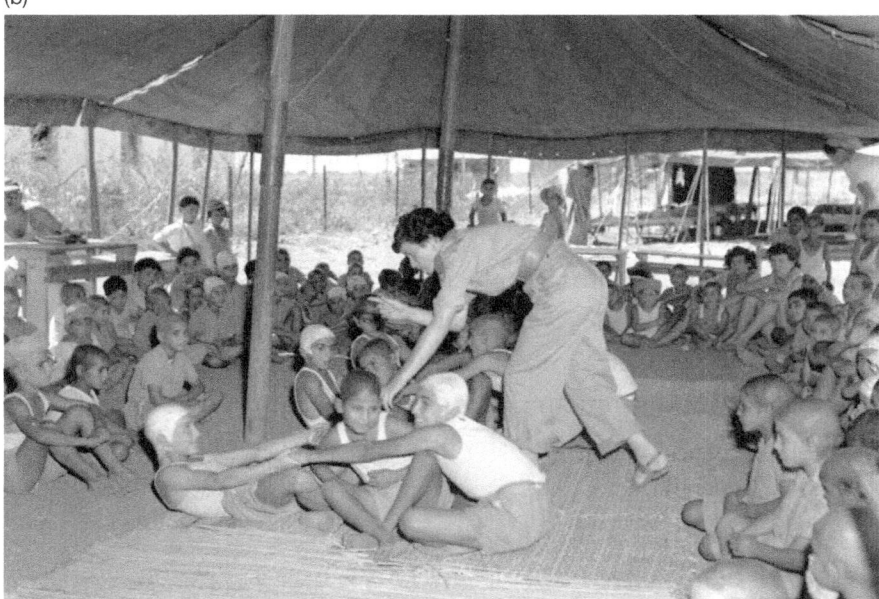

Figure 9.6 Female soldiers working with children with ringworm, 1951
Courtesy of the IDF Archives.

Hadassah radiology institute in Jerusalem (until 1959). In 1953, the Tel HaShomer Hospital near Tel Aviv (today the Sheba University Medical Center) opened an institute to treat children with ringworm, which was designed to treat sick children in Tel Aviv and the vicinity; there, in 1960, some 1,500 children underwent treatment.[83]

Parallel to operation of the organized machinery for treating ringworm, Hadassah published a document sent to all medical institutions in Israel treating ringworm that set forth the following standing regulations:

1. Regular examinations by school nurses.
2. Taking hair samples from children suspected as being infected with ringworm and sending the hairs for microscopic examination in the laboratory.
3. Sending sick children for treatment with irradiation (the Kienböck–Adamson method [3 to 5 days of irradiation]); smearing the head with Vaseline for about 3 weeks; manual epilation; smearing *colifonium* (a mixture of glue and wax) and waxing of remaining hair; and smearing the head with an iodine solution for 4 to 5 weeks after hair loss.
4. After the treatment, the children are kept in quarantine in an organized framework (the Schneller camp, Shaar HaAliyah camp) or in the family domicile.
5. The Ministry of Health will underwrite the treatment in collaboration with the Jewish Agency, Hadassah, and the GSF.
6. Monthly payment in accordance with the number of patients is made to the institutions and to the private doctors who have been authorized by the Ministry of Health to carry out irradiation against ringworm.[84]

Hadassah's instructions for treating ringworm were standing orders in all the medical institutions in Israel, both public and private. They were enforced by Hadassah, which even conducted periodic visits at these institutions.

Establishment of a hospital for trachoma and ringworm in the Shaar HaAliyah immigrant intake camp

In January 1952, a trachoma and ringworm treatment hospital was opened within the central immigrant intake camp in the State of Israel—Shaar HaAliyah, south of the city of Haifa—as a substitute for the temporary hubs that operated at the outset after declaration of statehood. It was established to deal with the many children with ringworm who were arriving as immigrants to Israel. The management and administration of the camp was entrusted to the Jewish Agency, which was responsible for organizing immigration to Israel. The number of trachoma patients stood at 68,000 children; they were the largest group of sick persons that concerned the Ministry of Health.[85] The number of ringworm cases designated for treatment was approximately a fourth the number of trachoma cases, and therefore ringworm was considered a secondary problem. It is not surprising, therefore, that trachoma was viewed as the largest medical problem at the time, and most of the attention of health agents was directed first of all to treating trachoma.

The underlying assumption behind opening a hospital at Shaar HaAliyah was that concentrating all resources for treating trachoma and ringworm in one place would improve and maximize the effectiveness of treatment. In addition, it was preferable to treat sick children immediately after they arrived and before they entered the country's school system in order to prevent the spread of the disease among the general population. In addition to the medical examination setup that was the primary objective of the service, health officials at Shaar HaAliyah had to provide first aid and medical care for sick immigrants until they recovered and left the camp. However, in the initial deployment in setting up the camp, the following was not taken into account: (a) all the medical needs and (b) the number of sick persons in need of lengthy care who would need to stay in the camp with their families for a number of weeks. This created serious crowding and pressure on the camp's services and on the immigrants themselves, since the policy for release of patients—set in advance—envisioned that arriving families would remain only a week. Even if the number of children with ringworm was low compared to those with trachoma or compared to other diseases treated at the camp, ringworm treatment was more lengthy (sometimes up to 6 weeks in duration).

The decision to establish a national center for treatment of trachoma and ringworm patients in the Shaar HaAliyah camp was a logical move in light of prevailing conditions at the time. The underlying assumption of the Ministry of Health was that it would be possible to concentrate in the Shaar HaAliyah camp the immigrants with trachoma and ringworm arriving at the intake camp and that Shaar HaAliyah would also become a national center for treating these disease. Children from the veteran Jewish community in Israel would also be sent for treatment there, alongside children from the transit camps and anyone else who needed such treatment. Another underlying assumption was that establishing a national center for treating trachoma and ringworm would contribute to the organized eradication of both of these diseases in the country as a whole.

Two x-ray machines were donated for the Shaar HaAliyah camp by UNICEF, and the United Nations agency even promised to take care of providing spare parts. UNICEF's contribution to a mass treatment campaign against ringworm in Israel was part of a worldwide policy of the organization to eradicate infectious diseases that afflicted children and mothers. Parallel to Israel, UNICEF operated similar programs to eradicate ringworm in Yugoslavia (Serbia; see Chapter 6)[86] and in Syria.[87]

An agreement for UNICEF aid to the government of Israel was signed in late 1948 and led to the arrival in 1952 of the x-ray machines that were installed in the Shaar HaAliyah hospital.[88] UNICEF assisted in ringworm treatment and also underwrote the operations of *Tipat Chalav* ("a drop of milk") mother and child clinics for early detection (as much as possible) of infectious diseases (tuberculosis, trachoma, syphilis, and ringworm) among mothers and children.[89]

In parallel with the treatment of immigrant children with ringworm in the camp, the Ministry of Health conducted tests for ringworm in all public kindergartens and schools. The hair of children suspected of being affected was sent for laboratory examination. If ringworm was confirmed, they were sent in organized groups for a week of radiation therapy at the Shaar HaAliyah camp. Parents were asked to approve sending their children for intensive radiation therapy. The children were usually sent in groups of 10, accompanied by a nurse or a paramedic. All the children were rechecked in Shaar HaAliyah before irradiation.

The camp reports often stated that, in the course of this preliminary hair examination, some children were found to be completely healthy; they were kept in the camp, separated from the group they arrived with, until transport back home could be arranged. Sometimes they had to remain in the camp for a full week due to lack of transport. Shula Tzarfati, a public health nurse from the Ashkelon region whose job was to escort sick children going to Shaar HaAliyah for treatment, said:

> Only children whose disease was substantiated at Shaar HaAliyah by the doctor on site underwent treatment. There were no preventive treatment or *en bloc* of classrooms, only of children whose disease had been confirmed . . . All the trips to Shaar HaAliyah and back were in lorries with up to 10 children. There were never trips in trucks.[90]

Strict observance in carrying out microscopic examination of each child's hair prior to treatment was a Hadassah directive. That is, medical supervision of treatment for ringworm at Shaar HaAliyah was in the hands of Hadassah Hospital in Jerusalem, and personally in the hands of Dostrovsky and Drukmann, who were joined later by Dr. Frederic Raubitchek,[91] also from Hadassah. The trio visited the Shaar HaAliyah Hospital regularly, sent professional reports to the Ministry of Health, oversaw the work of the physicians there, and served as consultants to the Ministry of Health on ringworm. They also oversaw the work of private doctors, and those who failed to meet the criteria they set were removed from the list of doctors authorized to treat ringworm on behalf of the Ministry of Health.

The protocols for treating ringworm were set by the dermatology department of Hadassah (Professor Dostrovsky, Dr. Raubitchek, and Dr. Sagher).

Dr. Sagher wrote after one of his visits to the Shaar HaAliyah Hospital that "the organization and treatment were built in this camp in accordance with the experience gained in previous camps such as the Schneller camp and Rosh HaAyin" (two camps administered by Hadassah). On the page of directives for treating ringworm sent by Dr. Sagher to Dr. Yaffe (deputy director-general of the Ministry of Health), the stages of treatment were set out in detail:

1. The diagnosis of the department must be verified by a microscopic examination prior to giving therapy and should not rely on clinical diagnosis only.
2. Examination of the heads of all family members.
3. An internal examination of children up to age 12 before irradiation is recommended.
4. Irradiation with x-ray.
5. At the completion of irradiation, smearing of Vaseline day after day until epilation, which is approximately 14 to 17 days. (During this time, it is possible to shampoo the head once, twice a week in warm water and soap, but this is not imperative.)
5a. The correct time for epilation will be set by a doctor via an attempt to remove a hair with tweezers. If the hair comes out easily, it is possible to follow through with epilation. One should also ensure disinfection of the cap and also of bed linen.
6. Thorough epilation of the hair by a heated mixture of 450 gr. Coli + 75 gr. Cera Alba. After the treatment, cleaning the head with benzene and smearing of Pasta Zinci to soothe the skin.
6a. The next day, a careful examination by a doctor, and if necessary black spots and individual [remaining] hairs with tweezers must be removed.
7. Begin a sequence of spreading Iod . Tinct. 10% Iod. daily for 6 days, and before each sequence [session] examination of the head by a doctor.
8. In the event of *trichophytia* (ringworm), 3 sequences [applications] of Iod.

9. Between each sequence, smear with Pasta Zinci and the next day shampoo in warm water and soap and before beginning the new sequence, examination by the doctor.
10. Upon conclusion, the infected [child] must come for a doctor's examination after 1-2-3-4-4 weeks.

Remarks:

a. From the setting of the diagnosis until completion of the therapy the head of the infected [child] needs to be bandaged.
b. From the setting of the diagnosis until completion of healing, the infected [child] is not permitted to be in the company of children such as school, a children's daycare, and so forth.
c. Hygiene directives to prevent spread of the disease are presented in minute detail to the family.
> The examination is carried out at the Ministry of Health by a professional nurse in this realm.
> The examination at the Ministry of Health is carried out meticulously as cited above.[92]

The therapy period lasted approximately 6 weeks, in groups of 150 children each; irradiation treatment was given to children aged 3 and above (this stipulation was set by Hadassah physicians who oversaw treatment); children under the age of 3 were treated by smearing the scalp with a salve and wrapping the head in a clean kerchief (without irradiation). After services for follow-up and complementary medical care were set up in the community, the period spent in Shaar HaAliyah was shortened to a week, after which the child was sent home and treated locally by a specially trained public health nurse. During this period, children could return to their own school, provided they wore a head covering.

In other words, as already mentioned, children were sent to be cured only after it was certified by microscopic examination of their hair that they were indeed infected with ringworm. After verification and diagnosis, the child's hair was cut and they were sent for irradiation. After children were completely cured, they were examined by a doctor and only then was the decision made whether to release them. The irradiation of children who had received irradiation abroad was suspended until exact details were received about previous treatments. More than once Leah Weissberger—the head nurse and the wife of the chief administrator of the Shaar HaAliyah camp, Yehuda Weissberger—complained that she had to postpone treatment of children due to absence of information about prior irradiation. She requested that immigration certificates together with health certificates be transferred with the children infected with ringworm, because otherwise it would not be possible to treat them.[93] The principle was that children would not be treated if no information was available on whether they had been irradiated previously or not.

This practice applied to all children and youth, whether or not their parents were present in the Shaar HaAliyah camp, whether they were waiting for completion of treatment or had already been transferred to one of the transit camps, or whether the patient was a member of a youth group immigrating to Israel without family that belonged to a settlement "nucleus" destined to settle as a group in a particular kibbutz, farm, etc. In general, it was preferred that parents stay in the camp until their children were cured, but the Ministry of Health, given the high cost of extending the stay of such families, preferred that the families be sent on to their destination (a *ma'abara* or a new farm or village) and have the children join them at a later date. More than once, there were heated discussions between Sh. Halevy (deputy director-general of Hadassah) and the Immigrants Medical Service personnel and the medical staff at Shaar HaAliyah regarding the accrued costs of caring for the families of the children under treatment.[94] Each side stood firm on its position, and no unified policy on this issue was reached.

After release from the camp, the children's follow-up was carried out by doctors serving their place of residence. A child released from the camp received a referral letter to the family doctor with recommendations for follow-up treatment or monitoring.

Not everyone was happy with the establishment of the Shaar HaAliyah Hospital. Dr. Weille from Hadera, who up until this point had received referrals from the Ministry of Health of children in need of treatment in her private radiology institute, suffered from the drop in the number of patients and therefore began to treat primarily children from the Arab sector in her area. Dr. Itzkowitch, who had treated children in his radiology institute in Haifa on behalf of the Ministry of Health, facing a dwindling clientele, began to treat children from Acre and Arab villages in the Galilee who lacked any specialized facility for treating ringworm in their vicinity. Dr. Weille strove from time to time to convince the Ministry of Health to renew referrals of children for treatment at her practice, parallel to irradiation being conducted at the Shaar HaAliyah camp, but the suggestion was turned down. All irradiation operations were now concentrated exclusively at Shaar HaAliyah.

In 1953, the Shaar HaAliyah Hospital received a new irradiation machine (a donation from UNICEF). Following the donation, one of the machines at their disposal was transferred to the Tel HaShomer Hospital (Sheba Medical Center) near Tel Aviv, which at the time was being transformed from a military hospital into a government hospital (for civilians). The treatment given to children with ringworm at Tel HaShomer was also carried out under the supervision of Hadassah doctors (Dostrovsky and Drukmann).

Hundreds of children from veteran settlements in Israel, including kibbutz children who had become infected with ringworm, were sent for treatment at Shaar HaAliyah. In general, the kibbutz children were examined in their schools, and hair samples of those suspected of having ringworm were sent for examination in a lab (Figure 9.7). Parents of infected children were told they must have their children treated at Shaar HaAliyah. Dr. Mirko Brill,[95] a dermatologist for the GSF in Jezreel Valley settlements, stated that in addition to children in the *ma'abarot* in the valley, many children in veteran villages and kibbutz settlements had been treated for ringworm.[96] In a survey of schoolchildren in the Afula area,[97] Brill found that 4% of the children were infected with ringworm; in approximately 40% of them, the disease had been lengthy, and the other 60% were new infections. According to Brill, infection was spread primarily via combs and barbers' hair clippers. In his opinion, after ambulatory treatment

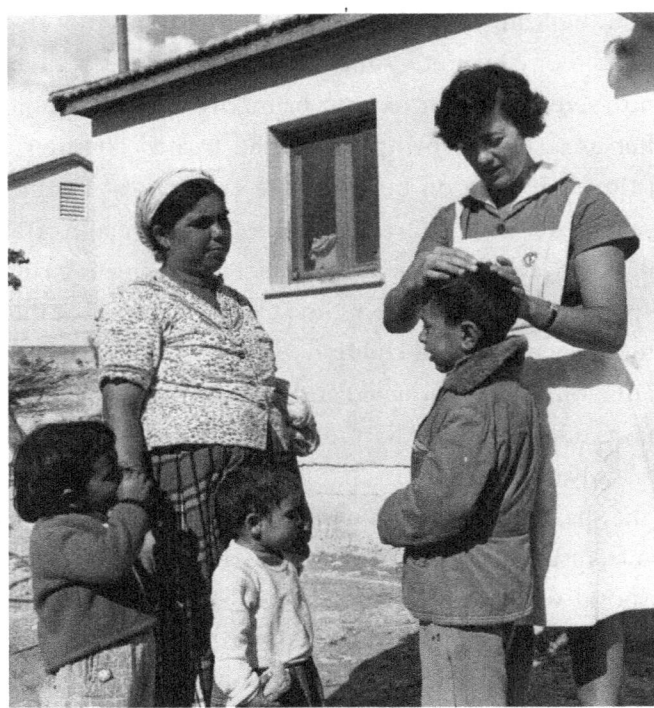

Figure 9.7 Checking scalps for lice and ringworm in a new community established by immigrants in the 1950s
Courtesy of the JDC Archives, New York, NY.

at Shaar HaAliyah, there were more cases of reinfection compared to local treatment that was more uniform—ongoing.

According to the Ministry of Health's Epidemiology Unit, from 1949 to 1954 a total of 2,354 immigrants were treated at Shaar HaAliyah (some of them at Dr. Itzkovitch's institute in Haifa); of them, 1,183 were immigrants from Morocco, 179 from Persia, 30 from Tripoli, 235 from Yemen, and 351 from Iraq; in addition, there were 167 immigrants from other countries.[98] In 1959, it was reported that 1,346 persons had been treated with irradiation for ringworm at Shaar HaAliyah, 199 at Tel HaShomer, and 43 at other places; the majority of patients (734) were immigrants from North Africa, 162 from Persia, 74 from IrAQ: and 45 from Yemen; other immigrants were listed as being from Turkey, Romania, India, and other countries.[99]

Yeduda Weissberger (chief administrator of the Shaar HaAliyah Hospital) reported that from 1952 to 1956, 5,000 children had been treated. According to a report sent to UNICEF, 1,500 children a year were treated at Shaar HaAliyah with irradiation. Up until irradiation treatment for ringworm stopped in 1960, a total of 12,000 children had been treated with irradiation.[100]

Treatment with irradiation for ringworm by the GSF

The GSF was the key health organization in the State of Israel from the beginning (and remains so to this day).[101] As such, it absorbed a substantial share of immigrants in terms of their health care needs. Among other things, the GSF ran two centers for ringworm treatment—one in Tel Aviv, the other in Haifa.[102] With establishment of the State of Israel, the GSF collaborated in formulating a national plan to "organize the war on venereal disease and social dermatoses" (including the war on ringworm), a plan in which all public health bodies in the State of Israel participated.[103] In the framework of collaboration on a national scale of all health agents, and according to directives of the Ministry of Health (as already noted), in February 1950 every person with ringworm was required to receive treatment (irradiation, as was standard procedure), and receipt of treatment was a necessary condition for a child to return to school or to kindergarten. As part of this collaboration, immigrant children who were not members of the GSF were also sent to GSF radiology centers in Tel Aviv and Haifa. From 1947 to 1960 the clinic in Tel Aviv treated 4,000 children, the majority of whom were not GSF members but rather children of new immigrants who were treated under an arrangement between the GSF and the Ministry of Health.

Treatment for ringworm at the GSF was not given in a residential setting as in Shaar HaAliyah; rather, the patients had to make daily visits to the treatment center and complementary treatment was conducted at community clinics. More than once, difficulties arose due to the distance of these centers from the patients' homes and the problems involved in transporting them daily to treatment centers. On the other hand, the cost of treatment was low since the children remained at home during the entire treatment period, and neither the GSF nor the Ministry of Health had to bear the expense of food and lodging.

Children with ringworm from the Jerusalem area who were members of the GSF were sent for treatment at Hadassah, at GSF expense. The opening of the Shaar HaAliyah Hospital enabled the GSF to reach an arrangement with the Ministry of Health by which children who were GSF members but lived far from the GSF's radiology centers would be sent for treatment at Shaar HaAliyah.

With the changes in operational arrangements at the Shaar HaAliyah Hospital (following establishment of a network of local follow-up services), the period spent at the hospital for treatment was cut from 6 weeks (the time until hair regrowth began) to only a week. Thus, the GSF could send a larger number of children with ringworm to Shaar HaAliyah, while the complementary treatment was carried out in the various community clinics operated by the GSF.

Although at the outset of 1952 treatment with irradiation against ringworm was compulsory and underwritten by the state, the Ministry of Health noted in its follow-up forms which of the children treated for ringworm in the various centers were insured by the GSF, apparently not only as part of recording personal data and follow-up but also in order to settle accounts between the state and the GSF regarding expenditures and services rendered in the treatment of immigrants. In addition, in follow-up forms sent to regional offices of the Ministry of Health, the nurse supervisor who managed the registry was required to note separately how many of the children treated were insured by the GSF. Thus, for example, a report of children with ringworm in 1956 stated that out of 2,254 children treated at Shaar HaAliyah, 906 were insured by the GSF.[104] A Ministry of Health report that estimated the outlay for treatment of ringworm in 1956 stated that GSF nurses conducted approximately 25% of all the work of nurses for ringworm, particularly complementary treatment after irradiation in the GSF's clinics.[105]

Those insured by the other sick funds operating in Israel[106] were not noted, and no documents were found that mentioned whether there were special agreements between them and the Ministry of Health. In the archives of the smaller sick funds, there are many documents that testify that children under the care of the smaller funds were sent for irradiation treatment at Shaar HaAliyah or, as an alternative, to private doctors with whom the funds had a service-provider agreement. The weight and size of the role of the GSF in health services in Shaar HaAliyah and in immigrant communities was much greater. As a result, the GSF (like Hadassah) became an important partner in curing ringworm at the Shaar HaAliyah Hospital, and the Ministry of Health would consult the GSF and engage it in decision-making on this issue.[107]

TREATMENT AGAINST RINGWORM IN THE ARAB SECTOR

Ringworm was also one of the most prevalent problems among children in the Arab sector in Eretz-Israel, both in the Mandate period and after establishment of Israel.[108] Crowded living conditions, lack of sanitation services and lack of running water (particularly in Arab villages), lack of health services, and apathy or indifference to ringworm and lack of treatment for it increased the number of children infected from year to year. With the expansion of treatment of ringworm to the children of new immigrants arriving in Israel in the 1950s, Arab families and Arab entities (primarily in the north of the country) requested ringworm treatment to eradicate the disease among Arab children as well.

The first requests came from the municipality of Acre,[109] which identified the spread of ringworm among its schoolchildren, followed by health and education entities in Nazareth and Arab villages in the Galilee. Requests from the Arab public that their children receive treatment at Shaar HaAliyah or within another framework operated by the Ministry of Health were rejected due to the existing demand for such services and apprehensions in combining Arab and Jewish children in the same treatment framework.[110] Economically established Arab families sent their children to private irradiation institutes that operated primarily in Haifa and Tel Aviv.[111]

In light of the numerous appeals for treatment against ringworm in the Arab sector, and out of understanding that the disease could not be eradicated without treatment of all children in Israel, the Ministry of Health decided to establish a center for irradiation treatment for ringworm in Nazareth. The center was opened in late 1956 and operated until 1960. It was directed by Dr. Simon Rosenblut,[112] a Ministry of Health physician, and operated under the supervision of the dermatology and radiology departments of Hadassah. Some of the examinations to diagnose ringworm were carried out in the Hadassah lab in Jerusalem. From 1957 to 1960, it was reported that 3,700 Arab children were treated with irradiation for ringworm. This was the only center in Israel that provided public-medical services for Arab children with ringworm.[113] A central issue that the Nazareth center had to deal with was whether children would come to the center. Since most of the infected children lived in agricultural villages, the treatments were scheduled in seasons when they were not required to help in the orchards and fields. Furthermore, most of the villages did not have paved access roads, making it difficult for residents to get to Nazareth in the winter. Consequently, time windows when treatment was feasible were short in duration and were set according to the seasons. The treatment center in Nazareth was closed when irradiation was replaced by griseofulvin. Treatment with this medicine was given to Jews and Arab alike, with financial assistance from UNICEF.[114]

CLOSURE OF THE CAMP FOR TREATMENT OF RINGWORM

In December 1959 the daily newspaper *HaAretz* published the following announcement: "Success of a new method in treating ringworm in Hadassah: On a new medical treatment against ringworm that will replace the accepted treatment with irradiation." The discovery of griseofulvin in place of treatment with irradiation led to the closure of the Shaar HaAliyah Hospital.[115] In the years of its operation, 12,000 ringworm patients had been treated in the hospital, most of them children.

In February 1962, the Shaar HaAliyah intake camp, which had a staff of 400 (including the hospital staff), was closed for good. According to an article in the daily newspaper *Davar*, the camp, which had been opened by the Jewish Agency in 1949, and though which more than 390,000 immigrants had been processed and screened, had completed its role. The total of immigrants treated for ringworm among the immigrant population that went through Shaar HaAliyah stood at 3%.[116] At the same time, the Ministry of Health began vigorous preparations for a national campaign to eradicate ringworm using griseofulvin; a new era had dawned in the treatment of ringworm.

During the 1960s, ringworm continued to be a key problem among Israeli children, but now it was treated in the various communities with medication. As a result, many private and public radiology institutes that had conducted irradiation for ringworm were closed.[117] The government of Israel, with assistance from UNICEF, conducted a mass campaign to eradicate ringworm with griseofulvin among all children in Israel, both Jewish and Arab.[118] Improved standards of living, improvements in health and education, and greater awareness of hygiene led to the almost complete eradication of the disease among children in Israel, but it still broke out from time to time among groups with a low standard of living or lack of awareness of hygiene. The disease was treated accordingly without isolating the infected child from society.

SUMMARY

There were three primary stages in irradiation treatment for ringworm in the Jewish community in Eretz-Israel and in the State of Israel. The first was between 1935 and 1948 during the British Mandate period, when treatment of ringworm was carried out under the leadership of Hadassah, in keeping with the Kienböck–Adamson treatment protocol, which was the standard and leading medical protocol worldwide at the time. Affected children were identified in educational institutions and sent for treatment at radiology centers in Jerusalem, Tel Aviv, and Haifa and at private institutes. Most of the funding for ringworm treatment during the Mandate period was received from Jewish philanthropic organizations and from the public sick funds. Records of the time reveal that some 5,000 children were treated throughout the Jewish community in Eretz-Israel under British Mandate, most by the public health network.

The second stage in the war on ringworm was conducted from 1948 to 1951 with the arrival of the first mass waves of immigrants to Israel after the establishment of statehood. Public health officials in Israel realized that ringworm was one of the most prevalent diseases among the children of new immigrants, and that the best way to deal with it was to organize irradiation treatment for ringworm via specialized frameworks (the Schneller camp, the Rosh HaAyin camp) or via agreements with private practitioners. That is, supervision and medical training were carried out by the Hadassah Medical Federation, which had treated ringworm since the days of the Mandate.

The third stage was from 1952 to 1960, when state officials concluded that from a cost perspective and the quality and effectiveness of treatment, it was preferable to concentrate those infected with ringworm in one place where they could be treated according to a uniform protocol and in an organized fashion. For this, a central hospital was established at the intake and screening camp for new immigrants at Shaar HaAliyah, south of Haifa, where children from throughout the country were sent for irradiation treatment. Secondary centers for treatment were operated by the GSF and Hadassah—public health organizations that operated a countrywide network that assisted in irradiation treatment, and in follow-up complementary treatment, while Hadassah oversaw all operations. Such irradiation treatments were given until 1960, when griseofulvin replaced irradiation.

The documents of the Ministry of Finance, Health and Welfare in the Israel State Archives, Hadassah reports, the Shaar HaAliyah portfolio in the Central Zionist Archives, and documents of the GSF can provide data to reconstruct the number of children treated for ringworm during this period: at Shaar HaAliyah, some 12,000 children (Table 9.1); at the GSF clinic in Tel Aviv, some 4,200 children and several hundred more at the GSF's radiology institute in Haifa; at the irradiation institute in Nazareth and at the clinics of private physicians, some 4,500 Arab children; at Hadassah and its institutions, some 3,800 children (at the Schneller camp, Hadassah Hospital in Jerusalem, the Hadassah Hospital in Tel Aviv, and the Rosh HaAyin camp); at the Tel HaShomer Hospital (a government hospital run by the Ministry of Health), 1,500 children; and by private physicians, approximately 1,000 children. The total number of patients irradiated for ringworm from 1948 to 1960 was between 26,000 and 27,000 Jewish and Arab children.[119] Estimating the actual number of ringworm patients in Israel during this period is very important in light of the public controversy over this matter raised in the years that followed.

Table 9.1 NUMBER OF PATIENTS IRRADIATED FOR RINGWORM AT SHAAR HAALIYAH, 1952–1960

Year	Number irradiated
1952	295
1953	725
1954	1,334
1955	1,717
1956	2,800
1957	2,160
1958	1,742
1959	1,346
1960	429
Total	12,548

Statistical data on ringworm and favus in 1959, Ministry of Health, Epidemiology Unit. Israel State Archive G-5088/9-

NOTES

1. Dr. Arieh Dostrovsky (1887–1975) was born in Russia, studied medicine in Breslow, Vienna, Basel, and Paris, and immigrated to Mandate Israel in 1919. He was a physician in the American Zionist Medical Unit (which grew to become the Hadassah Medical Federation). He was the first professor of dermatology in Israel and was head of the dermatology and venereal diseases department of Hadassah Hospital in Jerusalem. He was the first dean of Hadassah's medical school in Jerusalem. He founded and headed the Dermatologists Union in Israel. Levy N, Levy Y. Rofeiha shel Eretz-Israel 1799–1948 [The Doctors of the Land of Israel 1799–1948]. Zichron Yaakov, 2008:143.
2. Dostrovsky A. Ringworm in Jerusalem's Schools. 1928, Central Zionist Archives, Jerusalem (henceforth, CZA), J113/1434.
3. The geographic region of the present State of Israel was, prior to its establishment in 1948, called Eretz- Israel (the biblical name of the Holy Land, the "Land of Israel").
4. "Law for Compensation of Scalp Ringworm Victims, 1994," *Rishumot* (Knesset Record), Book of Statutes, 1478, 4 August 1994. Full version (in Hebrew) at: https://www.health.gov.il/LegislationLibrary/Gazezet_01.pdf
5. Eretz-Israel was conquered by the British in December 1917. In September 1922, Britain received from the League of Nations the Mandate for Palestine on its behalf. The American Zionist Medical Unit was founded as an emergency setup organized to rehabilitate health and welfare institutions of the Jewish community in Eretz-Israel that had been decimated in World War I. In 1921, the ad hoc taskforce became a permanent local health organization, the Hadassah Medical Federation. See: Shvarts S, Shehory-Rubin Z. Hadassah for the Health of the People. Tel Aviv: Samuel Watchman's Sons Inc. & Dekel Academic Press; 2012.
6. Shvarts S, Brown T. Kupat Holim, Dr. Isaac Max Rubinow, and the American Zionist Medical Unit's experiment to establish health care services in Palestine 1918–1923. *Bull Hist Med.* 1998;72(1):28–46.
7. Berachiahu M. Beit ha-Sefer veha-Talmid b-Eretz-Israel [The School and the Pupil in Eretz-Israel]. Jerusalem: 1926;4, 17.
8. Uprooting hair using tar, thick sticky sugar-based pastes, pincers, or tweezers.
9. Dr. Mordechai Berachiahu (1882–1959) studied medicine in Switzerland (MD in 1910). In 1912 he immigrated to Eretz-Israel and worked as a doctor at the Hebrew High School in Tel Aviv. He founded the school hygiene department for Hadassah and was one of the leaders in the field of hygiene and preventive medicine in educational institutions as well as stations for the treatment of children in stressful situations (Levy and Levy, 153).
10. Dostrovsky A. Achuz ha-Cholim b-Gazezet bein Talmidei Batai ha-Sefeer l'fee Batei Sefer b-Reishit ha-Shanah (lifnai ha-Ripu'i) ooba-Sof ha-Shanah (achrei ha-Riopu'i) b-meshech 1920-1921 [Percentage of Ringworm Patients among School Pupils, by School at the Beginning of the Year (Prior to Cure) and at the End of the Year (After Cure) during 1920-21], p. 1, CZA, J113/1434. Dostrovsky stated that in educational facilities in Jerusalem that did not operate under the auspices of the Education Committee, there were 517 pupils with ringworm.

11. Ibid.
12. Dostrovsky A. Avodat ha-Machlekah ha-Hygi'enit shel Batei ha-Sefer: ha-Milchamah b-Malchalot ha-Or ha-Midabkot [The Work of the Schools' Hygiene Department: The War against Contagious Dermatological Diseases]. *HaChinuch*. 1926;9:101.
13. Gorwitz Y. ha-Briut ba-Batei ha-Sefer b-Eretz-Israel [Health in the Schools in Eretz-Israel]. *Doar HaYom*, 9 July 1924, p. 2.
14. Ibid.; Iskovitch Y. Yehudi M'tzura [Pariah Jew]. *Doar HaYom*, 19 August 1932, p. 6.
15. Shvarts and Shehory-Rubin, 91–109.
16. Levy and Levy, 206.
17. Letter (no name) to Hadassah Management, Supplies Department, ordering supplies for the radiology lab from Siemens, 24 March 1925, in the portfolio Hadassah Engineer B. Ziloni Correspondence 1925–1932, Israeli Radiology Union Historical Archive, Hadassah Ein Karem. Courtesy of Professor Jacob Sosna.
18. *Doar HaYom*, 5 December 1924, p. 2.
19. Dr. Avraham (Adolf) Drukmann (1895–1964), a graduate of the medical school in Vienna, immigrated to Eretz-Israel in 1925 and with establishment, joined the radiology department of Hadassah. In 1933, he was appointed to head Hadassah's radiology department and in 1938 became a professor of radiology at the Hebrew University and one of the founders of the school of medicine in 1949 in Jerusalem. See Levy and Levy, 171.
20. The use of *colifonium* for hair removal was conventional in most European countries, primarily in France, and followed traditional practices of removing ringworm-infected hair using tar or a sugar-based sticky solution. Dostrovsky A. Ringworm in Jerusalem's Schools. 1928 CZA Jerusalem , J113/1434.
21. Dostrovsky, Work of the Schools' Hygiene Department, 102–103.
22. Ibid., 102.
23. Ibid., 98.
24. Ibid., 102.
25. Dostrowsky A. Das Phänomen der herdöfrmigen Haarhypertrophie nach Röntgenepilation [The phenomenon of hereditary hair hypertrophy after x-ray epilation]. *Archiv Dermatol Syphilis*. 1931;162:739–761.
26. Berachiahu, School and the Pupil, 4, 17.
27. Berachiahu to Hadassah Management, 4 April 1928, CZA, J113/1434.
28. Memorandum, Dr. Berachiahu to the Head Management of Hadassah in Jerusalem, 22 March 1932, CZA, S6/346.
29. Berachiahu M. Avodat ha-Machlekah ha-Hygienah shel Batei ha-Sefer: Skirah Clalit shel Hitpatchut ha-Avodah [The Work of the School Hygiene Department: A General Survey]. *HaChinuch*. 1926;9:185.
30. Itskovitch, 6.
31. Halamish A. A New Look at Immigration of Jews from Yemen to Mandatory Palestine. *Israeli Studies*. 2006;11:62–64.
32. Dostrovsky A. al Ripu'i Machanot ha-Or veha-Min b-Eretz-Israel (On Curing Dermatological and Venereal Diseases in Eretz-Israel), Hadassah portfolios J113/5422, undated document CZA, J113/5422.

33. On the health cards of the Immigration and Work Department of the Jewish Agency, in clause 4–5, a doctor was required to examine the cardholder and record whether the candidate for immigration had a dermatologic or venereal disease. CZA, S6/1457.
34. Gurevitch L. Twenty-Five Years of OZE, 1912–1937. Paris; 1937:88–101; Wolman L. Medical Welfare Activities Among Jews in Poland 1919–1939. Warsaw; 1939. See also Chapter 5.
35. Dr. A. Katznelson to Dr. Y. Davidson, Immigration Office, Tel-Aviv, 14 October 1934, CZA, S4/1131. On criteria for immigration of Yemenite Jews, see details in Halamish, 59–78.
36. Letter, Dr. Berachiahu to the School Hygiene Department, Memorandum No. 19, 11 December 1941, the Oded Yarkoni Archive of the History of Petach Tikvah, Petach Tikvah 1/13-518.
37. Dr. P. Weill, Hadassah director in Safed, to Hadassah Management in Jerusalem, regarding a schoolgirl from the Alliance School whose parents refused to send her for irradiation treatment, 27 January 1939, CZA, J113/2292.
38. Berachiahu to Hadassah Management, April 4, 1928, CZA, J113/1434.
39. Dr. P. Novick to the Public Medicine Department of Hadassah, 10 March 1942; Dr. Brumberg to the Health Department of the Jewish National Council (*Vaad HaLeumi*, the Jewish community's self-governing body during the Mandate period), 16 March 1942, CZA J113/2298.
40. This responsibility was given to the two by the Israeli Ministry of Health at the close of the Mandate and declaration of independence of the State of Israel, and they were the professional-medical agents overseeing all treatments in Israel against ringworm employing irradiation, up until 1960. Minutes from a meeting on October 30, 1951, at the Strauss Center, Jerusalem, signed by Dr. Jenny Thaustein, director of the Ministry of Health's Mother & Child Department, Social Medicine Branch, Sheba Archive, Sheba Medical Center, Tel-HaShomer, Ramat Gan.
41. Weill.
42. Dostrovsky A, et al. Tinea Capitis, An Epidemiologic, Therapeutic and Laboratory Investigation of 6300 Cases. *J Invest Dermatol*. 1955;24:195–200; Drukmann A. Künstliche Erzeugung des Phänomens der herdförmigen Haarhypertrophie nach Röntgen Epilation [Artificial generation of the phenomenon of herd-shaped hair hypertrophy after x-ray epilation]. *Archiv Dermatol Syphilis*. 1932;167:174–178.
43. Correspondence of the local Jewish community governing council in Tiberias (*Vaad HaKehilah HaIvrit*) to the Public Medicine Department of Hadassah Medical Federation, March–October 1942, CZA, J113/2298.
44. Dr. Ernst Feilchenfeld (1895–1966) studied medicine in Freiburg, with a specialization in dermatology and venereal diseases, and worked in Tel Aviv with a specialized practice in ringworm. From 1956 to 1959 he was the chief physician at the Ministry of Health's Center for Treatment of Ringworm in Nazareth and treated the Arab population. Levy and Levy, 332.
45. Feilchenfeld E. Erfahrungen bei Behandlung und nachgehender Fürsorge bei Tinea capitis in 30 Jahren [Experience in treatment and follow-up care for tinea capitis in 30 years]. *Dermatol Wochenschr*. 1959;1:14–20.
46. Dostrovsky, Percentage of Ringworm Patients.

47. The General Sick Fund (GSF, today Clalit Health Services) was and still is the largest public health organization in Israel. GSF was founded in 1911 and operated until 1995 as part of the General Federation of Laborer in Israel. In 1948, with the establishment of the state, over 70% of the residents were members of or insured by the GSF. After the enactment of the National Health Insurance Law in Israel in 1994, their number fell to about 52% of the total population of the country, Jews and minorities alike. Shvarts S. The Workers' Health Fund in Eretz Israel. University of Rochester, NY, and Boydell & Brewer Press, UK; 2002.
48. Sefer ha-Rofim: Rishimat ha-Rofim Chevrei ha-Histadrut ha-Refuit ha-Ivrit b-Eretz-Israel [Physicians' Registry: List of Doctors Members of the Hebrew Medical Federation in Eretz-Israel]. Tel Aviv; 1941.
49. Tosefet Machalot Min b-Rishimat ha-Machalot ha-Midabkot, Hoda'ah al Gazezet [An Addition to Venereal Diseases on the List of Contagious Diseases, Proclamation on Ringworm]. *Harefuah*. 1951;40. The British demanded only that venereal diseases be reported, perhaps because they did not often deal with treatment against ringworm.
50. Drukmann to Hadassah Management, 24 August 1946, CZA J113/2085; in European countries, in England, and in the United States there was no uniform or agreed-upon policy regarding an obligation to report cases of ringworm to health authorities, and it is possible that this also contributed to Mandate authorities not demanding reporting of ringworm cases.
51. Yaski C. Machalat ha-Or b-Beit ha-Cholim ha-Universita'i Hadassah [Dermatological Diseases in the Hadassah University Hospital]. *Harefuah*. 1947;32:2.
52. When there were technical breakdowns at the Hadassah radiology institute, in order to prevent the children under treatment from missing many schooldays, Hadassah decided to send the children for irradiation at private institutes until the machinery was fixed. Drukmann to Hadassah Management, 24 August 1946, CZA J113/2085.
53. In late 1944, the Jewish Agency established the Immigrants Medical Service in order to care for immigrants who came to Eretz-Israel with the close of the Second World War, appointing Dr. Theodor Grushka to serve as director. Until 1946, the Service operated as a special department of the Jewish Agency, and on October 1, 1946, its management was transferred to Hadassah, which took charge until October 1948. In November 1948, it was decided that the Service would be transformed into a governmental agency, under the administration of the Ministry of Health. See: the Knesset Library, Protokol Vaadat ha-Sherutim ha-Tziburi'im [Protocol of Public Services], the Provisional Council of State, 7 November 1948, p. 3.
54. Halevi HS. Skirah al Peulot ha-Sherut ha-Refu'i le-Olim b-meshech shnat ha-Taktziv 1947/8 [Survey of Operations of the Immigrants Medical Service during the Fiscal Year 1946/7]. Tel Aviv Municipality Historical Archive, 4–1486.
55. Dostrovsky et al., Tinea Capitis.
56. 1940 Public Health Ordinance, Clause 11(A), Amendment 1949, Ben Gurion Heritage Institute Archive, Sde Boker. Special thanks to Dr. Rami Dycian for his assistance regarding amendments to the Public Health Ordinance.

57. Public Health Ordinance, 1949 Amendment, Ben-Gurion Heritage Institute, Sde Boker.
58. Tochnit ha-Avodah shel ha-Mador le-Milchamah b-Machalot Min ve-Machalot Or Sotzialiot [Work Plan of the Section for the War on Venereal Disease and Social Dermatoses]. Ministry of Health, 1950. Lavon Institute for Labour Movement Research Archive, IV-243-3-138.
59. Ordinance Corpus No. 98, 25 Iyar, 12 February 1950, p. 943.
60. Public Health Ordinance, 1949 Amendment; Ordinance Corpus No. 98.
61. It was cited only in a few sentences on p. 12 of the plan.
62. 15 Chodshei Sherut be-Misrad ha-Briut [15 Months Service in the Ministry of Health]. *Davar*, 6 December 1950, p. 2.
63. Dr. Felix Sagher (1908–1981) was born in Austro-Hungary and studied medicine in Prague, where he specialized in dermatology. He immigrated to Israel in 1938 and underwent specialized training in the United States in 1947–1948 in the treatment of leprosy. From 1958, he was a professor of dermatology at the Faculty of Medicine in Jerusalem. He is considered a world-renowned expert in leprosy and was an advisor to the World Health Organization on this subject. See: Levy and Levy, 208.
64. The "special medicine" could be obtained "from nurse Dvorah." From a letter to all the residents of the Jerusalem Corridor from Nurse Dvorah, no date, CZA S84/220.
65. Letter from Dr. Sagher to Dr. Kalman Mann, deputy director-general of Hadassah, 21 November 1949, CZA, J 2566-113. The practice of isolating children with ringworm in separate classrooms or even in separate schools began in France (see Chapter 3), where children with ringworm were sent to separate schools adjacent to the hospitals where they were being treated. A similar practice existed in the United States, and during the great ringworm epidemic in the 1940s in the Jewish community in New York, the New York Education Authority established special schools for pupils with ringworm (see Chapter 8).
66. Dr. Yosef Meir (1890–1953) was the first medical director of the GSF (1929–1948) and from 1948 to 1950 was the first director-general of the Ministry of Health. He studied medicine in Vienna, immigrated to Eretz-Israel in 1922, and specialized in pulmonary diseases, primarily tuberculosis. He was a core member of the National Council's (the self-governing body of the Jewish community during the British Mandate) Medical Central Committee. Levy and Levy, 275.
67. Levy-Lebhar G, Levy-Lebhar JP. L'épilation en serie des teigne du cuir chevelu par la radiothérapie. *Journal de radiologie, d'électrologie & archives de lectricite medicale*. 1953:630. Dr. Levy-Lebhar was chief radiologist at the ringworm treatment center in the Jewish community in Casablanca. In his article he cited the differences between the strains of fungi that caused ringworm among European children and among Middle Eastern and North African children. This difference led to the use of epilation employing a waxy substance to complete the treatment against ringworm in Israel and in North Africa, in contrast to the absence of this additional measure when treating children with ringworm in Europe. Dr. Mirko Brill was a dermatologist who immigrated to Israel from Yugoslavia, where he had participated in a UNICEF campaign to eradicate ringworm in the 1950s. In Israel he treated children with ringworm as a General Health Fund doctor in the Jezreel

Valley. He claimed that the ringworm fungus in Israel required mechanical means of epilatoin after irradiation, using *colifonium* (wax) and tweezers.
68. The 54th session of the 2nd Knesset (Tuesday, 12 February 1952). Jerusalem, Knesset, 1–4 p.m.
69. Dr. Mann to the head of the Tiberias Municipality, 27 December 1949, CZA J 2566-113.
70. Dostrovsky to Ministry of Health Management Jerusalem, Beer Sheva Health Bureau, to Hadassah Management, 6 January 1955, CZA, J 2566-113.
71. *Alopecia* = balding. *Atrophic dermatitis* = thinning of the upper layers of the skin that makes the skin more fragile and susceptible to ulceration.
72. The American Jewish Joint Distribution Committee, also known as the Joint or the JDC, is a Jewish relief organization based in New York City.
73. Drukmann's words about treatment in Morocco related to the treatment for ringworm carried out in Fez. Similar letters of complaint were also sent by other doctors. The Israeli Ministry of Heath's lack of authority regarding irradiation treatment against ringworm being carried out by the Jewish health organization OSE with funding from the Joint, in essence, blocked the ability of Israel to influence and stop treatments such as this in Fez. A letter to this effect on irradiation treatment in Fez is in the Israel State Archives, Gimmel-5088/1.
74. Drukmann to Dr. Davis, Hadassah director Jerusalem, 22 May 1950, CZA, 24405/113.
75. The *ma'abara*, a transit village, had relatively more solid temporary housing, mostly tin shanties. In the first years of statehood, there were 225 such transit camps that sheltered more than 220,500 newcomers, 80% of them Jewish refugees from Arab countries.
76. Reports of the number of children treated with irradiation at Rosh HaAyin are hazy, and therefore the numbers stated here are the maximums and minimums, as they appear in correspondence.
77. Documents in the archives of the Israel Electric Company reveal that there were problems with the electric power supply to Rosh HaAyin and as a result there was difficulty operating the radiology institute. Thanks to Mr. David Ben Ephraim, director of the department of Project Execution at the Israel Electric Company, who researched this issue for us in the company's archives.
78. This campaign involved sending children from the *ma'abarot* to live temporarily with individual families and to stay at youth villages during the unusually harsh and bitter winter of 1950–1951. In addition, the Army set up a special camp for children with trachoma adjacent to an Air Force base south of the city of Rechovot, run by the Israeli Air Force.
79. Alfei Yaldei Olim Nirshamim l-Korat Gag [Thousands of Immigrant Children are Signing Up for "Roof Over their Heads"]. *Davar*, 26 November 1950, p. 1. Hosting the children in various frameworks included not only food and lodging but also social activities, plays, celebrations, assistance with schoolwork, and more.
80. A document on the subject of closure of the Schneller camp, 12 July 1953, Israel State Archives, Gimmel-5087/5.
81. CZA, Hadassah portfolio J 2566-113.

82. Letter from the sick fund in Jerusalem to the Ministry of Health presenting a summary of treatment at Dr. Izmojik's practice, Israel State Archives, Gimmel-5088/9. Dr. Avraham Izmojik (1901–1960) was born in Paris. He operated a private radiology institute in Jerusalem and worked with Hadassah and the Leumit Sick Fund. Levy and Levy, 91.
83. Various correspondence on the subject of irradiation at Tel HaShomer, Israel State Archives, Gimmel 5088/3.
84. Approximately 20 private physicians were authorized at the outset of the 1950s to treat children with ringworm in Jerusalem, Tel Aviv, Haifa, Tiberias, Nazareth, Rechovot, Rishon le-Zion, Natanya, and Hadera under an agreement with the Ministry of Health, Hadassah, or the GSF. Most, if not all, were dermatologists or radiologists with private radiology institutes. All the doctors operated under the professional supervision of Hadassah. If doctors failed to operate according to the Hadassah's instructions, their work on Hadassah's behalf was suspended.
85. Grushka T. Sherutei ha-Briut b-Israel 1950/1951 [Health Services in Israel 1950/1951]. *Megamot*. 1968;3:298.
86. Shvarts S, Sevo G, Tasic M, Shani M, Sadetzki S. The Tinea Capitis Campaign in Serbia in the 1950s. *Lancet Infect Dis*. 2010;10:571–576. See more on this topic in Chapter 6.
87. UNICEF Archives, CF/HST/MON/1989-003.
88. Agreement between the United Nations International Children's Emergency Fund [UNICEF] and the Provisional Government of Israel, 20 September 1948, UNICEF Archives, NYC. The request on the part of the Israeli government for assistance, and its agreement to the aid program set forth by UNICEF, was not only executed due to exigencies of the time but also rested on confidence in the organization's motives and expertise from a longtime acquaintance with UNICEF's founder, Dr. Ludwik Rajchman. Rajchman, a Polish epidemiologist of Jewish origins and the founder and director of UNICEF, had strong ties with the heads of the Joint. Thus, it was only natural that with the establishment of the State of Israel, and with the arrival of mass immigration that brought a host of health problems that had to be addressed, the government of Israel viewed Rajchman and UNICEF as a major and friendly agent for aid. A letter (without a full signature) from the Department of [Jewish] National Institutions (*Machleikah l-Moshdot Le'umi'im*) to the Minister of Foreign Affairs, 22 August 1948, relates to the tie with Dr. Rajchman and UNICEF, CZA F 49/2007.
89. A countrywide network of public nursing stations that monitored pregnancies and infant care, promoted education in hygiene and childcare, administered inoculations, and monitored early childhood development.
90. Shula Tzarfati, Ashdod, interview, October 10, 2010.
91. Dr. Frederic Raubitchek (1908–1964) was born in Prague, where he studied medicine with a specialty in dermatology and venereal diseases. He immigrated to Eretz-Israel in 1939 and joined the dermatology department of Hadassah in 1945. For a short period, he headed the dermatology department of Ichelov Hospital in Tel Aviv. See Levy N, Levy Y. Rofeiha shel Eretz-Israel 1799–1948 [The Doctors of the Land of Israel 1799–1948] (2nd ed.). Zichron Yaakov; 2012:380.

92. Instructions of Professor Zagheir for treatment of ringworm, as sent to Dr. Yaffe, 27 September 1955, Israel National Archives 23/425. The content is quoted verbatim.
93. Leah Weissberger to Dr. Spiro, Jerusalem, 1953, Tebenkin Kibbutz HaMe'uchad Movement Archive—Ramat Efal, Temp. 1/196-15.
94. Ch. Sh. Halevy (deputy director-general of Hadassah) was appointed the first deputy director-general of the Ministry of Health.
95. Dr. Brill was chief of one of the hospitals for ringworm in Yugoslavia at the time of the ringworm campaign conducted there. See note 23 and Shvarts et al.
96. Brill M. al ha-Pitriot (Mikozot shel ha-Or) ve-al ha-Tipul b-Hem b-Yishuvei ha-Olim shel ha-Emek [On Fungi (Mycoses of the Dermis) and on their Treatment in Immigrant Settlements of the Emek]. *Dapim Refui'im*. 1968;11:311–316.
97. Afula, a small city that is the "capital" of the Jezreel Valley, absorbed a large number of new immigrants.
98. Dr. Pachthold, Bikoret Refu'it al ha-Aliyah, 1948–1956 [Medical Supervision of the Immigration 1948–1956]. Israel State Archives, Gimmel 4247/3.
99. Nitunim Statisti'im shel Gazezet ve-Ya'eret b-1959 [Statistical Data of Ringworm and *Favus* in 1959]. Ministry of Health, Epidemiology Unit, Israel State Archives, Gimmel 5088/9.
100. Cohen Y. Epidemologia shel Gazezet b-Israel [Epidemiology of Ringworm in Israel]. *Harefuah*. 1968;58(8):16–17.
101. Shvarts S. Health and Zionism. University of Rochester, NY, and Boydell & Brewer Press, UK; 2008. In 2019 about 52% of the Israeli citizens were insured by the GSF.
102. A radiology institute on Yavneh Street (opened in 1951) and the Sick Fund clinic adjacent to it, on nearby Ibn Sina' Street.
103. Tochnit ha-Avodah shel ha-Mador le-Milchamah b-Machalot Min ve-Machalot Or Sotzialiot [Work Plan of the Section for the War on Venereal Disease and Social Dermatoses], 12/10 1950, Lavon Institute for Labour Movement Research Archive IV-138-243.
104. Monthly accounts on treatment for ringworm and favus, October 1955, October 1956, and February 1957, Israel State Archives, Gimmel-5088/7.
105. Ha'arachat Hotzaot ha-Tipul neged Gazezet b-1956 [Estimation of Outlays of the Treatment for Ringworm in 1956], Dr. Yaakov Cohen, Ministry of Health, August 1957, Israel State Archives, Gimmel-5088/7.
106. Until 1975 there were six small public health funds in Israel (each providing health services to 5% of the population). In 1975 they merged into four public health funds, and in 1994 they all entered the framework of the National Health Insurance Law enacted in Israel.
107. The full cooperation of the GSF in formulating policy on treating ringworm emanated primarily from the fact that the GSF was the dominant player in providing health services and the largest health organization in Israel, serving close to 70% of Israel's population. It had opened local clinics in all the new immigrant settlements and *ma'abarot* and treated the overwhelming majority of new immigrants. It should be kept in mind that this policy of "bringing doctors to the people" in local clinics, rather than "sending people to the doctors," was not an ad hoc solution to the exigencies of the times; this pattern has been part of the GSF's

108. unique structure and part of the Fund's corporate culture since its founding in 1911.
108. Dr. Ernst Feilchenfeld noted that in 1934 he treated 100 Arabs and 20 Jews in his private clinic in Tel Aviv. He stressed that ringworm was endemic among Arab residents in the country. See: Feilchenfeld, 16.
109. In the days of the British Mandate, the municipality of Acre (whose population was overwhelmingly Arab) reached an agreement with the GSF that the Fund would operate a network of health services in the city's schools, including treatment with irradiation against ringworm. The establishment of statehood, and formulation of a national policy for treating ringworm, brought to a close the agreement between the municipality and the GSF, and the city turned to state authorities with the demand that treatment against ringworm for all schoolchildren in their jurisdiction continue, in keeping with the new policy.
110. At the time, feelings and ethnic tensions ran high in the aftermath of a horrific war in 1948–49 initiated by the local Arab population, from which the country was still recovering, coupled with the influx of some 680,000 immigrant Jews (most between 1948 and 1957) as a result of the departure, evacuation, flight, or expulsion of 850,000 Jews from Muslim countries in response to the establishment of Israel. Both the war and the burden of absorbing the immigrants served as a backdrop to apprehensions that a tinderbox would result from bringing local Arabs and Jews from Arab countries together at this time, in the same treatment setting. Moreover, emotions and existing pressure on health services tied to both events probably also played a role in priority setting and rejection of the appeal.
111. Feilchenfeld.
112. Dr. Simon Rosenblut, born in Poland, studied medicine in Switzerland (Zurich, 1936) and was a specialist in dermatology and public health. He worked as a doctor in Poland, was a Holocaust survivor, and immigrated to Israel in 1957. At the outset, he was a public health physician in Afula, and in December 1957 he was appointed to head the irradiation center for ringworm treatment in Nazareth for children of minorities.
113. Rosenblut S. Nisiyon le-Chisul ha-Gazezet ha-Endemit b-Kerev Bnei ha-Meeyutim b-Tzfon ha-Aretz [An Attempt to Liquidate Endemic Ringworm among Members of Minorities in the North of the Country]. *Briut HaTzibur.* 1968;6:449–461.
114. UNICEF and Israel, 1948-1985, HIST/66/Rev/1, 315739:3, UNICEF Archives.
115. Hatzlacha le-Shitah Chadashah be-Tipul Gazezet b-Hadassah [Success of a New Method in Treating Ringworm at Hadassah]. *HaAretz.* 15 December 1949.
116. Op. cit.
117. Despite the use of irradiation treatment for ringworm ceased in 1960, this treatment continued to be the accepted treatment for a host of other diseases. For example, the Zamenhof radiology institute of the General Health Fund in Tel Aviv continue to use irradiation for other diseases up until the 1970s.
118. Op. cit., note 67.
119. Bar Oz A. me-Achorei 'ha-Me'ah Elef' shel Parashat h-Gazezet [Behind the "One Hundred Thousand" of the Ringworm Affair]. *Harefuah.* (10)159:637–641.

10

"Think before you act"

Ringworm research in Israel, 1965–1995

SIEGAL SADETZKI-JACKOBSON

BACKGROUND

The aim of the Israeli tinea capitis (TC) studies is to assess the late health effects of childhood exposure to ionizing radiation of the head and neck region. The research is based on a population exposed to radiation in the 1950s for TC treatment. When the comprehensive study began, it focused on examining the risk of developing cancer among irradiated subjects, but over the years it has expanded to examine various other health outcomes.

The TC studies in Israel are based on a large study population and are conducted using reliable data sources (e.g., national morbidity records, personal interviews, and samples of biological material for DNA testing). The study is performed using up-to-date methods accepted in leading radiation studies. The studies include an individual assessment of radiation doses for 13,158 subjects, based on the original records of irradiation, so that the definition of exposure is validated, and the estimated risk of morbidity in these studies comprises quantitative data, expressed as excess risk per radiation unit. The study designs include follow-up (prospective) and case–control (retrospective) studies. The comparison populations (non-exposed subjects or controls who did not manifest morbidity) were matched for sociodemographic characteristics with exposed or affected subjects respectively.

In recent years the studies have been extended, as mentioned, to examine genetic sensitivity to radiation, using the innovative research tools of genetic epidemiology. In addition, interactions between radiation and other risk factors, both genetic and environmental (such as smoking), were investigated.

The studies' results have been implemented in legislation and in the formulation of appropriate medical guidelines for irradiated subjects. Thus, this research and its implementation serve as an informative model for illustrating epidemiology at each of its stages, from postulation of the scientific hypothesis, through the research in all its aspects, up to the elaboration of a health policy. The results of these studies help to refine the risk assessment by addressing specific questions like dose, age at exposure, gender, time elapsed between exposure and development of disease (latency period), and additional factors.

SCIENTISTS WHO CONTRIBUTED TO THE TC STUDIES

For the past 15 years TC studies have been conducted under the leadership and responsibility of the author of this chapter, Professor Siegal Sadetzki-Jackobson. The research represents a team project that has involved many scientists over the years. Among these, Angela Chetrit's significantly contributed to the data analysis and Dr. Abraham Werner, who began work as a medical physicist in the oncology department at the Chaim Sheba Medical Center in 1964, made an appreciable contribution in estimating the doses of radiation to which the subjects were exposed. Many additional scientists took part in the studies, contributing their share as part of their academic careers by preparing theses for master's and PhD degrees. An additional support team, without which it would have been impossible to conduct this important scientific work, comprised professionals from many varied disciplines, including nurses, interviewers, and fieldwork supervisors who recruited the study subjects and collected data; encoders and computer typists, who refined and completed the data; computer personnel and statisticians, who analyzed the data; and the supportive secretarial team.

The founding father of the "TC studies," as they are popularly known, or using their more formal title "Studies on the Health Effects of Exposure to Ionizing Radiation Used to Treat Tinea Capitis," was the late Professor Baruch Modan. Professor Modan was an outstanding scientist, among the initiators and foremost proponents of the discipline of epidemiology in Israel. For most of his academic and professional life, from 1966 to 2000, he was director of the Department of Clinical Epidemiology at the Chaim Sheba Medical Center, Tel HaShomer, and he transformed it into an exemplary venue for research, counseling, teaching, and training in the field of epidemiology. During his brilliant academic career, Professor Modan published more than 330 original articles on public health and epidemiology (in particular on cancer and late effects of radiation, as well as on the evaluation of health services, cardiovascular diseases, health policy, and aging).

From 1977 to 1984, Professor Modan was Deputy Director of the Ministry of Health, and subsequently its director. In this capacity, he initiated the Population Health Act in 1982, which mandated reporting of cancer cases to the National Cancer Registry.[1] This act was designed to ensure full and up-to-date reporting on new cases of cancer and enables the assessment of risk of developing cancer among various sectors of the population in Israel, including the population irradiated for TC.[2]

Professor Modan was born in Poland in 1932 and immigrated to Israel with his family in 1940. He completed his medical studies in 1958 at the Hebrew University in Jerusalem. From 1961 to 1964 he was at the School of Public Health at Johns Hopkins University in the United States, where he obtained his doctoral degree in public health, focusing on the association between radiation treatment for polycythemia vera and the development of leukemia. As a result, he began to take an interest in the effects of exposure to ionizing radiation on the development of cancer.[3]

In 1980 Professor Modan published an article in the *American Journal of Epidemiology* on the role of migrant studies in understanding the etiology[4] of cancer.[5] In the introduction he described the start of the TC studies (and perhaps the initiation of the discipline of epidemiology in Israel altogether) as follows:

> I first came to Hopkins because of a "migrant study." A very amateurish analysis of death certificates in Israel for the 1950–58 period—done as part of my MD thesis—revealed an increased leukemia rate in the 0–14 age-group among the Asian- and African-born... Looking for a plausible explanation, the question of previous exposure to therapeutic scalp radiation for tinea capitis, which was prevalent among this population, was raised. Meeting Abraham Lilienfeld,[6] I showed him the findings. His reaction that this was an interesting epidemiologic observation was a big surprise to me, since to my knowledge, leukemia was not considered an infectious disease, so why use the term "epidemiology"?[7] The response was "Come and see," and here I am—19 years later.

When he returned to Israel he continued to take an interest in the health effects of ionizing radiation, using the study population of subjects who had received therapeutic radiation for TC in Israel. The research program Modan aimed to implement entailed a comparison between the incidence[8] rates of cancer in irradiated subjects and those who had not been exposed to radiation. To this end he began to collect the treatment records of subjects irradiated for TC, to identify individuals who had received this treatment, and to seek appropriate populations for comparison. This constituted the original TC cohort (the "Modan cohort"), marking the start of the Israeli TC studies.

A prominent investigator who made a substantial contribution to the TC studies from 1974 to 1986 was Dr. Elaine Ron (1943–2010).[9] In 1980 she was awarded a doctorate by the Tel Aviv University for her thesis on risk factors for developing cancer and other late health effects in children following scalp irradiation for TC.[10]

THE ISRAELI TC STUDY: A FOLLOW-UP STUDY TO ASSESS MORBIDITY RISK—THE "MODAN COHORT"

Study population

In 1965 Professor Modan began a study aimed at assessing the possible influence of exposure to ionizing radiation given for treatment of TC on the risk of developing cancer. Out of about 20,000 individuals (Jews,[11] mostly new immigrants from North African countries [Morocco, Tunisia, Algeria, and Libya] and Asia [mainly from Iran, IrAQ: and Yemen]) who were treated with ionizing radiation in Israel, 16,473 original medical records were located from the archives of the medical institutions where the treatment was performed. Recorded in these files were the first name and family name of the patient, father's name, gender, year of birth, country of birth, and year of immigration to Israel.

Details of the irradiation performed for treating TC included date of treatment, irradiated field (the scalp was divided into three or five irradiation fields), body site irradiated, distance between the source of radiation and the skin at the irradiated site (tube–skin distance [TSD]), type of filter used, degree of irradiation in the roentgen tube,[12] the superficial dose (measured in rads on the skin), number of rads/minute,[13] and total duration of irradiation in minutes.[14] (An example of an original record appears in the Appendix to this chapter.)

Because the records did not include ID numbers,[15] the treated subjects were identified by searching the population registers by name, date of birth, and father's name. Once a subject (unique) was identified according to the demographic data mentioned, his/her ID number was recorded and the person was considered identified with certainty as having been irradiated for TC. All the individuals identified were entered in a data file that included demographic data, number of treatments, and date and location of first treatment.

This method of retrieval obviously did not allow for complete identification of all those treated, because sometimes the available details fitted more than one individual. For example, more than one individual answered to the description Cohen, Abraham, son of Cohen, Yaakov, born in Morocco in 1950. Because in such cases it was not possible to identify a single individual with certainty, such subjects were not included in the study population. Hence, persons with common family names, such as Cohen and Levy, were excluded in advance from the study, and no attempt was made to trace them individually. Due to this difficulty in authenticating the identity of the patient by name, name of father, and place and date of birth, Arab patients were not included in the compilation.

In addition, in order to compose a uniform research sample, individuals aged more than 15 years at the time of treatment were excluded (TC usually disappears spontaneously at older ages; see Chapter 1), as were European-born children (a minority among those treated) and individuals irradiated before 1949. This decision was made on scientific grounds, since a group composed of too few individuals (such as few adult irradiated subjects) does not have high enough statistical power for a reliable analysis of the findings.

A total of 12,386 subjects met the criteria for inclusion, of whom 88% were traced through the Central Population Registry. The final study population, known as the Modan cohort, includes 10,834 individuals identified by name who received ionizing radiation[16] (Figure 10.1). Mean age at the time of irradiation was 7.1 ± 3.1 years; 54% of the children were 5 to 9 years old at treatment, 23% were 10 to 15, and 23% were 0 to 4.

It should be noted that there is a controversy about using radiation in babies. Consequently, in the Modan cohort there are only four children under the age of 1 year who were irradiated, 3.8% who were treated at age 1 to 2 years, and 19.35% who were irradiated at ages 4 or 5. The gender ratio was similar (49% and 51% adjusted).

Most of the subjects irradiated were born in North Africa (59%), 20% were born in Asia, and 21% were born in Israel (most of them born to parents newly immigrated from North Africa and Asia).

An attempt was made to match each individual in the irradiated group with individuals from two comparison groups, as follows (see Figure 10.1):

Ringworm research in Israel

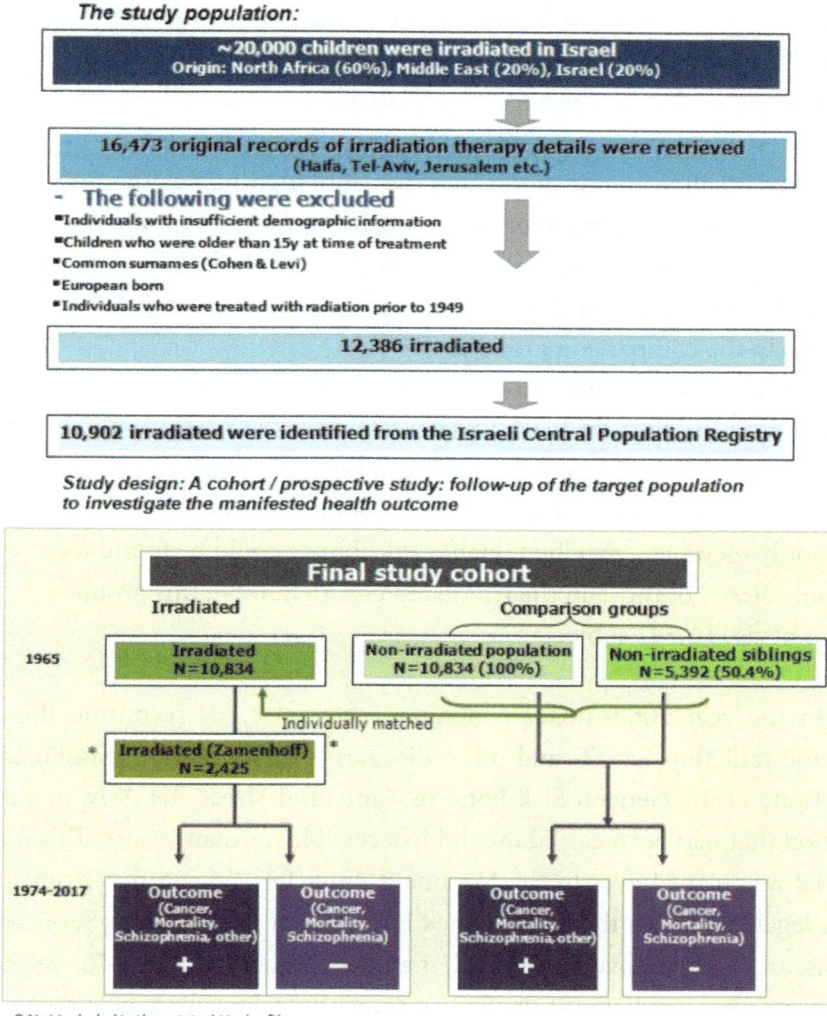

Figure 10.1 Flowchart

- *General population*—composed of 10,834 non-irradiated individuals, matched individually by gender, age (±2 years), country of birth, and date at immigration, to a subject in the irradiated group. It is important to note that while the level of verification regarding those who underwent irradiation is high, the fact that a given individual was found in the population register and was not found among those irradiated is not grounds for concluding that they were not irradiated. It is possible that some of these individuals were irradiated abroad, or even in Israel but lacked positive identification, and therefore their name does not appear in the Modan cohort as having been exposed. In other words, the Modan cohort contains, to a certain extent, flaws in classification (of people who were irradiated but were registered among the comparison group).

- *Family*—composed of non-irradiated siblings (brothers and sisters of irradiated subjects), matched by age (± 5 years), with a preference for siblings of the same gender as the exposed subjects. Because this was a contagious disease often affecting several family members, matched unaffected siblings could be found for only 50.4% of those in the irradiated group. In total, this group comprised 5,392 subjects.

In the year 2000, boxes containing original cards recording therapeutic radiation for TC and other diseases were found at the radiology institute of the General Sick Fund in Zamenhof Street, Tel Aviv, in a location that had been closed off and inaccessible for many years. This material was turned over to the National Center for Ringworm Victims by the legal counsel of the General Sick Fund (today Clalit Health Services). This archival discovery revealed that between 1944 and 1970, 38,795 patients were irradiated at the Fund's Zamenhof Clinic for a wide range of dermatologic ailments, including acne, herpes zoster, scabies, various skin inflammations, and more. Only 4,188 of these patients were irradiated for ringworm.[17]

From 2001 to 2003, 2,425 individuals who had received therapeutic irradiation for TC were identified with certainty from these records, and they were added to the "expanded Modan cohort." The identification process was similar to that used for the original subjects in the Modan cohort, using the same criteria for inclusion or exclusion (see Figure 10.1).

Study methodology

The study design chosen by Professor Modan for this research is known as follow-up (prospective). By this method, subjects exposed to the suspected risk factor, as well as individuals not exposed to it (the comparison group), are followed up. The results of the study are based on comparing the incidence rates of the health outcome under investigation (in this case, cancer) between the two groups. If there is no difference in the rate of the health outcome between the two groups, it is concluded that the investigated exposure factor (in this case, radiation) is not a risk factor for this effect. If the rate of the health outcome is found to be lower in the exposed versus the non-exposed group, it is concluded that the exposure constitutes a protective factor against the effect. When the rate of the effect is higher in the exposed group, it is concluded that exposure is a risk factor for the health outcome studied (see Figure 10.1).

Evaluation of the rate of the main health outcome in this study—development of cancer—was based on the Israel National Cancer Registry, which, as mentioned, was set up in 1960. Periodic quality control of the data revealed that the completeness of ascertainment for solid tumors approached 95%. Thus, one could say that in ringworm research, the information about development of cancer is full and complete, and there are no subcategories of cancer that were diagnosed among the research population that are not known to the researchers.[18]

Information on the cancer patient population was obtained by linking the Modan cohort with the cancer registry, using ID numbers and additional demographic data (name, gender, and year of birth) to verify the identification. For the linkage and identification of tumors the reviewers were unaware of whether the subject belonged to the exposed or the comparison groups (blinded). In the first linkage, updated to January 1, 1973, the information was supplemented with data from death certificates for the years preceding the establishment of the cancer registry (1949–1959). This updating allowed for the addition of cases of solid tumors as cause of death. Furthermore, the vital status of all subjects was checked against the population registry.[19]

Dosimetry

One of the outstanding advantages of the TC research is that the data include an estimate of average radiation dose for the whole research population as well as individual dosimetry estimates for each subject and for each organ. In 1968, and subsequently in 1971, the first papers by the Israeli TC research group were published. In these papers, Werner and Modan described the technical details involved in irradiation treatment of the subjects and estimated the radiation dose absorbed by different body organs, in particular the brain, skull, and thyroid gland.[20]

Most treatments for the patients in the Modan cohort were given soon after immigration to Israel, at a number of venues (Shaar HaAliyah in Haifa, Tel HaShomer in the center of the country, Hadassah University Hospital in Jerusalem, and additional locations). The therapeutic procedure followed the Kienböck–Adamson technique[21] in almost identical fashion at the different locations. After cutting the hair to a length of about 0.5 cm, the scalp was divided into five fields, each of which was irradiated on 1 of 5 consecutive days. Irradiation was performed by means of a superficial x-ray machine, by which penetration of the rays is relatively not high (75–100 kV). Air exposure at a focal skin distance (FSD) of 25 to 30 cm ranged between 350 and 400 roentgen per field,[22] depending on age.[23] Following irradiation, the children wore a hat or a sterile bandage for 18 to 21 days. Complete scalp epilation was subsequently performed by means of a wax cap, and the hair showed regrowth some 6 weeks later. This procedure was used in most of the children; about 10% were recalled for further therapeutic cycles (two to four cycles) using the method described above.[24]

Dosimetry estimates were performed on an anthropomorphic phantom, using the original x-ray machine, under the original therapeutic conditions. The phantom was constructed from a child-size skull (circumference about 50 cm) covered with a tissue-like substance. The findings indicated that the outer layer of the brain absorbed a dose of 121 to 139 rad,[25] while deeper layers (2.5 cm) absorbed about 8% to 20% less (95–121 rad); deeper still, in the area of the pituitary gland, a dose of 48 to 66 rad was absorbed. The posterior part of the skull absorbed more radiation than the anterior, and the left side of the brain more than the right.[26]

Estimates of average radiation dose absorbed by the different organs (in rad or cGy) was as follows:

152.0 ± 51.6 to the brain
9.4 ± 4.1 to the thyroid
78.2 ± 24.4 to the salivary glands
422.3 ± 139.3 to bone marrow in the skull
67.5 ± 26.4 to total bone marrow
50.8 ± 16.2 to the eye
1.73 ± 0.7 to the breast

The teeth absorbed 20 to 40 rad; the highest dose was absorbed by the posterior teeth. Average dose absorbed by the scalp skin was 6.1 and 6.8 rad for those who received a single treatment and for all subjects irradiated, respectively.[27] These radiation doses constitute part of the data recorded to date in the TC study file. These estimates are based on the dosimetry calculated by Dr. Werner during the 1960s as well as on personal average calculations performed by Dr. Marilyn Stovall, both during the 1980s and at the end of the 2000s (for the Zamenhof subjects). Following is the method of calculating the irradiation data, as described by Dr. Stovall:[28]

> Staff at the University of Texas M.D. Anderson Cancer Center supported these studies by providing dosimetry data since 1987 at the request of Elaine Ron at the Radiation Epidemiology Branch of the National Cancer Institute. The dosimetry data were based on data published by several investigators.[29] These data were measured in anthropomorphic child phantoms, using the cap to minimize radiation dispersing that localized the five treatment fields of the Adamson-Kienbock technique as well as face shielding. In addition, we made measurements in a water phantom using a Philips superficial X-ray machine at 70 kVp with a HVL of 1.1 mm AI [a superficial beam that doesn't penetrate deeply]. These water phantom measurements

were used to confirm the initial thyroid dosimetry and to expand the dosimetry to other ages and other organs, such as breast and teeth. We also analyzed the uncertainties in the dosimetry, which included patient age and size, machine calibration, patient movement during treatment, and variation in machine parameters.[30]

Individual dose for each organ was also estimated. We did not receive the detailed radiation records for individual patients; however, we did receive a summary from each center with standard treatment parameters and some sample records from Zamenhoff. Within each center, we assumed that all patients received the same exposure to each field and calculated doses to various organs for each patient based on the number of courses each patient received.

The question of accuracy in dosimetry estimates used in the TC studies is fundamental in evaluating the risk of developing cancer per radiation unit, as performed in later studies.[31] The suspicion of lack of precision in dosimetry estimates arose from situations such as movement of the child during treatment, or deviation from the accepted treatment guidelines. The possibility of lack of precision in estimating the exposure dose on the findings of the TC studies was examined by Schafer et al.,[32] who concluded that such measurement errors in dosimetry have only a negligible effect on risk calculations and the dose–response curve.

Findings

Risk assessment for tumor development in the irradiated area

The initial findings were published by Modan et al. in the *Lancet* in 1974.[33] The elevated rates of head and neck tumors in irradiated subjects versus the non-irradiated groups (general population and siblings) were already apparent from this early publication. This result was based on 27 cases of tumors (in the head and neck region alone) in the irradiated subjects versus eight cases in the comparison groups (six in the general population and two in siblings). High incidence rates in the exposed group versus the non-exposed groups were observed for brain tumors (eight cases in the irradiated group vs. two in the comparison groups), thyroid tumors (15 cases, of which 12 occurred among the irradiated), and salivary gland tumors (four cases, all in the irradiated group). In the discussion section of the article, the authors wrote, "As far as we can ascertain, ours is the first report to definitely demonstrate a role for ionizing radiation in the etiology of brain tumors in humans." Over the years, additional articles were published in which the follow-up period was extended and information was obtained on the risk of cancer in specific sites.[34]

Thyroid tumors

During the first study period, thyroid tumors represented the majority of the tumors diagnosed in the study group (15/35) and the risk of developing such tumors among the irradiated subjects was sixfold higher than in the comparison groups. Hence, Professor Modan decided to expand the study of this subject. It was thus decided to link the study population with surgical records from all hospitals in Israel to discover additional cases of cancer as well as benign tumors (adenomas) of the thyroid, which might not have been reported to the cancer registry. The findings indicated that exposure to radiation increased the risk of developing not only malignant thyroid tumors but also benign tumors.[35]

Because thyroid tumors span a broad spectrum in terms of the type of affected cell and the extent of damage (histologic grade), a supplementary study was conducted to validate the histologic diagnoses of the tumors as defined in the study (based on data from the cancer registry). For that purpose, the histologic data from 59 of the 68 subjects (irradiated and non-irradiated) were re-examined. The findings pointed to a 90% agreement between the original diagnosis and the one obtained in the study. Four out of 27 cases initially diagnosed as malignant were reclassified as benign (14.8% rate of misdiagnosis). Because the lack of agreement was similar for the irradiated and the comparison groups, the relative risk[36] shown for the association between radiation and tumor development was not significantly affected by classification errors.[37]

The magnitude of the risk of developing thyroid tumors among the irradiated subjects was updated by Ron et al. in a 1989 article[38] and subsequently by Sadetzki et al.[39] In the latter study, the effect of low-dose radiation absorbed by the thyroid (4.5–49.5 cGy) on the risk of developing thyroid cancer was investigated, based on 159 tumors (an additional 100 tumors since the previous data analysis, and an additional 144 tumors since the initial analysis). This data analysis was performed up to 54 years after the time of exposure. The excess relative risk per radiation unit (excess relative risk per Gray [ERR/Gy]) for the whole group reached 20.2 (95% confidence interval [CI], 11.8–32.3[40]). The risk was found to increase with higher doses of radiation and with earlier ages at exposure. The elevated risk began to appear 10 to 19 years after the radiotherapy, peaked at 20 to 30 years after exposure, and decreased slightly 40 years after exposure (although it remained significantly high even after this period). The elevated risk was observed for both papillary and follicular tumors. It should be mentioned that the risk estimate found in this study was two to 18 times greater than that estimated in similar studies, although it was within the confidence limits obtained in a pooled analysis conducted on this subject.[41] Since then, the data from the TC studies were also shared and contributed to a more recent pooled analysis.[42]

These findings concerned the researchers, who wondered whether they should try to locate the irradiated populations for early detection of tumors that might have developed in the thyroid. The question of the need for a foundation for early detection of such tumors among those undergoing screening was raised a number of times over the years. This complex matter was also discussed throughout the world in regard to exposure to radiation in various circumstances, including the disaster at the Chernobyl power plant in the Ukraine in April 1986 and at Fukushima in Japan in March 2011.

Brain tumors

Toward the end of the 1980s, the first article dealing in detail with the individual risk of developing brain tumors after radiotherapy for TC in childhood was published in the *New England Journal of Medicine*.[43] Based on 60 brain tumors diagnosed over a period of 30 years, the risk of developing nervous system tumors in the head and neck region was found to be 8.4 times greater among subjects exposed to radiation (95% CI, 4.8–14.8) than in the comparison groups. Increased risks were most apparent for meningiomas (mostly benign brain tumors), for which the relative risk (RR) was 9.5 (95% CI, 3.5–25.7); gliomas (tumors of the brain tissue, which are usually malignant), RR = 2.6 (95% CI, 0.8–8.6); nerve sheath tumors, RR = 33.1 (95% CI, 9.4–116.6); and "other neural tumors," RR = 6.0 (95% CI, 1.5–23.5). These findings indicated a dose–response association,[44] with the RR approaching 20 after estimated doses of 2.5 Gy. The findings indicated that radiation doses of 1 to 2 Gy (considered a medium dose) could significantly increase the risk of developing neural tumors.

The possible role of the radiation treatment given for TC performed in Israel during the 1950s in the development of meningiomas was also reported by a group of physicians from the neurosurgery department at Hadassah University Hospital in Jerusalem.[45] As early as 1972, Beller et al. described the clinical features of a series of 16 patients diagnosed with intracranial meningiomas who had previously received ionizing radiation for treatment of TC. The latency period from exposure to diagnosis ranged from 22 to 45 years. In this article the investigators noted that ionizing radiation was considered the treatment of choice for TC, and they cited the 1969 article by Munk et al. describing five cases of meningioma following radiotherapy for TC.[46] In their discussion Beller et al. pointed out that according to reports by Davidoff et al. in 1938,[47] the meningeal tissue reacts to irradiation with different degrees of inflammatory response. Consequently, the authors adopted Zulch's hypothesis[48] that "misregeneration" of the tissue following trauma or inflammation could be a possible cause for development of tumors. With regard to the dose effect, the authors cited the 1964 article by Fabrikant et al.[49] suggesting that in tumor formation, the type and the degree of tissue alteration were more important than the radiation dose. Today it is know that the development of a tumor after exposure to radiation occurs primarily due to damage to genetic material in the cell (DNA); if this damage does not repair itself and destruction of the damaged cell does not occur, it is liable to trigger a malignant process.

Beller et al. estimated that 15,000 individuals in Israel had received radiotherapy for TC between 1948 and 1951. They noted that the original radiotherapy records were not accessible and thus the individual doses received could not be assessed. In their conclusion, they suggested that if exposure to radiation were indeed associated with the development of intracranial meningiomas, many more cases of such tumors could be expected in the future.

In 1983 a group of investigators led by Professor Soffer published an article comparing a series of 42 cases of radiation-induced meningiomas with 84 meningiomas that were not radiogenic.[50] This series comprised all the intracranial meningiomas that had developed following radiotherapy for TC in childhood diagnosed at the Hadassah University Hospital during the years 1952 to 1981. Analysis of these data indicated that although it was not possible to distinguish between radiation-induced and "spontaneous" tumors at the individual level, there were appreciable differences between the groups regarding the location and aggressiveness of the tumors.

In 1984, another team of Israeli neurosurgeons published a clinical and histopathologic description of 201 cerebral meningiomas operated on during the years 1978 to 1982 at the Rabin Medical Center in the center of the country.[51] Forty-three patients in this group reported having undergone ionizing radiation of the head region in the past, most of them for TC. The findings of this study, too, indicated differences between the radiation-induced tumor group and the "spontaneous" group.

One needs to clarify that there is a significant different between (1) the comparative epidemiologic research carried out by Modan (in 1974) in which analytic methods showed an elevated risk of developing a meningioma following radiation and (2) the theoretical research studies reported by Beller et al. (in 1972). The theoretical research was a preliminary and important clinical observation that raised assumptions that required factual and quantitative reinforcement that epidemiologic research can provide.

Research on the effects of irradiation on the development of brain tumors in general, and meningiomas in particular, was expanded at a later date by Sadetzki et al. In any case, it is important to stress that in the 1980s up until the first decade of the 21st century, the medical community was divided about whether brain tissues and the meninges are sensitive to ionizing radiation.

Breast cancer

A complex and interesting subject, still under debate today, is the possibility that the minimal dose absorbed in the breast region (16 mGy) could have caused an increased risk of breast cancer among women irradiated in childhood for TC. This possibility was first discussed toward the end of the 1980s, again in the *Lancet*.[52] The findings at that time pointed to a significantly higher risk of developing breast cancer during the years 1982 to 1986 among women who had undergone radiotherapy for TC when they were 5 to 9 years old (RR > 12; 95% CI, 3.16–46.7).

Modan and colleagues were skeptical about these findings, emphasizing that they should be interpreted with caution as they may have been due to chance alone. In this regard, the hypothesis was raised that for some reason (coincidentally), the incidence of breast cancer was very low among the comparison group with which the girls irradiated at age 5 to 9 years were paired (0 cases compared to 10 cases diagnosed among those irradiated). Therefore, the distribution of the incidence of breast cancer among the irradiated group compared to the RR of breast cancer among the comparison group of the same age showed a significantly higher RR.

This explanation seems to discount the possibility of a true excess of breast cancer among the irradiated women and supports the idea that the findings were due to an artifact and not a true association. Another possibility proposed by the authors was that the results could have been due to inaccurate estimates of the radiation dose absorbed in the breast.

Parallel to this, the researchers cited a number of postulations that could explain the finding biologically, despite the low dosages of irradiation, if indeed the results are true. These explanations include arguments that breast tissue is known to be sensitive to radiation (although existing proof is correlated with higher levels of radiation) and it is possible that young breast tissue (around the onset of puberty) is particularly sensitive to radiation. Or, alternatively, the radiation absorbed in the area of the hypophysis[53] in the brain (48–66 mGy) could have an effect on the incidence of breast cancer due to damage to the endocrine axis, which would impact the secretion of hormones, including prolactin, and thus disrupt ovulation and the menstrual cycle. The researchers recommended continued study of this matter in order to further establish the findings and verify the data. In this matter as well, further study was conducted at later periods, and many discussions were conducted at the Ministry of Health on this issue. Although an additional risk of developing breast cancer was found among those irradiated and the findings were replicated in subsequent analysis of the data, breast cancer is not considered grounds for compensation under the ringworm law.

Skin cancer
Radiation-associated skin neoplasms are a recognized phenomenon, observed both in experimental animals and in human studies. At the same time, not all radiation studies have demonstrated an association between ionizing radiation and the development of skin tumors, and it has been claimed that the association has been observed only in Caucasians. Consequently, the TC studies provided an opportunity to examine the effect of radiation on subjects with medium skin color (ranging from light to dark).

To examine this question, investigators reviewed the records of the pathology departments at all Israeli hospitals (22 at the time) for the results of biopsies performed and diagnosed as benign[54] or malignant skin tumors in the head and neck region for the years 1950 to 1980. The malignant tumors were divided into melanoma and non-melanoma[55] tumors. More than 2 million records were reviewed; 59,000 of them were considered suitable for linkage with the study population (by age and country of origin, similar to those in the Modan cohort).[56]

A diagnosis of any skin tumor was made in 58 individuals in the irradiated group, 16 in the general-population comparison group, and six in the non-irradiated sibling group. Melanoma was diagnosed in two individuals in the exposed group and one only in the comparison groups, and the excess risk of developing this malignancy following irradiation was not significant (RR = 3.0; 95% CI, 0.3–33.1). Conversely, the risk of developing non-melanoma cancer and the risk of developing benign skin tumors were significantly higher in the irradiated group versus the comparison groups (RR = 4.2; 95% CI, 2.3–7.6 and RR = 3.5; 95% CI, 1.4–9.1, for these tumors, respectively).

Most of the non-melanoma malignant rumors were basal cell carcinomas (BCC): 98% (41/42) in the irradiated group and 87% (13/15) in the non-irradiated groups. Further data analysis was performed regarding these tumors to reveal additional factors that could have influenced the risk. The results indicated that the linear dose–response curve was appropriate in describing the risk ($p < 0.01$); the risk per radiation unit increased significantly with decreasing age at exposure and was similar for both genders and for the different ethnic origins.

In general, it is known that the incidence of skin tumors differs between different ethnic groups and that in Israel, Jews of North African and Asian origin show relatively lower rates of these disorders. In an attempt to ascertain the individual factors that may have caused skin cancer following radiation exposure among certain individuals in the TC study (and not in others), a nested case–control[57,58] study was conducted examining the physical and behavioral characteristics that could have influenced the development of the disease.[59]

In a multivariate analysis, two main factors emerged that may have been responsible for the appearance of skin cancer: (1) a higher radiation dose, as expressed by a higher frequency of radiation skin damage among the irradiated and (2) more frequent exposure to the sun (tanning). It is important to note that despite the above, all types of malignant tumors (including melanomas that, as noted, are not related in any way to radiation) are among the morbidities eligible for compensation under the ringworm law.

Salivary gland tumors

The salivary gland was another specific site of cancer for which a significant association with irradiation was determined.[60] Focused research of such tumors found that the incidence of malignant tumors of the salivary gland was 4.5 times higher among irradiated individuals than among the comparison group, and the incidence of benign tumors was 2.6 times higher. There was a clear dose–response association for both types of tumors.

Hematologic neoplasms

A separate report dealing with hematologic cancer was not published in the context of the TC studies, at least up until 2017. However, a data analysis expressing the risk of developing such cancers at various periods was included in the framework of various studies on other tumors discussed above. A data analysis updated to 1981, in which the incidence of leukemia in the irradiated group was compared with that in the two comparison groups (general population and siblings), revealed an RR of 2.6 (95% CI, 1.30–5.29).[61] In the update to 2002, the relative risk decreased to 1.34 and was not statistically significant (95% CI, 0.78–2.29) (unpublished data). It is interesting to note that no association between radiotherapy and lymphoma was demonstrated in the TC studies (up to 1981, RR = 0.91; 95% CI, 0.52–1.59; and in the 2002 update, RR = 0.78; 95% CI, 0.55–1.11). Here as well, there is a discrepancy between clinical studies and what is stipulated in the ringworm law.

GENERAL FINDINGS ASSOCIATED WITH CANCER DEVELOPMENT

Over the years, additional risk assessments were performed for which the follow-up period was extended and the influence of individual factors such as gender, age at exposure, and ethnic origin on the development of cancer was discussed. In interpreting the findings of these studies, various hypotheses were raised to explain the findings. These hypotheses formed the basis for further scientific investigation in later studies.

For example, in the update published in 1984,[62] exceptionally high rates of thyroid gland neoplasms were found in subjects born in North Africa, especially those from Morocco and Tunisia (vs. those born in Asia and Israel). Two hypotheses were put forward by the investigators as possible explanations for this phenomenon. The first was that this group may have absorbed higher doses than those estimated by the investigators. In this context Ron and Modan pointed out for the first time that radiotherapy was also commonly administered in Morocco, so part of this subpopulation may have been treated in their country of origin before immigrating to Israel. If this assumption is valid, then the radiation dose recorded for these subjects (including only the dose they absorbed in Israel) is lower than the actual total radiation dose they had absorbed. This also gave rise to the possibility that some of the subjects in the comparison group had actually been exposed to radiation.[63]

The second hypothesis discussed by the authors in the context of the excess risk for developing cancer apparently observed in the subjects of North African origin was that this population may have a greater genetic susceptibility to developing cancer. They might be more sensitive to radiation as a result of being carriers of a specific gene mutation (ATM [ataxia telangiectasia mutation]) that suppresses cancer (tumor suppressor gene[64]) and plays a key role in the control of cell division, apoptosis,[65] and the reaction to DNA damage, such as reparation of double-stranded breaks that characterize radiation damage. A homozygous mutation[66] of this gene causes the serious disease ataxia telangiectasia, which is characterized, among other phenomena, by neurodegeneration, cerebral ataxia, and also sensitivity to ionizing radiation and an increased risk of developing tumors following exposure.[67] It is known that among Jews of Moroccan origin (who constitute a major part of the population treated by radiotherapy for TC), there are relatively high rates of carriers and individuals affected with this disease compared with the general population. It is estimated that 1.2% of this population is heterozygous[68] for a founder mutation[69] at this gene.[70] Hence, the authors proposed that an interaction[71] between sensitivity to radiation and a predisposition to developing cancer among heterozygotes for the ATM gene could be responsible for the elevated risk of developing cancer among North African immigrants in the TC-treated subjects. However, the authors stated they were skeptical about this hypothesis.

An additional finding of a suspected higher susceptibility to radiogenic tumors among women led investigators to the hypothesis that a radiation dose of 48 to 66 rad absorbed by the pituitary gland could result in hormonal changes that enhance the development of brain tumors.[72] They pointed out the difficulty of distinguishing between benign and malignant brain tumors in most studies and emphasized the importance of accurate data analysis on this issue. Although the finding of elevated risk among women was not confirmed in the later studies, in the in-depth discussion mentioned above, the authors emphasized the importance of various host factors and their possible influence on the risk involved in radiation exposure. They thus proposed that further data should be collected on hormonal function, comorbidity, and inherited diseases in the study population. At this stage it was proposed to conduct a survey that included distribution of postal questionnaires to about 10% of the population in order to expand the data collected for this study.

Assessment of the Risk of Other Health Outcomes (Mortality, Hormonal Disturbances, Early Cataract Formation, and Mental Function)

Assessment of cerebral function, cognitive effects, and mental processes

In 1980 an article was published evaluating cerebral function in subjects irradiated in childhood, assessed using visual evoked response (VER).[73] This test examines mainly the cortical response to direct visual stimulation. At that time decreased amplitude in VER had been observed in experimental animals and patients who had undergone ionizing radiation for brain neoplasms (and were subjected to high doses of radiation). In this study, 44 irradiated subjects were compared with 57 non-irradiated controls, matched for age (range 20–35 years) and ethnic origin. The findings demonstrated significant differences between the VER averages of the study groups. The authors concluded that these differences could reflect delayed functional damage to the central nervous system, caused by radiation exposure to the immature human brain. The left hemisphere appeared to be more involved, consistent with the fact that the children had received, on average, higher doses of x-rays to the left side of the brain, as shown in the simulated phantom models.[74] The major differences observed were in sub-cortical response, a finding that could also indicate damage to the visual system. The investigators pointed out that the subjects were unaware that the findings could be associated with the radiotherapy they had undergone in childhood, that all subjects were healthy and not on medication, and that, to the best of their knowledge, TC does not in itself cause neurotoxic changes, even in severe cases.

In an additional study that reviewed electroencephalographic (EEG) responses in 44 irradiated subjects and 59 non-irradiated individuals, differences between the two groups were observed, especially with regard to distribution of β-waves.[75]

In the early 1980s, 20 years after exposure, Ron, Modan, and colleagues sought to assess the effects of irradiation on the central nervous system using a number of mental parameters.[76] While not all the comparisons were statistically significant, there seemed to be a consistent trend for irradiated subjects to exhibit signs of central nervous system impairment more often than either comparison group. Irradiated children scored lower in scholastic aptitude tests scores,[77] intelligence quotient (IQ), and psychological test results.

From 1966 to 1970, 38% of the irradiated children took the scholastic aptitude test, compared with 46% and 44% in the sibling and general-population comparison groups, respectively ($p < 0.005$). The mean scores were 59.4, 61.2, and 61.0, respectively. The teachers' evaluation scores agreed with this grading. It is interesting to note that the scores for the children who received multiple treatment doses were on average slightly lower than those who received a single treatment, but the difference was not significant.

Unrelated to irradiation, children born in Israel had higher scores than those born abroad; those who had immigrated at an early age (1–5 years) scored higher than those who immigrated later (6–8 years); and boys scored higher than girls. The authors pointed out that these findings suggested that immigrant children adapted relatively slowly to the Israeli educational system.

As a direct index of mental function, IQ tests performed before mobilization to military service were compared in the study groups. On comparing the scores required for officer training it appeared that the percentage of eligible candidates was lower in the exposed (irradiated) group than in the matched groups of siblings or the general population ($p < 0.005$ and $p < 0.001$, respectively). In addition, two psychological tests were performed, as used by the Army to predict leadership potential. In these tests, too, the irradiated group fared less well, although the differences were not statistically significant. Moreover, it was found that more individuals in the irradiated group were exempted from military service on psychological grounds. The exposed (irradiated) group completed fewer school grades and had an increased risk for mental hospital admission for certain disease categories, and there seemed to be a slightly higher frequency of mental retardation in this group.

At the time of this study, 351 subjects from the Modan cohort had been admitted at one time or another to psychiatric hospitals (151 irradiated subjects, 137 in the general population, and 63 in the sibling group). Mean age at hospitalization was 19.5, 20.2, and 20.5 years, respectively. These findings indicated that the risk of psychiatric hospitalization was 10% and 20% higher in the irradiated group, compared with the general-population and the sibling comparison groups, respectively. The disease categories for which higher rates of admission were recorded included epilepsy, observation, and mental retardation. The association with irradiation was strengthened by the findings in the group that was irradiated more than once.

Two hundred sixteen persons (0.8%) in the Modan cohort were diagnosed as mentally retarded (compared to the 1–3% incidence cited in the world literature of that time). Of these, 94 were from the irradiated group, 64 from the general-population comparison group, and 58 from the sibling comparison group. Familial retardation was observed in four irradiated/sibling pairs.

These findings led the investigators to conclude that although no single measure of mental function was sufficient in itself to point to a general agreement on a causal relationship between irradiation and mental effects, it was clear that a broad range of indices, both objective and subjective, consistently demonstrated signs of impairment in mental function among irradiated subjects versus the control groups, leading to the conclusion that irradiation of the immature brain could damage the central nervous system.

These findings undoubtedly point to the need for further study of the effects of early exposure to radiation on various (and late) cognitive parameters in the TC study population, including psychological impairment such as depression and anxiety, memory impairment, Alzheimer's disease or early development of senile dementia, psychiatric disturbances, and more. A study examining specifically the possible association between exposure to radiation and schizophrenia was conducted at a later date.

Mortality

After an average follow-up period of 26 years, when the mean age of the tinea-affected subjects was only 33 years, a study was conducted to assess the effect of radiation on mortality.[78] This was done by linking the identity numbers listed in the Modan cohort with the Israel population registry. In another study conducted at about the same time, the percentage of individuals lost to follow-up through emigration was assessed (based on population registry data that also included leaving the country). According to this estimate (updated to 1982), 5% of the study population had emigrated, with no significant difference between the different study groups.[79]

In the mortality follow-up,[80] 609 deaths occurring between 1950 and 1982 were reviewed (individual cause of death was recorded for 569 of them). Mean age at death was 23 years in the irradiated group and 27 and 25 in the general-population and the sibling comparison groups, respectively (range 6–43 years). The period elapsed between irradiation and death ranged from 2 to 28 years, with no significant differences between the study groups: Average time elapsed between exposure and death was

16.3 years for the irradiated subjects, 18.9 years for the general-population comparison group, and 16.7 years for the sibling comparison group.

Comparison of mortality rates among irradiated subjects with those in the general population of Israel showed a 30% excess (specific mortality rates adjusted for age, gender, and ethnic origin; SSMR = 1.3; 95% CI, 1.1–1.4). It is important to note that the mortality rates for the two comparison groups in the study (general population and siblings) did not differ significantly from those for the general Israeli population. Thus, there was a 30% elevated risk of mortality in the irradiated group compared with the general-population comparison group and a 10% increase with respect to the sibling comparison group.

Excess mortality was due mainly to death from neoplastic diseases (tumors of the head and neck region and leukemia) and unknown causes. Overall, 40% of all cancer deaths among irradiated subjects were radiogenic (70% for head and neck tumors and 57% for leukemia). Mortality rates for other neoplastic diseases were similar for the irradiated group and for the comparison groups. Unrelated to irradiation, 50% of the causes of death were external, mainly traffic accidents (16%) or other accidents, such as drowning, burns, or falls (11%), or events related to military service (21%). Mortality in males was twice as high as in females. The gender difference in mortality rates was particularly prominent for the external causes, these rates being fourfold higher among males, while deaths from disease were only 1.2 times higher.

The investigators suggested that an estimate of the actual impact of irradiation on mortality should be performed at a later date to take into account the increasing age of the study population. These findings undoubtedly indicated that the elevated risk of mortality and its causes among irradiated subjects should be re-examined as they reach the age ranges for death from natural causes.

Hormonal disturbances and reduced fertility
Hormonal disturbances and impaired fertility are recognized side effects of ionizing radiation at relatively high doses of 0.75 to 6.0 Gy to the testes and 4 to 10 Gy to the ovaries. But the consequences of low-dose

irradiation of the gonads[81] and medium- to high-dose irradiation of the brain in childhood (and hence its effect on the endocrine axis: pituitary–hypothalamus–gonad) are not clear.

Hence, within the framework of the TC studies it was decided to conduct a study to assess the effect of brain exposure to ionizing radiation in childhood on the level of fertility and on the hormonal status of both males and females. The target population for this study included 3,215 irradiated subjects who had same-gender siblings (in addition to the comparison population of the same gender, matched to all the irradiated subjects). Accordingly, during the years 1987 to 1990, 7,660 individuals from the three study groups were interviewed (1,266 irradiated females and 1,339 males, and a similar number of non-irradiated matched controls [siblings and general population]). This sample constituted 80% of the target population.

Data collection for this extensive study was performed by personal interviews and comprised demographic data (including family status and age at first marriage), occupational data, information on current and past health status (including hospital admissions), smoking habits, and anthropometric parameters (height and weight). Fertility disturbances and hormonal status were assessed by collecting information about age at menarche and menstrual regularity for the females, and age at first shaving for males, as well as a detailed obstetric history of the female interviewees or the spouses of the men (number of pregnancies, deliveries, abortions, age at first childbirth, fertility problems and their treatment if relevant, and contraceptive use). Age of irradiated subjects at the time of the interviews was 30 to 52 years (mean 39.2 ± 4.1). The rate of unmarried individuals was less than 5%, and the average years of schooling of all the interviewees was 10 years.

The data were analyzed using the univariate and multivariate conditional logistic regression model. This model assessed the risk of developing hormonal disturbances with each of the life events studied, along a time axis (e.g., age at menarche precedes age at first childbirth). The analysis was performed separately for males and females, while comparing the irradiated group with the sibling group and the general population.

The detailed findings of this study are still being elaborated prior to submission for publication. It may be mentioned that on the whole no differences in the frequency of most study parameters were observed between the irradiated subjects and the comparison groups. The relative risk was very close to 1, and the confidence interval in most cases was very narrow, suggesting a lack of association between exposure to ionizing radiation and the health effects or events studied. Exceptions were the age at first marriage (which was significantly higher among the irradiated women relative to the comparison groups) and the number of live births (which was higher among the wives of the irradiated males relative to their comparison groups).

Cataract

Damage to the lens, including opacity, is a known side effect of exposure to ionizing radiation. In the late 1990s extensive eye examinations were performed (including slit-lamp photography of the cortical, nuclear, and posterior subcapsular lens) for 81 irradiated subjects in the Modan cohort to detect early cataract formation. The examination was performed by a professional ophthalmologist (Professor Orna Geier) at a hospital in central Israel. Age of the irradiated subjects at the time of examination ranged from 45 to 57 years (mean 50.2 ± 2.8), and a third had received more than one radiation treatment. The estimated dose of radiation absorbed by the eyes was 61.2 ± 28.6 Gy. Opacity was classified as 0 = no opacity, 1 = early opacity, and 2 = pronounced opacity, with cataract defined as grade 1 or more.

The incidence of cataract in this group was 29.6% (20.3% cortical, 14.3% posterior subcapsular, and 6.3% nuclear). While the incidence of cataract (of all types) was similar in males and females, a negative association with educational level was found. The incidence of cortical cataract was elevated in subjects who reported diabetes compared with non-diabetics (57% vs. 17%, $p = 0.01$).

While no association was detected between age at exposure and development of cataract of any type, there was a positive association between the dose of radiation and the appearance of cortical cataract (an excess of

2% in risk for each Gy unit of radiation, adjusted for diabetes, educational level, and gender). These findings, which agree with reports in the scientific literature, hint at a higher incidence of cortical cataract in a relatively young population following early exposure to ionizing radiation.

This study was not published because of the relatively small sample and especially because of low compliance of the comparison groups of non-irradiated subjects, who declined to attend the examinations performed at the medical center.

CONCLUSIONS

Ionizing radiation from natural sources (cosmic radiation, the sun, and various radioactive elements in the earth and in rocks, such as potassium, uranium, thorium, and especially radon gas) has accompanied humanity from time immemorial. During the 20th century, since the discovery of x-rays by Wilhelm Konrad Roentgen in 1895, and the subsequent discovery of radioactivity by Henri Becquerel in 1896, additional artificial sources of radiation have been added for various purposes, including war, industry, and medicine, and the segment occupied by medical radiation is ever on the increase.

During the years of research described in this chapter, the causal association between exposure to ionizing radiation and the development of neoplastic diseases has been clearly recognized. From this viewpoint, the TC research has added to the series of studies performed during those years throughout the world in terms of understanding the damage caused by ionizing radiation. These studies began with observations and case studies and expanded into analytic research that included the follow-up studies on the survivors of the atomic bombs released on Hiroshima and Nagasaki in 1945 (focusing on medium- and low-dose radiation) and studies conducted after fallout and nuclear accidents such as those of the Marshall Islands and Chernobyl. An appreciable number of studies dealt with populations exposed to medical irradiation, including diagnostic radiation (low-dose) and therapeutic radiation for the treatment of benign disease (medium-dose) and malignant disease (high-dose). Additional studies dealt with workers exposed to occupational radiation and environmental radiation from natural sources, especially exposure to radon gas in residential environments (low-level chronic radiation).

Experimental studies to examine the effect of radiation on the formation of tumors were conducted mainly after World War II and established biologic mechanisms explaining carcinogenic damage. Hence, the role of ionizing radiation as a cancer initiator, acting directly through damage to cellular genetic material, was explained by the destruction of links in the DNA strands or indirectly by releasing free radicals.[82] Such damage can lead to cell death or cause mutations or other genetic alterations, which, unless repaired, can cause tumors in exposed tissues.

The TC studies have made a considerable and invaluable contribution to knowledge on this subject. Indeed, they were ground-breaking in a number of fields, including recognition of the importance of ionizing radiation in the development of brain tumors (a controversial subject for many years) and awareness of the effect of low-dose radiation on tumors of the thyroid, an organ whose sensitivity to higher-dose radiation was recognized relatively early.

The TC studies began as a scientific project, but at a relatively early stage, the investigators raised additional health and ethical questions regarding the irradiated population. At first these questions focused on medical aspects only (the need for timely action for early detection of morbidity that might arise from radiotherapy), but subsequently complex social and legal questions were raised. These questions gave rise to the Ringworm Victims Compensation Law, that passed in 1994 based on the results of the studies described in this chapter. The law necessitated continuation and expansion of the scientific research which indeed developed under the supervision of the author of this chapter to include the investigation of more health outcomes using wider range of methodologies and study design.

APPENDIX A

Appendix A: **Photocopy of original clinical record of Tinea capitis treatment**

The 1951 clinical record documents the personal details of a male patient born in Israel in 1945, showing a diagnosis of Trichophytis (Tinea Capitis), and recording 3 treatments to the head region, the TSD (Tube-Source Distance), the dose given per minute, and the duration of each treatment in minutes.

NOTES

1. The Cancer Registry in Israel has operated since 1960 and today includes report on cases of malignancy in Israel and cases of meningiomas (primarily benign tumors of the meninges).
2. Knesset Record (*Reshumot*) Ordinances Compilation 4335 11/4/1982. *Takanot Bri'ut ha-Am—Divu'ach ve-Meida Miyuchad al Machalat ha-Sartan 1982* (Public Health Regulations—Report and Special Data on Cancer 1982), Jerusalem, pp. 833–834.
3. Modan B, Lilienfeld AM. Polycythemia vera and leukemia: The role of radiation treatment. Medicine, 1965, 44:305–344.
4. Etiology = study of causes or factors; causality.
5. Modan B. Role of migrant studies in understanding the etiology of cancer. Am J Epidemiol, 1980.
6. Abraham Lilienfeld (1920–1984) was a renowned oncologist and a pioneer in the epidemiologic methodology of chronic diseases. In 1950 he joined the faculty of Johns Hopkins Medical School in the department of hygiene and public health. He was appointed assistant professor of epidemiology in 1952, and in 1970 he was appointed professor and head of the epidemiology department.
7. The discipline of epidemiology dealt initially with the study of infectious diseases, leading to the association of the word "epidemiology" with infectious disease.
8. Incidence rates = number of new cases of a specific disease appearing within a defined period of time in a given population. This figure expresses the individual risk of developing the disease.
9. Dr. Ron was a leading epidemiologist in the field of the association between ionizing radiation and cancer in general, and its effects on the thyroid gland in particular. On her return to the United States she worked in the Radiation Epidemiology Branch of the National Cancer Institute (NCI), where she headed the department from 1997 to 2002. She conducted and participated in many important studies on radiation throughout the world, among them a follow-up of patients who had received I-131 for hyperthyroidism, a follow-up of children in the United States who had been irradiated for benign diseases of the head and neck, a follow-up of individuals who had been exposed to I-131 from nuclear experiments conducted in Nevada, a follow-up of the effects of exposure after the nuclear disaster at Chernobyl, and a follow-up of survivors of the atomic bombs dropped on Hiroshima and Nagasaki in Japan in World War II. These studies formed the basis of recommendations for protection against low-dose radiation in the workplace and for the general population, as formulated in the mid-1990s. Dr. Ron wrote more than 200 scientific articles and participated in numerous national and international committees dealing with assessment of the health effects of radiation.
10. Ron E. Benign and Malignant Thyroid Neoplasms Following Scalp Irradiation in Childhood. PhD thesis, Tel Aviv University, 1980:262.
11. This figure, quoted in Modan's article (as well as in direct conversation with him) is his estimate of the number of Jews treated with irradiation against ringworm in Israel in the 1950s. In addition, during the corresponding period, Arab children

were also treated in Israel, but this population was not included in ringworm research.
12. The amount of radiation in the x-ray tube is determined by power (kilovolts) and current (milliamperes).
13. Number of rads/minute expresses the intensity of irradiation measured usually in exposure units (Gray or rad) per minute or per hour, depending on the source. For the definition of rad, see note 29.
14. The superficial dose is calculated by multiplying the number of rads/minute by the duration (in minutes) of irradiation.
15. Each Israeli citizen is given a nine-digit identity number that serves to identify him/her uniquely in all official state records.
16. Modan B, Baidatz D, Mart H, et al. Radiation-induced head and neck tumors. Lancet, 1974, 1:277–279; Sadetzki S, Chetrit A, Freedman L, et al. Long-term follow-up for brain tumor development following childhood exposure to ionizing radiation for tinea capitis. Radiat Res, 2005, 163:424–432.
17. See also: Bar Oz A. me-Achorei ha-Me'ah Elef shel Parashat ha-Gazezet (Behind the 100,000 in the Ringworm Episode). Harefuah, 2016, 155:637–641.
18. Fishler Y, Keinan-Boker L, Ifrah A (Eds.). The Israel National Cancer Registry: Completeness and Timeliness of the Data. Israel Center for Disease Control, Israel Ministry of Health, Publication #365, February 2017.
19. Modan et al., 1974.
20. Werner A, Modan B, Davidoff D. Doses to brain, skull and thyroid, following x-ray therapy for tinea capitis. Phys Med Biol, 1968, 13:247–258; Werner A, Modan B. A direct method of measuring total radiation dose to the brain using the Fricke dosimeter. IAEA-SM-143, 1970, 12:435–443.
21. Adamson HG. A simplified method of x ray application for the cure of ringworm of the scalp: Kienböck's method. Lancet. 1909, 173(4472):1378–1380 (Originally published as Volume 1, Issue 4472).
22. Routine x-ray examination uses x-rays emitted from a tube, within the range of 120 electron-volts (eV) to 120 kilo electron volts (KeV). X-rays can penetrate objects and are thus most useful for diagnostic purposes. A roentgen unit is the amount of ionizing radiation in the air.
23. Werner and Modan; Professor A. Verner, telephone conversation, July 25, 2011.
24. Modan et al., 1974; Werner et al., 1968.
25. Radiation absorbed dose (rad) is the unit of energy absorbed from ionizing radiation by living tissues. In the case of x-rays or γ rays, 1 roentgen unit = 0.94 rad. The rad was replaced as the accepted scientific unit by the Gray (Gy). 100 rad = 1 Gy.
26. Werner et al., 1968.
27. Ron E, Modan B, Preston D, et al. Radiation-induced skin carcinomas of the head and neck. Radiat Res, 1991, 125:318–325.
28. Stovall, Marilyn, correspondence dated November 2001.
29. Schultz RJ, Albert RE. Dose to organs of the head from the x-ray treatment of tinea capitis. Arch Environ Health, 1968, 17; Lee W, Youmans HD. Doses to the Central Nervous System of Children Resulting from X-ray Therapy for Tinea Capitis. U.S. Department of Health, Education, and Welfare, BRH/DBE, 70–4, 1970; Modan B,

Ron E, Werner A. Thyroid cancer following scalp irradiation. Radiology, 1977, 123; Harley NH, Kolber AB, Shore RE, et al. The skin dose and response for the head and neck in patients irradiated with x-ray for tinea capitis. Epidemiology Applied to Health Physics, CONF-83010, 1983.
30. Lubin JH, Schafer DW, Ron E, et al. A reanalysis of thyroid neoplasms in the Israeli Tinea Capitis Study accounting for dose uncertainties. Radiat Research, 2004, 161:359–368.
31. Sadetzki et al., 2005; Sadetzki S, Chetrit A, Lubina A, et al. Risk of thyroid cancer following childhood exposure to ionizing radiation for tinea capitis. J Clin Endocrin Metabol, 2006, 91:4798–4804.
32. Schafer DW, Lubin JH, Ron E, et al. Thyroid cancer following scalp irradiation: A reanalysis accounting for uncertainty in dosimetry. Biometrics, 2001, 57:689–697
33. Modan et al., 1974.
34. Ron E, Modan B. Benign and malignant thyroid neoplasms after childhood irradiation for tinea capitis. J Natl Cancer Inst, 1980, 65:7–11; Ron E, Modan B, Boice JD Jr, et al. Tumors of the brain and nervous system after radiotherapy in childhood. N Engl J Med, 1988, 319:1033–1039; Modan B, Chetrit A, Alfandary E, Katz L. Increased risk of breast cancer after low-dose irradiation. Lancet, 1989, 1:629–631; Ron E, Modan B, Preston D, et al. Thyroid neoplasia following low-dose radiation in childhood. Radiat Res, 1989, 120:516–531; Modan B, Chetrit A, Alfandary E, et al. Increased risk of salivary gland tumors after low-dose irradiation. Laryngoscope, 1998, 108:1095–1097; Sadetzki et al., 2005, 2006.
35. Ron and Modan, 1980.
36. Relative risk (RR) is defined as the ratio between the incidence rate of a disease in the exposed group compared with the comparison group. When the RR is higher than 1 (statistically significant), the exposure constitutes a risk factor for the disease studied. When it is less than 1 (statistically significant), it constitutes a protective factor against the studied disease. When the RR equals 1 (approximately), the risk factor does not affect the risk of morbidity.
37. Ron E, Griffel B, Liban E, Modan B. Histopathologic reproducibility of thyroid disease in an epidemiologic study. Cancer, 1986, 57:1056–1059.
38. Ron et al., 1989.
39. Sadetzki et al., 2006.
40. Confidence interval (CI) is an accepted index for estimating the statistical significance and degree of accuracy of the parameter (e.g., point estimate of risk) obtained in the study. It describes a range of values determined by the degree of presumed random variability in the data, within which the value of the parameter is thought to lie, with specified level of confidence.
41. Ron E, Lubin JH, Shore RE, et al. Thyroid cancer after exposure to external radiation: A pooled analysis of seven studies. Radiat Res, 1995, 141:259–277.
42. Lubin JH, Adams MJ, Shore R, et al. Thyroid cancer following childhood low-dose radiation exposure: A pooled analysis of nine cohorts. J Clin Endocrinol Metab, 2017, 102:2575–2583.
43. Ron et al., Tumors of the brain, 1988.

44. Dose response means that a rise in the dosage of exposure (to radiation, e.g.) will result in a rise in response being observed (risk of developing brain tumors, e.g.).
45. Beller AJ, Feinsod M, Sahar A. The possible relationship between small-dose irradiation to the scalp and intracranial meningiomas. Neurochirurgia, 1972, 4:135–143.
46. Munk J, Peyser E, Gruszkiewicz J. Radiation-induced intracranial meningiomas. Clin Radiol, 1969, 20:90–94.
47. Davidoff LM, Dyke CG, Elsberg CA, Tarlov I. The effect of radiation applied directly to the brain and spinal cord. Radiology, 1938, 31:451–463.
48. Zülch KI. Brain Tumors—Their Biology and Pathology. New York: Springer; 1957.
49. Fabrikant JJ, Dickson RJ, Fetter BF. Mechanisms of radiation carcinogenesis at the clinical level. Br J Cancer, 1964, 13:459–477.
50. Soffer D, Pittaluga S, Feiner M, Beller AJ. Intracranial meningiomas following low-dose irradiation to the head. J Neurosurg, 1983, 59:1048–1053.
51. Rubinstein AB, Shalit MN, Cohen ML, et al. Radiation-induced cerebral meningioma: A recognizable entity. J Neurosurg, 1984, 61:966–971.
52. Modan et al., 1989.
53. The hypophysis is the pituitary gland located at the base of the skull within the sella turcica. Its primary function is secretion of hormones, including growth hormone (Heprolactin), which causes the breast to produce milk, and TSH or thyrotropin, which activates the pituitary gland to produce the hormone thyroxine.
54. These tumors included the following diagnoses: benign sweat gland adenomas, basal cell benign tumors, dermatofibroma, benign nevi, and skin cylindromas.
55. These tumors included the following diagnoses: epithelial cell cancer, squamous cell carcinoma, and basal cell carcinoma.
56. Ron et al., 1991.
57. A case–control study, also called a retrospective study, is one in which the studied population is composed of cases (individuals who manifest the health effect studied) and controls (unaffected individuals who are representative of the population from which the cases were drawn). In such a study the investigators estimate the rate of the studied risk factors among the two groups.
58. "Nested" means a case–control study in which the study population (patients manifesting the studied disease (skin cancer), and controls free of this disease are identified in an existing cohort.
59. Modan B, Alfandary E, Shapiro D, et al. Factors affecting the development of skin cancer after scalp irradiation. Radiat Res, 1993, 134:125–128.
60. Modan et al., 1998.
61. Modan et al., 1989.
62. Ron E, Modan B. Thyroid and other neoplasms following childhood scalp irradiation. In: Boice JD Jr, Fraumeni JF Jr (Eds.), Radiation Carcinogenesis: Epidemiology and Biological Significance. New York: Raven Press; 1984:139–151.
63. Underestimation of the radiation among exposed individuals and/or misclassification of some individuals from the comparison groups as non-exposed, although they had been exposed, will lead to a decrease in the RR describing the effect of radiation. Thus, these possibilities do not nullify the study findings obtained. In such a case, the real risk of an association between irradiation and the

studied effect is greater than revealed in the study. That is, the real risk has been underestimated, not overestimated.
64. A tumor suppressor gene or anti-oncogenic gene prevents the cell from initiating the neoplastic process. When this gene is damaged, a decrease or loss of the coded protein results, and the cell can progress to neoplastic changes. This process generally occurs in conjunction with additional genetic alterations.
65. Apoptosis is programmed cell death resulting from harm or damage to cellular DNA, setting off a complex and graduated process during which a large number of proteins and enzymes interact and cause cell death.
66. Homozygous mutation is the presence of the same mutation in both alleles of a specific gene.
67. Lavin MF. Ataxia-telangiectasia: From a rare disorder to a paradigm for cell signalling and cancer. Nat Rev Mol Cell Biol, 2008, 9:759–769. Erratum in: Nat Rev Mol Cell Biol, 2008, 9(12).
68. Heterozygosity is the presence of two different alleles at the same locus on the paired chromosomes.
69. A founder mutation is a mutation that occurred in a forefather of a homogeneous population (a particular ethnic group) and was transmitted to the offspring. If the mutation is nonlethal, it may recur relatively frequently in such a population
70. Gilad S, Bar-Shira A, Harnik R, et al. Ataxia-telangiectasia: Founder effect among North African Jews. Hum Molec Genet, 1996, 5:2033–2037.
71. An interaction involves differences in the tested effect of a specific factor at various levels of another factor. Interaction takes place when the incidence of a disease in the presence of two or more risk factors diverges from the incidence expected from the action of each factor separately. The effect of each individual variable on the dependent variable is termed the "main effect."
72. Ron and Modan, 1984.
73. Yaar I, Ron E, Modan M, et al. Long-term cerebral effects of small doses of X-irradiation in childhood as manifested in adult visual evoked responses. Ann Neurol, 1980, 8:261–268.
74. See Chapter 2.
75. Yaar I, Ron E, Modan B, et al. Long-lasting cerebral functional changes following moderate-dose X-radiation treatment to the scalp in childhood: An electroencephalographic power, spectral study. J Neurol Neurosurg Psychiatry, 1982, 45:166–169.
76. Ron E, Modan B, Floro S, et al. Mental function following scalp irradiation during childhood. Am J Epidemiol, 1982, 116:149–160.
77. Scholastic aptitude tests were conducted on all eighth-grade pupils in the educational system in Israel during the late 1960s. These tests assessed, among other parameters, cognitive capacities, and served to channel the pupils into different streams in secondary school. They were a prime criterion for assessment of the size of the grant given for school fees (high-stakes tests), and this determined the fate of the pupils.
78. Ron et al., Mortality after radiotherapy, 1988.

79. Ron et al., 1991.
80. Ron et al., Mortality after radiotherapy, 1988.
81. Gonads are the organs in which reproductive cells are produced—testicles in males, ovaries in females.
82. Preston RJ. Radiation biology. Health Phys, 2004, 87:3–14.

11

The muted voices of the ringworm patients and their families worldwide

LIAT HOFFER

Baldness that robbed me of my childhood; that robbed me of my smile, my happiness. Baldness that prevented me from running in the street and playing like every other child. [She's] bald! [She's] bald: The calls of the children still resonate in my tormented head. Baldness that caused my family such numerous expenses and despite difficulties making a livelihood, bought me a wig so I could look better. This didn't prevent the fear and anxiety of "What will become of me?" and the feeling of not being a mother, not to hold a baby.

(X. has been bald since childhood as the result of ringworm irradiation treatment in the 1950s.)

INTRODUCTION

Modern medicine ascribes great importance to the human-social dimension of the patient and views this as an important element in dealing with the disease, any disease.[1] Psychiatrist George Engel, founder of the bio-psychosocial model,[2] argued that biologic, psychological (including thoughts, feelings, and behaviors), and social elements have a significant impact on the health status of a person undergoing treatment.[3]

This model, first presented in 1977, can serve as a way to understand the personal, social, and environmental aspects that ringworm involves, and the impact of the x-ray treatment that the children received. On the surface, it would appear that ringworm, which is known as a very contagious dermatologic disease,[4] is similar to other contagious diseases whose treatment included quarantine and special attention. However, unlike other diseases, ringworm carries a stigma that is not medical: It has been associated with filth, poverty, ignorance, and low social standing.[5] Bladin, in his article "The Surprising Treatment of Ringworm in a Hospital in Nantes at the Outset of the 20th Century," described ringworm patients as "engendering feelings of trepidation and disgust."[6] Other sources noted that the disease led to social ostracism.[7] The negative connotation of word *parech* in Yiddish for ringworm (an insulting word for baldness) was used as an epithet for children with ringworm and became a synonym for ringworm among Eastern European Jews.[8] Dr. Levy Lebhar, the chief radiologist at the OZE clinic in Casablanca, who treated Jewish children with ringworm, labeled the children "dirty, from the lowest [social] classes."[9] Within the Jewish community during the British Mandate period and after establishment of the State of Israel, ringworm carried a social stigma that was expressed in the daily press and in medical communication. Ringworm patients were described as "leper-like," and in many cases the descriptions were accompanied by fear of contagion that was liable to tag the child as inferior and "trichophytonic" (from the Latin term for the ringworm fungus).[10] Moreover, due to the prominent clinical signs on the children's heads—scars, bald spots, and open sores—it was impossible to hide the ailment. Ringworm was therefore viewed as an epidemic that needed to be addressed and eradicated. Because of such negative attitudes, those who contracted the disease carried with them painful and traumatic memories from the period of their illness and its treatment—memoires that in most cases had a negative impact on their peace of mind and caused difficulties throughout their lives.

One could argue that had such ringworm children been treated in keeping with the criteria of the bio-psychosocial model, the trauma of treatment might not have been so deeply etched in their psyche and would not have become a constant presence throughout their lives, or might not have placed such a heavy a burden on their personal, family, and social development. Thus, this chapter seeks to provide a space where the muted voices of former ringworm children and their families around the world can be shared, so that their feelings and the personal hardships and distress they have experienced and grappled with over the years can become part of the public medical discourse. The hardships and distress that these patients from around the world express in this chapter reflect shared experiences that bridge the diversity of their national and cultural backgrounds. This chapter is designed to describe what is missing from discourse on ringworm—the human perspective.

The voices of ringworm children from different countries in the world have been compiled from various archives, personal correspondence, email exchanges, interviews, and personal testimonies sent to the author of the chapter, covering uncharted territory.[11] Efforts have been made to preserve the original tone/style of the letters verbatim as much as possible.

UNITED STATES

The number of children in the United States treated with irradiation for various diseases until the 1960s is estimated to range from 2 million to 4 million.[12] Irradiation was most commonly used for acne and enlarged glands in the neck.[13] The number of children estimated to have undergone irradiation treatment for ringworm in America is between 20,000 and 50,000.[14]

By the mid-1960s, researchers in the United States had already found additional health risks among those irradiated for ringworm in childhood, as well as a higher incidence of emotional disorders.[15] However, despite mention of an emotional dimension in research during the 1960s, it appears that such findings were pushed aside and the emotional distress of ringworm children remained unnoticed and unaddressed.

Barbara Beck Hess

I was born on February 26, 1939, and was raised in Oregon[16] *... In the summer of 1942, I petted my aunt's kitten and I put it on my head, although my aunt warned me not to touch the kitten because it had ringworm. Later, I developed ringworm on the hairline above the eyebrows. My mother told me that she took me to the doctors for 13 months in order to cure me. During this period my sister was infected from me with ringworm. In addition, at the end of this period, my mother was pregnant and was worried that the baby would contract ringworm too.*

This was a period of anxiety for me. I remember I was tense in the doctor's office and when he shaved my head, I yelled and struggled. I remember the blood and the fear. My mother told me that the doctors continued to give me prescriptions for salves, but I had a reaction to the salves before the ringworm could be cured ... My next memories were my mother taking me into the basement of the house and putting on my head wide strips of sticky tape, and then pulling the tape and trying to pull out the hair roots to finish off the source of the ringworm. My mother would cry and I would cry together with her.

The children of the neighbors (except my aunt) didn't play with me for a year. They called me "the kid with ringworm on her head" and worse than that ... She [my mother] made me hats from the toe part of socks, and added bells to them. She also tried to dress me with kerchiefs around my exposed head. The only homes that were willing to accept me were those of my grandmother and grandfather and the houses of my aunts ... I only remember the fear that my head would be shaved, or getting treated with the strips of sticky tape. In one of my last "treatments," I remember my father and mother holding me over the side of the bathtub, and discussing how to put the iodine on my head so it would stay. In the end they poured it on my head and wrapped my head in a bandana. They told me that my entire head was covered with water blisters from the treatment. I remember it was horribly painful . . . .

My mother had read about irradiation treatment for ringworm and finally found a doctor or a technician who agreed to treat me and my sister. I don't have any recollection how many times he irradiated the ringworm or how many visits we had in the clinic. What I do remember is the doctor said to my mother that I and my sister would never have hair again. I can only surmise how this impacted on my mother.

I began first grade in January 1945. My hair began to sprout again . . . I haven't a clue how my hair would look without the epilation, but my hair is very thin and okay since then. I haven't any idea how it was before the treatment.

I learned from a nurse who worked with me in 1982 that people who received irradiation such as I received need to go for annual checkups for cancer of the thyroid gland and there are certain people who developed brain cancer following treatment.

My childhood was difficult and this [was] due to difficulty trusting my parents and other children after this experience of 13 months or more, with a sense of maltreatment and torture.[17]

Barbara's son

My name is Mathew Beck.[18] *I am the second son of Barbara. I read my mother's description of the ringworm matter, which brought tears to my eyes. I heard many stories about her education, but I didn't know the full details of this matter. As she noted, she had other tough periods in her life, some less destructive and some perhaps a bit more so. In the end, I am very thankful for the host of warm and generous memories that I have of my mother who raised me. I know she went through some complex times with the four of us, but she prevailed. And I know I am a better person thanks to her.*

Sharon Hoare Orfinik

I received treatment with irradiation at NYU Medical Center at the outset of the 1950s when I was in third grade, for ringworm of the scalp.[19] I always believed that this treatment was the factor behind my thin hair and that it [the treatment] contributed to the skin cancer on my scalp that I was recently diagnosed with.

I was born in 1943 and today I am a retiree living in Panama, Florida. I was in a private Catholic school up until eighth grade and the only one in the whole class who contracted ringworm. We had a lot of feral cats that were roaming the open areas where we were living, and the results were that I contracted ringworm from one of the cats. Since I was only 7 or 8 at the time, my memory is foggy. I do remember that it was my mother who noticed the affliction and she was the one who took me to the doctor in the city where we lived. He instructed her to take me to the medical center of New York University for treatment. We lived in a small town outside the city, and therefore we had to take the train into the city in order to receive treatment.

My treatment was built at the beginning on shaving the hair from my head, and afterwards to take my head and quickly pluck it [the hair] out. Afterwards a blue ointment was spread on my scalp and we were sent home with instruction how to use the salve daily . . . I also don't remember how many times we traveled to the city or how many irradiations there were. I was scared and I remained in the room alone during the treatment and I would cry from the intense pain on the way home afterwards. I also remember my mother sewing me a cap to cover my head which had two straps so to fix it firmly under my chin but at the same time, it was forbidden for me to return to school, for instance what was left of the school year, and to be in contact with other children, except for my three sisters.

I don't have a picture from that period, but I remember that I was ostracized. I was in isolation .

Allen Arnett

In 1946 when I was 5 years old I had a ringworm on my scalp. A doctor in Tyler, Texas, rubbed it with a cube of radioactive material, resulting in immediate hair loss, ringworm cure, and long-term health issues, including cancer. In 1974 I had a thyroidectomy and two radiation treatments

Dave Keilholtz

I received treatment in Lansing, Michigan. Because of my young age I don't remember much about the treatment. One thing I do remember is the fear that I would be sterile. I have five children, so much for that! I have never been contacted by anyone for any studies. I do remember having my head shaved and wearing a beanie cap. I was not allowed to attend school and missed one year of school.

Peter Baer

Thank you for forwarding excerpts of your articles which I read with great interest. I also took the liberty of scanning the web and seeing all of your literary contributions. I honestly had no idea of the magnitude of the "ringworm problem" until communicating with you. It's a blessing that the scope of your research and studies generate great value to many individuals both within your profession and to those like myself, who have been afflicted and kept in the dark regarding the long-term effects of their treatment . . .

   Be advised that I received radiation treatment for ringworm of the scalp in 1946 at the age of seven. The hospital was Kings County Hospital in Brooklyn, New York . . . I am now seventy-five years of age and in reasonably good health. I have had two very small basal cell carcinomas removed from my face. The first one was removed from my nose approximately 20 years ago at age 55. The second one was removed from my temple 5 years ago at age 70. Again, both were very small. I visit my dermatologist for a cancer screening twice a year.

ENGLAND

As in the United States, in England children with ringworm were identified at school and sent for treatment at public clinics (see Chapter 4) . In later years, there were no attempts to inform the public about possible health risks.[20]

Susan Lees wrote the following:

My father has suffered with brain tumors for the last 10 years at least, going through numerous treatments and surgery. He now suffers from epilepsy and has bruising to the frontal lobe as a result.

He has always said that he remembers as a very small child going to Canterbury Hospital on the bus with his mother and having radiation treatment on his head for ringworm. I spoke to my father today regarding his treatment and he said it was his mother that discovered his ringworm; apparently she used to do regular head checks for lice for him and his brothers. She took him to the doctor's, who made the diagnosis and referred him to Canterbury Hospital in Kent, where the treatment was carried out. He said his doctor at that time was situated on Buckland Avenue in Dover, Kent, Dover being the district in which they lived. My father has described extensively having to wear a hat because his hair had fallen out and the shield put over his head to cover the areas they did not want irradiated. He said they had to keep the treatment going and kept moving areas, as they said the ringworm had moved.

Now, not believing this to be possible, knowing the implications of such a treatment, I finally decided to have a look on the internet this evening because I thought as a child, they must have found cancer and protected him by telling him he had ringworm. Now reading all the articles, about the documentaries of what happened in Israel and eastern Europe, "I believe!" I am dumbfounded that they should have used such an extreme measure for a fungal infection and used it so universally too. It seems they used it as the doctors' dream cure-all, but at their victims' expense. I guess there is a very good chance this could be the reason my father is suffering now. It is quite saddening, and I hope you get every bit of help you need to obtain some (albeit belated) justice for the victims of this quick-fix ignorant solution to a problem that could have been remedied by safer, more traditional means given just a little more time.

Sorry for the wait and I hope it helps. I have been talking to my family since this all came to light and they are as shocked as I was.

The speaker's father died in July 2014 with secondary complications of the irradiation he received. Susan said her sister had talked with another family in the oncology department of the hospital where her father was hospitalized, who said that the health status of their father was almost identical, and he also had undergone the same ringworm treatment when he was a child. Susan wrote that the research into this topic was very important and that people need to know about the treatment and its results, not just basic details. She offered her assistance in publishing the research on social media.

PORTUGAL

In the early 1950s, the Portuguese government embarked on a campaign to eradicate ringworm, which had spread after the Second World War (see Chapter 7),[21] As part of treatment for preventing the disease, children were irradiated with the Kienböck–Adamson method.[22] According to current estimates the number of children irradiated was in the vicinity of 30,000.[23]

G.N.

I had two beautiful braids when they shaved my head. My aunt saved one and one my mother saved. This [shaving her head] caused great sorrow; I heard my parents weeping. I remember that I traveled to Porto [for treatment]. The trains were full, everyone traveling for the same purpose. . . . I did the irradiation treatment of the epilation and I wore a white scarf until the hair sprouted again. But the sprouting of the hair wasn't normal. I had straight hair, but it turned curly when it began to grow again. I had a full head of hair and now the hair is thin. I haven't cut the hair on top for 30 years and still my hair doesn't reach the middle of my back.

M.V.

I remember that I was making coffee when someone warned, "The head doctors are coming!" . . . It was my aunt who cut off my hair. And if it wasn't shameful enough that I was bald, my mother gave me a beating when I returned with the scarf.

C.H.

I was irradiated at age 4. Although I was small, I remember everything. I feel that as a result of the disease, my life changed and I never had a healthy life. When I would complain to my mother that I didn't feel well, my mother didn't care and would even hit me. I always had difficulty in crowds of people, difficulties finding work. I kept to myself the feeling of disgust that only I can understand.

SERBIA (YUGOSLAVIA)

According to current estimates, the number of children irradiated in Yugoslavia (Serbia) was in the vicinity of 50,000 to 94,000 as part of an organized UNICEF campaign at the request of the Yugoslavian government (see Chapter 8). Most of the irradiation was conducted at special ringworm hospitals.[24] The irradiation treatment carried out in Serbia to prevent the spread of ringworm was also conducted using the Kienböck–Adamson method.[25]

The testimony presented below is part of interviews conducted by Dr. Goren Sevo,[26] the first part of which focused on the personal experience of the patients in the social context, the second part on medical questions.

N.B.

I left the hospital with a funny-shaped hat. They told me it was forbidden to wet the skin underneath. Due to shame I spent almost a year confined to home. I failed school this year . . . I also remember headaches immediately after the irradiation.

O.P.

I remember that the children were treated badly there, and often bitten by the teachers of the facility where they were situated. I also remember that one child committed suicide in the facility and another child died there when they poured boiling-hot wax on his head. (This individual sued the hospital afterwards, but without success.)

T.G.

I even went to see a private doctor in order to confirm I was not ill, so I wouldn't be forced to be hospitalized. I had long hair, beautiful [and] blond. Thus I remember. But it didn't help. I had to go . . . I remember that hospitalization of children wasn't accompanied by a medical issuance of any kind. (While telling her story she pointed to the small amount of hair that remained, particularly on the back of the head.)

EASTERN EUROPE (POLAND, LATVIA, UKRAINE, ROMANIA)

Between 1921 and 1938 the Jewish organizations OZE and the Joint operated clinics to treat ringworm with irradiation throughout Jewish communities in Eastern Europe (see Chapter 5). According to the Jewish organizations' reports, 27,760 children in these Jewish communities were treated with irradiation.[27] Few testimonies remain from these ringworm children; many were murdered in the Holocaust and others have since died.

Jack Fields

I was born in Irshava in the province of Karpatia, Czechoslovakia, in 1925. At the age of six I contracted ringworm on my scalp. My mother took me to a larger city, where I was treated with radiation. Years later I noticed a small lump on my throat, which turned out to be located on my thyroid, and went to an endocrinologist. I was given a test by swallowing a radioactive pill. It showed that I had multiple modules, but no surgery was necessary. Since then I have been checked annually and my situation remains the same. I take no medication for this. Should you require any more information I would be happy to comply. A friend of mine has a similar situation but her experience resulted in thyroid cancer.

Nelly

My mother died in 1984. My uncle, my father's brother who is also my mother's cousin, died two years ago. Both had meningioma, which is a benign brain tumor. Both had radiotherapy for ringworm as children.

Sara V.

In 2009 Sara V. died. Her son buried her with the wig that she wore all her life to hide the baldness from irradiation for scalp ringworm that she had received as a child in Odessa (Ukraine).[28] Her son said he buried her with the wig at his mother's request, and that his mother never took it off, and her children never saw her without it on her head.

NORTH AFRICA

From 1947 to 1960 the Jewish organizations OZE and the JDC-Joint operated clinics for the treatment of ringworm with irradiation in North Africa, based on the Eastern European model.[29] The reports of the Jewish organizations show that 22,000 children were treated for ringworm, the majority from Jewish communities in French Morocco. Some 3,000 children were treated for ringworm in Tunis, Algeria and Libya.[30]
(See Chapter 5.)

D., Algiers

At the time they told me I had a sore, a little sore here [pointing to her head], and I need to be there. They shaved off all my hair and I was left bald. I remember that they were putting iodine and putting a kind of bandage and every morning they shampooed our heads. They spread on the iodine and then they did with the machine. You go through this like CT, You sit and some kind of machine goes zzzzzz on your head and you're forbidden to move. You're forbidden to move a muscle. I was 13 years old.

S: When you went out, did you return to the same place in the camp or return to the hospital?

In the camp. The custom was that it was forbidden to go to the camp where your parents were. Why? Because it was contagious . . . There was follow-up to see everything was OK . . . that the hair returned to sprout. But there were places where the hair didn't grow back in. Then they would say this was "because you moved in the machine." It was a kind of radio-activity, what they did—if you moved, then at this point [hair] wouldn't sprout . . . like here [points to a bald spot].

I felt chagrined because they removed all my hair and all the time I cried and they would tell me, "Don't cry. It will grow 'inside' [during treatment under quarantine]. You're still a little girl" and I didn't have a choice. I got used to it, until the hair sprouted [while] "inside."

I had very pretty hair—blond. And after this it grew a lot weaker [thinner]. I had full thick hair, "a head full of hair," and after this it was weak.

S.

When I was 5 I was infected and they determined that I had ringworm. We didn't say a word. We began a series of treatments that lasted a year plus, daily several hours in the morning, a taxi up and back, shaving hair. And every day that a hair sprouted, it was plucked out in order to make sure all hairs had been pulled out. After they finished this treatment, they spread boiling wax and removed it after a few minutes. I felt an earthquake and burns on the back of my head. Afterwards they spread a white salve and put on this gauze.

And thus I went around school with gauze on the head. I missed a lot of material [at school]. I cried, but no one came near me—so they wouldn't be infected from me. They kept me back a year and my studies deteriorated. Today I do housework; that's what I can do to support my children. Life isn't rosy.

In the end, out of all the treatment, I am bald on my entire head, thin hair that covers the scalp. Nothing can be done with the hair, I look awful and disgusting, I'm agitated, and I don't have any way to take care of [my] hair.

D.

I was born in Casablanca in Morocco. I underwent irradiation at age 5 in 1955. I remember as a small child how they told me not to move, I had terrible pain following the wax that they put on my head that burned my scalp and I was afraid to cry, just like I was afraid of the machine. My grandmother always warned me what the machine does to children who move.

I always went around with a cap on the head in order to hide the baldness, didn't go out of the house, and was very, very ashamed of my looks. As a result, I didn't have any girlfriends. I was forbidden to go to school so as not to infect the pupils. They ostracized me for years in the neighborhood, at school, and in the family. When my mother or my grandmother would visit family, I would stay at home because who wants to catch a harsh disease like ringworm?

Thus I grew up with lack of confidence, terrible fear, and a deep sense of inferiority. Afterwards, very thin hair began to sprout; the eyebrows and eyelashes almost didn't sprout at all. I have recurrent infections on [my] head and behind the ears . . .

I married lovelessly at an early age not to the man of my choice but rather to someone who accepted me as I looked. In the course of my marriage, I suffered from insults. Time and again my husband called me "bald one" at every opportunity and I would break down crying from the insult and pain.

At age 30 he finally left the house and left me with four little children, claiming my looks disgusted him, and so it was in my adult years. I still suffer from the baldness and disgusting look that destroyed my life as a child and as a woman. Without hair, without teeth, with pain and illness without end.

A 2016 study of the historical, medical, and psychosocial aspects of irradiation treatment for ringworm found that 71.25% of the women reported having a lifelong low self-image.

ISRAEL

From 1946 to 1960, 26,000 to 27,000 Jewish and Arab children were treated for ringworm at clinics, institutes, and hospitals and their branches, and by private physicians.[31] The treatment in Israel was similar to treatment during this period in Western countries, including the United States and Canada.

B.

I am B., age 50. I was negatively affected by irradiation I received in childhood . . . To this day I suffer as a result of those irradiations. Among other things, I suffer from hair loss—I'm essentially half-bald . . . I underwent various and sundry examinations to try and improve the situation. Without success. As well, I got another dermatological disease in the mouth that has no solution or cure ever . . .

As a result of all the suffering I endured, my joy of life and happiness and the depressions are indescribable. Here I am, a woman who suffers from lack of self-confidence that today can't be fixed. I can't forget the iodine they would smear on my head and irradiate and afterwards tear out [the hair].

The screams I would scream and nobody cared about me. Also, they didn't sign anyone [get a signed consent form] from a member of my family, and afterwards, I can't forget how the children would yell after me, "[She's] bald! Bald!" All my life I suffered due to the baldness.

Up until 2015, the State of Israel recognized for compensation 5,804 women in Israel as persons who suffered from baldness as a result of irradiation for ringworm in childhood. Among them, 4,087 had small bald patches and 1,717 suffered major permanent balding, partial or full.

The 2016 study mentioned earlier found that 70% of the 80 woman sampled mentioned the sense of depression they experience daily in light of their situation. Such a daily reality amplifies the suffering and the emotional state of these women.[32]

G.

I was born in 1941. I am single. I'm one of 13 brothers and sisters. In my childhood, I lived with my parents in Tel Aviv. To the best of my knowledge and recollections, out of all my sisters and brothers only several were affected by ringworm and underwent the treatment with irradiation. To the best of my recollections, at the time my entire family was summoned to undergo medical examinations in regard to ringworm, which was prevalent at the time in the country, and they also made examinations of my head.

Since I was a little girl, in kindergarten or the beginning of elementary school, I don't remember all the details . . . After the treatments I suffered and was ashamed to be with other children, and I was ostracized from them . . . After I underwent the treatment with irradiation on my head, I had sores on the head. My head itched without stop, and afterwards the hair on my head began to fall out and they made me bald. And, the skin on my scalp peeled. I would feel heat waves in my head, from which I suffer from time to time to this day. To this day [my scalp] is red and scarred due to the many burns that I received on the back of my head and on my head. I suffered and I suffer today at times from headaches. I had sores on the skin of my scalp that burned a lot . . . and since then to this day I wear a head scarf. And to this day I suffer from headaches and dizziness . . .

In the same period I studied at the nursing school in Tel Aviv. And I remember the jeers of the children from whom I kept my distance, and to this day I refrain from the company of people and I never married.

V.

I immigrated to Israel in 1955, when I was 13 years old. They sent me . . . in order to receive treatment to prevent ringworm and then they gave me electric radiation on the head, and after about a month I was sent home and since then, to today, I suffer from baldness on almost my entire head. And it's 21 years that I wear a false wig and it costs me a lot of money, and also suffering and unpleasantness in society.

G.

The treatment was carried out some time in 1950 or 1951. I don't remember the exact date. The treatment included irradiation, spreading a substance similar to honey on the head, a substance that would harden after the irradiation. The treatment staff removed it together with the hair . . . I went through this process a number of times until there wasn't any hair on my head . . . After the treatment we were sent home, bald of course, and after a number of months hair began to sprout . . .

Thus, life went on until the 1980s, when I turned to my family doctor and complained to him about a long list of medical problems from which I suffer for quite a long time. The family doctor referred me to the hospital. In a discussion I held with the doctor, I was asked by the doctor if I had ever undergone irradiation. Of course, I answered in the affirmative and told the doctor. Now it has become evident that there is a direct linkage between the treatment I underwent in my childhood and the functionality of the [thyroid] gland and my current health status.

Today I am bothered by many questions: Was I sick with ringworm? Why did they take only the children and not the adults as well? [Why] in the framework of the treatment didn't I see even one girl? Was the treatment given to all Israeli children or only new immigrants?. . . Today I go about things with melancholy eyes [without zest], with the knowledge that tomorrow morning a malignant tumor is liable to be discovered, and thus I'll end my life. If in the past I still had hope, today I'm left only with despair and anxiety that eats away at everything.

CONCLUSION

The main objective of this chapter is to provide a platform for the muted voices of former ringworm patients around the world to be heard. Most of the testimonies describe the treatment they underwent as harsh and traumatic, triggering a sense of fear, helplessness, and sadness. They recall feelings of embarrassment and shame, and painful memories of ridicule and rejection by peers and even by their immediate family. Sometimes their plight was accompanied by feelings of disappointment, shame, and anger regarding their caregivers. Their shared sense of distress is reflected in their comments contrasting the condition of their hair before and after treatment, and their feelings about their current lives as a result. Besides these sources of distress, there is also the shared worry about the health ramifications of the treatment. These feelings are strikingly similar between patients and their family members despite the geographic distances and cultural differences that divide them. It seems that their recollections and feelings represent a significant part of their lives and the lives of those surrounding them. These testimonies shed a new light on ringworm treatment, providing a more holistic view of the experience that has been overlooked by the medical community and revealing the almost uniform human distress experienced by these patients around the world.

NOTES

1. Liat Hoffer is a PhD candidate in Health Sciences at Ben Gurion University of the Negev. This chapter is dedicated to Barbara Hess from Oregon, who underwent irradiation for ringworm in the United States in 1943–1944, in recognition of her willingness to share with me her personal saga and the assistance of her family in writing this chapter.
2. Engel GL. The need for a new medical model: A challenge for biomedicine. *Science*, 1977, 196(4286):129–136. The model was first published in 1977 by George Engel from Rochester University, New York, and became a leading model within modern medicine.
3. Bowden G. The merit of sociological accounts of disorder: The attention-deficit/hyperactivity disorder case. *Health*, 2014, 18(4):422–438.
4. Blackwell W. Tinea capitis. In: Burns T, Breathnachs S, Cox N, Griffiths C (eds.), *Rook's Text Book of Dermatology*. 8th ed. Oxford: Wiley-Blackwell; 2010.
5. Tilles G. *Teignes et teigneux: Histoire médicale et sociale*. Paris: Springer Verlag; 2009; Tilles G. L'histoire inacheveé des enfants teigneux irradiés. *La Presse Medical*, 2008, 37(3):541–546.
6. Bladin G. Le surprenant traitement de la teigne dans un hospital nantais. *Histoire des sciences medicales*, 2009, XlIII(1):137–142 [quote on p. 137].
7. Kraut A. *Silent Travelers: Germs, Genes and the Immigrant Menace*. New York: Basic Books; 1994; Markel H. *Quarantine! East European Jewish Immigrant and the New York City Epidemics of 1892*. Baltimore: Johns Hopkins University Press; 1997;

Markel H, Stern AM. Which face? Whose nation? Immigration, public health, and the construction of disease at America's ports and borders, 1891–1928. *Am Behav Sci*, 1999, 42(9):1314–1331; Markel H, Stern AM. The foreignness of germs: The persistent association of immigrants and disease in American society. *Milbank Q*, 2002, 80(4):757–788.

8. Shvarts S, Romem P, Romem I, Shani M. The mass campaign to eradicate ringworm among the Jewish community in Eastern Europe 1921–1938. *Am J Public Health*, 2013, 103(4):e56–e66.
9. Lévy-Lebhar Par G. et J. P. Roentgen-épilation du cuir chevelu dans le traitement des teignes: Conclusions après 18000 irradiations dans une collectivité d'enfants (Casablanca). *Maroc Médical*, 1960, 39:82–84 .
10. Cohen Y. Epidemilogia shel Gazezet b-Israel (Epidemiology of Ringworm in Israel). *Public Health*, 1960, 58:16–18 [quote on p. 17].
11. Some of the voices remain anonymous at the request of the informants.
12. The maximum number irradiated in childhood—all cases, not just ringworm—is believed (based on various estimates) to be in the vicinity of 4 million children. Schmeck HM Jr . A cancer in young linked to x-rays. *New York Times*, September 16, 1960; Degroot LJ, Frohman LA, Kaplan EL, Refetoff S. *Radiation-Associated Thyroid Carcinoma* . Chicago: Grune & Stratton; 1977; Rosenthal S. *The Thyroid Cancer Book* . Canada: Your Health Press, a division of Sara Health, Inc. in association with Trafford Publishing; 2002 .
13. Crawford GM, Linkart RH II, Tiley RF. Roentgen therapy in acne. *N Engl J Med*, 1951, 245(19):726–728; Kaplan I. The treatment of female sterility with x-rays to the ovaries and pituitary with special reference to congenital abnormalities of the offspring. *Can Med Assoc J*, 1957, 76(1):43–46.
14. Albert RE, Omran AR. Follow-up study of patients treated by x-ray epilation for tinea capitis: Population, characteristic, post treatment and mortality experience . *Arch Environ Health*, 1968, 17(6):899–918; Omran AR, Shore RE, Markoff RA, Friedhoff A, Albert RE, Barr H, et al. Follow-up study of patients treated by x-ray epilation for tinea capitis: Psychiatric and psychometric evaluation. *Am J Public Health*, 1978, 68(6):561–567; Cipollaro AC, Kallos A. Measurement of gonadal radiations during treatment for tinea capitis. *NY State J Med*, 1959, 59(16):3033–3040.
15. Albert and Omran, 1968.
16. The letter was sent directly to the author of the chapter, underscoring that she had no objection to being identified by name.
17. Barbara Beck Hess (b. 1941) lives in Oregon with her family. During our correspondence, Barbara said the information I sent her helped her uncover additional details that she was unaware of concerning the treatment she received and its outcome. Barbara gave the author full permission to publish her personal story on behalf of the research and said she early awaits publication of the volume.
18. The letters were sent directly to the author of the chapter, and the senders expressed full consent to have the former patient's identity published.
19. The testimony was sent directly to one of the researchers, and the sender testified that she had no objection to having her identity published.

20. Homei A, Worboys M. Fungal disease in Britain and the United States 1850–2000. In *Mycoses and Modernity*. Palgrave Macmillan; 2013.
21. The testimonies in this section of the chapter are part of interviews conducted in Portugal by Dr. Paula Boaventura, a researcher of biomedical sciences at Porto University, Portugal.
22. See Chapter 2 for more information.
23. See Chapter 7.
24. Grin EI. Epidemiology and control of tinea capitis in Yugoslavia. *St. Johns Hosp Dermatol Soc*, 1961, 47:109–122.
25. Shvarts S, Sevo G, Tasic M, Shani M, Sadetzki S. The tinea capitis campaign in Serbia in the 1950s. *Lancet Infect Dis*, 2010, 10(8):571–576.
26. Dr. Goren Sevo, Gerontology Institute, Belgrade Serbia.
27. Shvarts S, Romem P, Romem Y, Shani M. Masa ha-Gazezet ha-Nishkachat shel OZE-TOZ Poland (The forgotten ringworm campaign of OZE-TOZ Poland). *Harefuah*, 2009, 148(4):125–129.
28. Shvarts et al., 2013.
29. Interviews conducted by Dr. Sachlav Stoler-Liss (Z"L, deceased) between 2007 and 2009, research #1217/04 funded by the Israeli Science Foundation.
30. Shvarts S. Chavat da'at shel Mumcheh b-Noseh ha-Yidiot veha-Diyun ha-Tikshorti odot Totza'ot ha-Tipool ba-Hakrana b-Holei Gazezet b-Israel (Expert Opinion by a Professional on the Topic of News and Media Discourse Regarding the Results of Irradiation Treatment of Ringworm Patients in Israel). Gertner Center for Epidemiology and Health Policy Research, Sheba Medical Center, Tel HaShomer, March 2015.
31. See Chapter 9 for more information.
32. Hooper L. Nashim sh-Hookranu k-Neged Machalat ha-Gazezet b-Shnot ha-50: Hebetim ha-HIstori'im, Refu'e'em v-Psichosotziali'im she ha-Tofa'a (Women Irradiated Against Ringworm in the 1950s: Historical, Medical and Psychosocial Aspects of the Phenomenon). Master's thesis, Ben Gurion University of the Negev—Beersheva, 2016.

INDEX

For the benefit of digital users, indexed terms that span two pages (e.g., 52–53) may, on occasion, appear on only one of those pages.

Figures and tables are indicated by *f* and *t* following the page numbers. Numbers followed by n. indicate endnotes.

Abraham, Phineas, 91
Academy of Medicine (France), 35–38
Achorion schoenleinii, 93
Adamson, H. G., 67
Afendi, Armanak, 252
Africa. *See* North Africa; *specific countries*
Age of Enlightenment, 4–5
ALARA ("as low a dose as reasonably achievable") concept, 21
Alder Smith, Herbert, 14, 88, 91–92
Algeria
 health ministry, 134–35
 Jewish community, 149
 ringworm treatment, 116, 138, 149–50, 343–44
Alibert, Jean-Louis, 2–3, 7, 31–32, 35*f*
Allen, Charles, 14
Alliance school network, 136, 139–40, 141–42
alopecia, 205–6, 206*t*, *See also* baldness
alopecia areata, 43, 58, 59*f*
American Hospital Association, 225
American Journal of Epidemiology, 296
American Medical Association (AMA), 225
American Roentgen Ray Society, 20–21
American Zionist Medical Unit (AZMU), 246–47

ancient Egypt, 2
Annals of Internal Medicine, 236–37
Arnett, Allen (former patient): testimony, 337
"as low a dose as reasonably achievable" (ALARA) concept, 21
ataxia telangiectasia mutation (ATM), 313
atomic bomb survivors, 206–7, 216–17, 321–22
Australia, xi–xii, 16–17
AZMU (American Zionist Medical Unit), 246–47

bacteriology, 86–87
Baer, Peter (former patient): testimony, 337–38
baldness. *See also* alopecia
 radiation-induced, 24, 63–66, 95, 102, 331–33, 343–44, 345, 346, 347–48
 ringworm children, 63–66, 146, 248, 249*f*, 250*f*
 ringworm patient testimonies, 331–33, 343–44, 345, 346, 347–48
 in Sabouraud radiotherapy of scalp ringworm, 63–66, 95
 scald-head, 78, 79–81
 stigma of, 205

Banstead Road School (Sutton, Surrey), 90
basal cell carcinoma (BCC)
  after ringworm irradiation, 199–203, 207–8, 311
  ringworm patient testimonies, 337–38
Bateman, Thomas, 4, 7
Bateson's Specific and Cuticura Soap, 110n.57
Bazin, Ernest, 39–41, 42f, 43–44
BCC. See basal cell carcinoma
Beatson's Ringworm Lotion, 110n.57
Beck, Matthew, 335–36
Becquerel, Henri, 321
Berachiahu, Mordechai, 248
Besnier, Ernest, 45f, 45, 47
Besredka, Alexander, 126
bio-psychosocial model of health, 332–33
Blackfriars Skin Hospital (London, England), 83
Blaxall, Frank, 92
brain tumors
  after ringworm irradiation, 200–3, 304–5, 306–9
  ringworm patient testimony, 338–39
breast cancer, 309–10
Bridge School (Witham, Essex), 90, 98–100
Brigadas Móveis de Profilaxia da Tinha (Mobile Teams for Tinea Prophylaxis), 190–91
Brill, Mirko, 275–76, 288–89n.67
British Medical Association, 22–23
British Roentgen Society, 20–21
Brocq, Louis, 67–68, 68f
Bromberg, Yehuda, 257
Brylcreem, 106–7
Buchan, William, 79–80

calotte (skullcap) or capellus piceus epilation, 3–4, 32–34
Canada
  radiation therapy for benign diseases, 215–16, 236–38
  radiation therapy for scalp ringworm, xi–xii

cancer
  breast, 309–10
  general findings, 312–14
  hematologic, 312
  radiation-induced, 20–21, 22, 24, 25–27, 309–10, 318, 322, 337
  risk factors, 216–17
  skin, 310–11
Canterbury Hospital (Kent, England), 338
carcinomatosis, 264
carotid sclerosis, 200–3
Carter, Henry, 101
Casablanca, Morocco
  Jewish population, 139–40
  ringworm treatment center, 139–48
  social-health centers, 155
cataracts, 320–21
Cazenave, Pierre Louis Alphée, 31, 41f
Celsus, Aulus Cornelius, 2, 3
Central Hospital for Ringworm Children, 56–59
Cera Alba., 272
cerebral function, 314–17
cerebrovascular accidents, 200–3
Chernobyl, 321–22
Chetrit, Angela, 294–95
children, ringworm, 227f, 248
  empiric treatment of, 35–39
  epithets for, 332–33
  former patient testimonies, 331–51
  at Hôpital Saint-Louis, Paris, 31–76, 54f, 57f
  Israeli healing campaign (1925–1960), xi–xii, 138, 164–65, 175–76, 245–92, 247f, 249f, 250f, 267f, 276f, 346
  medical treatment of, 39–46
  physician disregard for, 32–35
  radiation therapy for, 61–69, 63f–66f, 94–103, 98f, 99f, 105, 105t, 115–62, 121f, 122f, 123f, 124f, 140f, 141f, 155f, 163–79, 170f, 173f, 190–99, 193f, 331–51
  school for, 53–60, 55f, 56f
  in United Kingdom schools, 77–114
  in United States, 333–38

INDEX

Christ's Hospital School (London, England), 14, 80–81, 88
Clalit Health Services. *See* General Sick Fund (GSF)
cognitive effects, 314–17
Colcott Fox, Thomas, 92, 98–100
Coleridge, Samuel Taylor, 80–81
colifonium, 252–53, 262–63, 268, 272
Congress of French-Speaking Dermatologists, 47–48
Connecticut, 224
Cook's Antiseptic Soap, 88–89
cranial malformations, 194–95, 195*f*

Daniel, John, 11–12
Darier, J., 46–47
DCHSP. *See* Dispensário Central de Higiene Social
de Chauliac, Guy, 2–3, 7
Dee, Ivan, 218–19
Dennis, John, 22
depilation. *See also* epilation
  chemical methods, 105–6
  colifonium, 252–53, 262–63, 268, 272
  mechanical methods, 105–6
  radiation (*see* radiation therapy)
depilatory(-ies), 60
depression, 346
Dermatological Society of London, 86–87
dermatology, 81–84
Devergie, Alphonse, 31, 43*f*
Dispensário Central de Higiene Social (DCHSP) (Porto, Portugal)
  Brigadas Móveis de Profilaxia da Tinha (Mobile Team for Tinea Prophylaxis), 190–91
  tinea treatment, 182, 191–92, 191*t*, 199
Dore, Ernest, 102–3
dosimetry, 302–4
Dostrovsky, Arieh, 245–46, 262, 264–65
Downs Ringworm School (Sutton, Surrey), 90, 98–100
Drukmann, Avraham (Adolf), 252–54, 264
Duclaux, Emile, 47

Eastern Europe (Poland, Lithuania, Latvia, and Romania). *See also specific countries*
  historical background, 118
  JDC-Joint and OSE ringworm eradication campaign (1921–1938), 125*f*, 132–33, 139*f*, 140*f*, 141*f*, 256, 342
  Jewish community, 117–33, 332–33
  ringworm centers, 130–31
  ringworm patient testimonies, 342–43
Ebers Papyrus, 2
Ecole des Teigneux (Ecole Lailler), 53–60, 55*f*, 56*f*, 91–92
ectothrix, 92
Eddowes, Aldred, 89
Edison, Thomas, 21–22
education. *See also* school(s)
  ringworm effects, 77, 103–4
EEG (electroencephalography), 315
Egypt, 2–3, 215–16
Ein Karem, 262
Einstein, Albert, 126
electroencephalography (EEG), 315
Eliyahu Jewish Immigration Camp (Casablanca), 146
Elizabeth, Saint, 5*f*
Ellis Island, 163–64, 227*f*
endothrix, 92
Engel, George, 332
England
  ringworm cases, 105, 105*t*
  ringworm patient testimonies, 338–39
  ringworm research, 5–6
epidemics, childhood, 77
epidemiology, 92, 296
  American Journal of Epidemiology, 296
  of favus tinea, 190–91
  of tinea capitis, 186–90, 187*f*
epilation, 4, 60. *See also* depilation
  calotte (skullcap) or *capellus piceus*, 3–4, 32–34
  complementary, 140*f*, 153–54, 170–71, 172*f*, 262–63, 278

355

epilation (*cont.*)
  manual, 170–71, 172*f*, 248, 268
  radiation (*see* radiation therapy)
  side effects, 6
  traditional methods, 150
epithets, 332–33
Eretz-Israel
  Arab sector, 279–80
  Immigration Absorption Center, 256–57
  ringworm among new immigrants, 255–59
  ringworm eradication (1917–1948), 246–59, 247*f*
  school hygiene directives, 253
  x-ray treatment, 252–55
erythema skin units (ESU), 12
Etienne of Antioch, 2–3
Europe. *See also* Eastern Europe (Poland, Lithuania, Latvia, and Romania); *specific countries*
  Middle Ages, 2–3
  radiation therapy for benign diseases, 215–16
Evanston Hospital (Evanston, IL), 220–21
Evelina Hospital, 101, 102
eyes
  opacity, 320
  radiation absorbed, 320

favus
  clinical characteristics, 32, 34*f*, 93
  early classification, 7, 39–41
favus tinea
  clinical characteristics, 183–86, 184*f*
  epidemiology, 190–91
  radiation treatment of, 196, 199–208, 204*t*
FDA. *See* Food and Drug Administration
FDA Drug Bulletin, 230
Feilchenfeld, Ernst, 257–58
Felix, Cassius, 2–3
fertility, reduced, 318–20
Feulard, Henri, 56–57
Fields, Jack (former patient): testimony, 342

Fireman, Henry, 134
Flexner, Bernard, 119–20
Food and Drug Administration (FDA)
  Bureau of Radiological Health, 230
  FDA Drug Bulletin, 230
  public warning campaigns, 222–24, 230, 233–34
France
  Academy of Medicine, 35–38
  Jewish immigrant transit camps, 152–55
  ringworm research, 5–6
  ringworm treatment, xi–xii, 14–15, 35–39, 152–55, 154*f*, 155*f*
  school hygiene directives, 253
French Society for Dermatology and Syphilology, 47–48, 66
Freund, Leopold, 11–12, 61, 94
Frodsham, J. Mill, 83
fungal diseases
  early understanding of, 39–40, 78–79
  fungus germs, 85–87
  skin diseases, 81–84
  theory of, 81–84

Galen, Clarissimus, 2
Geier, Orna, 320
General Sick Fund (GSF)
  irradiation treatment of ringworm, 258–59, 266, 268, 277–79, 282–83, 283*t*
  Modan cohort study population, 300
  Zamenhof Clinic (Haifa, Israel), 258–59, 300, 303
George Washington University, 26–27
Germany, 5–6
Germolene, 102
germs, fungus, 85–87
Gibert, CM, 31, 32
Glasgow Western Infirmary, 84
gliomas, 306–7
The Globe and Mail, 236–37
Golden Age of ringworm, 46–50
Goldie Leigh Cottage Children's Homes (Woolwich), 104–5
Gonik, Alexander, 135
Grasshopper Ointment, 88–89

Great Britain, 77. *See also* United Kingdom
griseofulvin, 68–69, 198–99, 216, 280–81
Gruby, David, 2, 4, 40*f*
Grushka, Theodor, 287n.53
GSF. *See* General Sick Fund
Guy's Hospital, 101

Hadassah Hospital (Tel Aviv), 253–54, 258–59, 283
Hadassah Medical Federation
   irradiation treatment of ringworm, 24–25, 257, 281–83, 283*t*
   regulations for treating ringworm, 268
   ringworm eradication campaign, 246–51, 247*f*, 249*f*, 250*f*, 260–61, 262–66, 268
   School Hygiene Department, 252–53, 256, 257
Hadassah Radiology Institute, 252–54, 258, 266–68
Hadassah University Hospital (Jerusalem)
   irradiation treatment of ringworm, 17–18, 245, 258–59, 283, 302, 307–8
   radiation-induced meningioma, 307–8
   supervision of Shaar HaAliyah, 271
Hadassah Zionist Women's Federation, 246–48
hair growth, after irradiation treatment, 205–6, 253–54
hair loss. *See* baldness
hair removal. *See* depilation; epilation
Haklei, Zeev, 150
Halevi, Haim Shalom, 259, 262
half-value layer (HVL), 12
Hallier, Ernst, 86
Haly-Abbas, 2–3
Harefuah, 17–18
Hassan II, 149
head and neck tumors
   radiation-induced, 199–200
   risk assessment, 304–5, 306–7
health: bio-psychosocial model of, 332–33
health centers, 133, 134–35
health insurance, 278–79
Health Restorer Ointment, 88–89

hematologic neoplasms, 312
herpes tonsurant de Cazenave (tinea tonsurans), 39–40, 42
Hess, Barbara Beck (former patient): testimony, 334–36
Hippocrates, 2
Hiroshima, 206–7, 216–17, 321–22
history of radiation epilation for tinea capitis, 11–30
history of ringworm, 1–9
   first era, 2–4, 5*f*
   second era, 4–7
Holloway's Ointment, 110n.57
Holloway's Pills, 110n.57
Holzknecht, Guido, 112n.98
honey treatment, 3
Hôpital de la Couche (Paris, France), 31
Hôpital des Enfants-Malades (Paris, France), 56–57
Hôpital des Teigneux (Paris, France), 35–38
Hôpital des Vénériens (Paris, France), 31
Hôpital Sainte-Reine (Paris, France), 35–38
Hôpital Saint-Louis (Paris, France), 14–15, 91–92, 153, 191–92
   Central Hospital for Ringworm Children, 56–59
   Ecole des Teigneux (Ecole Lailler), 53–60, 55*f*, 56*f*, 91–92
   ringworm children, 31–76, 54*f*, 57*f*
   ringworm radiotherapy, 61–69, 63*f*–66*f*
Hôpital Trousseau (Paris, France), 56–57
hormonal disturbances, 318–20
Hospice du Nord (Paris, France), 31
Hospital Curry Cabral (Lisbon, Portugal), 192, 198–99
Hospital for Diseases of the Skin (London, England), 83
Hoxsey, Harry, 241–42n.67
humoralist doctrine, 32
Hutchinson, Jonathan, 47–48
HVL (half-value layer), 12
Hygienic and Medical Guide for the Primary School Teachers, 51–52
hyperparathyroidism, 207
hypophysis tumor, 207

ICRP (International Commission for Radiation Protection), 20–21
Illinois Hospital Association, 221–22
Illinois State Medical Society, 221–22
immigrants
  in Israel, 149, 152–53, 164, 255–59, 265f
  ringworm among, 151, 255–59
  transit camps, 146, 152–55, 265f
  Yemenite Jews, 151, 255, 256–57, 261–62, 263–65, 276, 297
Immigrants Medical Service, 259
intelligence quotient (IQ), 315, 316
International Advisory Committee on X-ray and Radium Protection, 20–21
International Commission for Radiation Protection (ICRP), 20–21
International Congress of Dermatology (1896), 47–48, 91–92
International Congress of Radiology (1925), 20–21
International Congress of Radiology (1928), 20–21
iodine tincture, 170–71, 192–93, 272
ionizing radiation. *See also* radiation therapy
  from natural sources, 321
isolation. *See also* quarantine conditions
  ringworm patient testimonies, 332–33, 337, 345, 347
  ringworm schools, 50–60, 87–93
  during ringworm treatment, 58–59
  social, 102–3, 119–20, 205, 248 (*see also* ostracism)
Israel
  Arab residents, 257–58
  Arab sector, 279–80
  British Mandate period, 246–59, 279–80, 281–82
  Eretz-Israel, 246–59, 279–80, 281–82
  immigrants and immigration, 149, 152–53, 164, 255–59, 265f
  Immigrants Medical Service, 274
  Immigration Absorption Center, 256–57
  Mandatory Public Health Ordinance(s), 260–61
  Ministry of Health, 136–37, 260–61, 263, 266, 268, 270–71, 274, 277, 278–79, 281, 295
  Modan cohort, 297–321, 299f
  National Cancer Registry, 295, 301
  National Center for Ringworm Victims, 300
  National Health Insurance Law, 291n.106
  Population Health Act, 295
  public health funds, 291n.106
  ringworm eradication campaign (1925–1960), xi–xii, 138, 164–65, 175–76, 245–92, 247f, 249f, 250f, 267f, 276f, 346
  ringworm infections, 17–18, 164, 250f, 255–59, 260–79
  ringworm patient testimonies, 346–48
  ringworm research (1965–1995), 217, 293–329
  Ringworm Victims Compensation Law, 246, 322
  Tipat Chalav ("a drop of milk") mother and child clinics, 270
  war on ringworm, 246
  war on venereal and social dermatological diseases, 260–61
  x-ray treatment, 252–55
Israeli Defense Forces (IDF), 265–66, 267f
Israel Society of Dermatology, 17–18
Italy, 16–17
Izmojik, Avraham, 266

Jerusalem
  private radiology institutes, 258
  ringworm, 248–49
Jewish Agency, 134, 136–37, 152–53, 268, 269, 281
Jewish community
  Eastern Europe (1921–1938), 117–33, 332–33
  Eliyahu Immigration Camp, 146
  immigrant transit camps, 146, 152–55, 265f
  Korat Gag campaign, 265–66
  Modan cohort, 297–321, 299f

INDEX

Moroccan, 148–49, 313
new immigrants, 255–59
North Africa (1947 to 1960), 133–55
ringworm in, 255–59, 282
Rosh HaAyin camp, 264–66, 271–72, 282–83
Schneller camp, 257–58, 265–68, 271–72, 282–83
Shaar HaAliyah camp, 151, 264, 268, 269–77, 280–81, 282, 283, 283t, 302
Yemenite immigrants, 151, 255, 256–57, 261–62, 263–65, 276, 297
Jewish National Council (JNC), 257
Johns Hopkins University, 295
Joint Distribution Committee (JDC)
budget, 127–28
current activities, 155
foundation, 119–20
funding, 134
objective, 119–20
ringworm eradication campaign in Eastern Europe (1921-1938), 115–33, 121f, 122f, 123f, 124f, 256, 342
ringworm eradication campaign in North Africa (1947 to 1960), 115–16, 133–55, 140f, 141f, 155f, 343
Journal of Cutaneous Medicine, 83–84

Kaplan, Ira, 15–16
Kassabian, Mihran, 22
Keilholtz, Dave (former patient): testimony, 337
Kienböck–Adamson (KA) technique
dosimetry, 303–4
scientific and historic aspects, 15–18, 22–23
use at Hôpital Saint-Louis, Paris, 67
use in Israel, 262–63, 268, 281–82, 302, 303–4
use in North Africa, 142
use in Portugal, 195, 339
use in Serbia, 164, 170–71
Kienböck, Robert, 67
Kings County Hospital (Brooklyn, New York), 337–38
Korat Gag campaign (IDF), 265–66

Lailler, Charles, 42, 44f, 44, 52–53, 58
La Maternelle (Casablanca), 139–40
Lamb, Charles, 80–81
Lancet, 80–81, 87–89, 94, 101–2, 165, 304–5, 309
Landsman, Bertha, 262
Latin America, 215–16
Latvia. *See* Eastern Europe
leeches, 22, 32
Lees, Susan, 338–39
leprosy *(tzaraʾat)*, 2
leukemia, 296
Libya
Jewish community, 151
Ministry of Health, 134–35
ringworm treatment, 116, 138, 151–52
Lilienfeld, Abraham, 296
Lister, Joseph, 85–86
Lithuania. *See* Eastern Europe
Liveing, Robert, 87–88
London, England, 14–15, 104–5
London Orphan Asylum, 80–81
London Times, 22
Longley, Walter, 101
lymphoma, 312

MacLeod, John, 97
magnetic resonance imaging (MRI), 26–27
Mahon brothers, 4, 35–39, 37f, 43–44
Mann, Kalman, 262
Mapother, Edward Dillon, 81–82
Markel, Howard, 93
Marseille, France
Jewish immigrant transit camps, 152–55
ringworm treatment, 152–55, 154f, 155f
Marshall Islands, 321–22
mass schooling, 77–114. *See also* school(s)
M'Call Anderson, Thomas, 84, 86
media coverage, xi, 220–21, 222–25, 223f, 229f, 231f, 232–35, 236–37, 237f
Medical College of Wisconsin, 222
medical malpractice, 220, 221f, 232–33
medical supervision, 50–51
Meir, Yosef, 262, 264
melanoma, 310–11

meningioma
  radiation-induced, 25–27, 199–203, 207, 307–8
  radiation patient testimonies, 343
mental processes, 314–17
mental retardation, 316
Mercurialis, Hieronymus, 2–3, 4, 6
mercurial lotion, 45–46
Michael Reese Hospital (Chicago, IL), 218f
  campaign to locate former radiation patients, xi, 218–25, 223f, 232–33, 234–35
  media coverage, xi, 220–21, 222–24, 223f, 232–33, 234–35
  medical malpractice suits, 220, 221f, 232–33
microbiology, 47
microscopic analysis, 4, 8f
microscopic fungus, 39–40, 47–48
Microsporon, 92
Microsporon audouinii, 92
Microsporon canis, 92–93
Microsporum canis, 183, 198–99
Microsporum felineum, 183
Middle Ages, 2–3, 4–5
Middle East, xi–xii, 16–17
Milton, John Laws, 83
Mobile Teams for Tinea Prophylaxis (Brigadas Móveis de Profilaxia da Tinha), 190–91
Modan, Baruch, 165, 295–96
Modan cohort, 297–321
  expanded, 300
  study population, 297–300, 299f
morbidity risk, 297–321
Morocco
  health centers, 116, 139–48
  health ministry, 134–35
  after independence, 148–49
  Jewish community, 138, 139–40, 312–13
  radiation therapy for benign diseases, 215–16
  radiation therapy for ringworm, xi–xii, 16–17, 116, 136–37, 138–49, 141f, 345
  ringworm infections, 139–40, 164
  ringworm patient testimony, 345

Morris, Malcolm, 90, 97
mortality, 317–18
MRI (magnetic resonance imaging), 26–27
Murillo, Bartolome Esteban: "Santa Isabela Reina de Hungria Curando a los Enfermos," 5f
Mycetes, 85
mycology, medical, 39–46, 47
mycoses, 2
Mycosis Hospital (Belgrade, Yugoslavia), 171–73

Nagasaki, 206–7, 216–17, 321–22
National Cancer Institute (NCI)
  campaign about radiation-related thyroid cancer, xi, 225–29, 226f, 229f, 231–32, 235, 236–37
  conference on late effects of head and neck radiation in infancy and childhood, 222–24
  media coverage and, 234
National Cancer Program (US), 222–24
National Cancer Registry (Israel), 295, 301
National Center for Ringworm Victims (Israel), 300
National Institute of Arthritis, Metabolism, and Digestive Disease (US), 234
National Society for the Protection of Children (N.S.P.C.C.), 102
NCI. *See* National Cancer Institute
NCI Act of 1971 (US), 231
nerve sheath tumors, 306–7
neurinoma, 207
New England Journal of Medicine, 306–7
Newman, George, 103–4
New York City, New York, 163–64
New York Times, 229f
New York University (NYU), 24, 217, 336
Noiré, Henri, 62, 94–95
North Africa. *See also specific countries*
  JDC-Joint and OSE ringworm eradication campaign (1947 to 1960), xi–xii, 16–17, 115–16, 133–55, 343
  ringworm patient testimonies, 340–41
  TTT prevalence, 134

Northern Ireland, 16–17
Northwestern Memorial Hospital (Chicago, IL), 220–21
N.S.P.C.C. (National Society for the Protection of Children), 102
nurses
    Israeli ringworm eradication campaign, 250f, 252–53, 266
    JDC-Joint and OSE ringworm eradication campaign, 128–29, 130–32, 143, 145

Orange's Universal Cerate and Vegetable Purifying Pills, 110n.57
Orfinik, Sharon Hoare (former patient): testimony, 336–37
Organization for Safeguarding the Health of Jews (*Obshchestvo Zdravookhraneniia Evreev* [OZE], OSE), 16–17
    foundation, 118–19
    funding, 134
    health centers, 133, 134–35, 155
    membership system, 129
    mission, 118–19
    operations, 119
    Polish Branch (TOZ), 115–16, 117–33, 121f, 156n.4
    ringworm centers, 116
    ringworm eradication campaign in Eastern Europe (1921–1938), 115–33, 121f, 122f, 123f, 124f, 125f, 256, 342
    ringworm eradication campaign in North Africa (1947 to 1960), 115–16, 133–55, 343
    welfare activities, 155
ostracism
    epithets, 332–33
    ringworm patient testimonies, 332–33, 337, 345, 347
    social isolation, 119–20, 205, 248
OxyContin, 233–34

Palestine/Eretz-Israel: ringworm eradication (1917–1948), 246–59
parotid carcinoma, 207
Pasta Zinci, 272, 273
Pasteur Institute, 47
patient testimonies, 331–51
Payne, Joseph, 89
pelade (alopecia areata), 43
Pennsylvania, 224
personal development, 79
physicians
    disregard for ringworm children, 32–35
    in primary schools, 50–53
Picker X-Ray Corp., 193–94
Pignot, Maurice, 94–95
Plinius Secundus, Gaius, 3
Plumbe, Samuel, 4, 41–42, 79, 80–81
Poland, 127–28. *See also* Eastern Europe
politics, 118, 230
porrigo decalvans (alopecia areata), 43
porrigo decalvans de Bateman (teigne achromateuse), 39–40
Porrigo favosa, 32
porrigo favosa et scutulata (favus), 39–40
Portugal
    Mobile Teams for Tinea Prophylaxis (Brigadas Móveis de Profilaxia da Tinha), 190–91
    ringworm epidemic, 181–90, 184f, 187f, 199, 208
    ringworm eradication campaign (1940–1970), 181–213, 193f, 215–16, 339
    ringworm patient testimonies, 339–40
primary schools, 50–53. *See also* school(s)
Prywes, Moshe, 133–34, 135
public health campaigns. *See also* ringworm eradication campaigns
    warning campaigns about radiation therapy, xi–xii, 222–24, 225–30, 226f, 233–34

quarantine conditions. *See also* isolation
    during radiation treatment, 120–25, 170, 268
    ringworm patient testimonies, 332–33, 337, 345, 347
Quinquaud, E., 45–46, 58–59

radiation
    "as low a dose as reasonably achievable"
        (ALARA) concept, 21
    erythema skin units (ESU), 12
    half-value layer (HVL), 12
    maximum permissible dose, 21
    protection against, 20–21
    recommended maximum
        exposure, 20–21
    tolerance dose, 21
radiation epilation. *See* radiation therapy
radiation therapy
    average dose absorbed, 303
    for benign diseases, 13, 215–16, 236–38
    cognitive effects, 314–17
    costs, 257
    cure rate, 197–98
    delayed effects of, 230
    depilation treatment, 94–107, 98f, 99f, 105t
    dosimetry, 302–4
    early years, 12–13
    epilation treatment, 14–19, 61–69
    health effects of, 293–329, 348
    high-dose, 13
    history of, xi, 11–30, 93–104
    hospitalization regimen, 198
    Israeli campaign (1925–1960), 245–92,
        247f, 249f, 250f, 267f, 276f, 303
    JDC-Joint and OSE campaigns, 115–62,
        121f, 122f, 123f, 124f, 125f
    Kienböck–Adamson (KA) technique,
        15–18, 22–23, 67, 142, 164, 170–71,
        193–94, 195, 262–63, 268, 281–82, 302,
        303–4, 339
    late effects of, xi, 175–76, 199–208, 201f,
        202f, 204t, 206t, 215–43, 231f
    long-term effects of, 13, 216–17
    low-dose, 306
    maximum dose, 121f
    mortality follow-up, 317–18
    OSE-TOZ campaign, 117–33
    patient testimonies, 331–51
    Portugal campaign (1940–1970), 181–
        213, 193f, 215–16
    psychosocial aspects, 345
    public health campaigns warning
        about, xi–xii, 222–24, 225–30,
        226f, 233–34
    recommended dose, 18–19
    as revolutionary, 93–104
    for ringworm, xi–xii, 61–69, 63f–66f,
        94–103, 98f, 99f, 105, 105t, 115–62,
        121f, 122f, 123f, 124f, 125f, 140f, 141f,
        154f, 155f, 163–79, 170f, 173f, 190–208,
        193f, 194f, 204t, 206t, 246–59, 268,
        277–80, 281–82, 283t, 293–329, 331–51
    risk assessment for other health
        outcomes, 314–21
    risk assessment for tumors, 304–12
    Sabouraud's method, 18, 61–69, 63f–
        66f, 94–95
    safe schedules, 22–23
    scientific aspects, 11–30
    Serbia campaign (1950s), xi–xii, 16–17,
        144, 163–79, 167f, 170f, 172f, 173f, 174f,
        215–16, 270, 341
    side effects, 21–25, 197, 253–54, 318–
        21, 331
    for tinea capitis, xi–xii, 11–30, 293–329
    UNICEF campaign, xi–xii, 135, 144,
        163–79, 167f, 170f, 172f, 173f, 174f, 215–
        16, 270, 275, 280
radiodermatitis, 61
radiology institutes, 258
Rajchman, Ludwik, 290n.88
Raubitchek, Frederic, 271
Rayer, Pierre François Olive, 32, 36f
Reichman, Ludwig, 120
Remak, Robert, 4
Renaissance era, 2–3, 4–5
Richard, Richard, 71n.25
ringworm
    complementary epilation treatment of,
        140f, 153–54, 262–63, 278
    decline, 104–7
    effects on education, 103–4
    effects on personal development, 79
    empiric treatment of, 35–39
    epithets for children with, 332–33
    as fungus disease, 85–87

INDEX

griseofulvin treatment of, 68–69, 198–99
history of, 1–9, 5*f*
Hôpital Saint-Louis, Paris children, 31–76, 54*f*, 57*f*
incidence of, 105
medical treatment of, 39–46
microscopic analysis of, 4, 8*f*
among new immigrants, 255–59
outbreaks, 80–81
patient testimonies, 331–51
prevalence of, 79–81, 103–4
radiation therapy for, 61–69, 63*f*–66*f*, 94–103, 98*f*, 99*f*, 105, 105*t*, 115–62, 121*f*, 122*f*, 123*f*, 124*f*, 125*f*, 140*f*, 141*f*, 154*f*, 155*f*, 163–79, 190–208, 193*f*, 194*f*, 204*t*, 206*t*, 246–59, 268, 277–80, 281–82, 283*t*, 293–329, 331–51
recommended treatment of, 12
research (Israel, 1965–1995), 293–329, 299*f*
of scalp (tinea capitis), xi–xii, 1–9, 11–30, 54*f*, 88–89, 182–99, 293–329, 331–51
in schools, 87–93
screening for, 50–53, 249*f*
social construction of, 61–69
treatment of, 68–69, 79–80, 88–89, 268, 279–80
treatment protocols, 271–73
ringworm (term), 77
ringworm centers, 116, 130–31
ringworm eradication campaigns. *See also* public health campaigns
Israel (1925–1960), xi–xii, 138, 164–65, 175–76, 245–92, 267*f*, 276*f*
JDC-Joint and OSE campaigns, 115–62, 121*f*, 122*f*, 123*f*, 124*f*, 125*f*
Portugal (1940–1970), 181–213, 193*f*, 215–16
Serbia (1950s), xi–xii, 16–17, 144, 163–79, 167*f*, 170*f*, 172*f*, 173*f*, 174*f*, 215–16, 270, 341
UNICEF, xi–xii, 135, 144, 163–79, 167*f*, 170*f*, 172*f*, 173*f*, 174*f*, 215–16, 270, 275, 280
ringworm research

history of, 5–6, 7
Israel (1965–1995), 293–329
Modan cohort, 297–321, 299*f*
ringworm schools, 87–93
Ringworm Victims Compensation Law (Israel), 246, 322
Riva, Nancy, 236
Roberts, Leslie, 92
Roentgen Society, 20–21
Roentgen, Wilhelm Conrad, 11–12, 61, 321
Rollins, William, 22
Roman Empire, 2
Romania. *See* Eastern Europe
Ron, Elaine, 296, 303–4
Rosenblut, Simon, 280
Rosh HaAyin camp, 264–66, 271–72, 282–83
Roux, Emile, 47
Royal Belfast Hospital, 16–17
Royal College of Surgeons, 83–84
Royal London and Westminster Infirmary for the Treatment of Cutaneous Diseases, 83
Royal Naval School, 80–81

Sabouraud agar, 49–50
Sabouraud–Noiré radiometer X, 62
Sabouraud, Raymond Jacques Adrien, 2, 4, 46–50, 48*f*, 49*f*
classification of ringworm, 92
at Hôpital Saint-Louis, Paris, 47, 58–59, 91–92
praise for radiotherapy, 62–63
radiotherapy of ringworm technique, 18, 61–69, 63*f*–66*f*, 94–95
Sadetzki-Jackobson, Siegal, 294–95
Sagher, Felix, 262–63, 264
salicylanilide, 151
salivary gland tumors, 304–5, 312
"Santa Isabela Reina de Hungria Curando a los Enfermos" (Murillo), 5*f*
scald-head, 78, 79–81
scalp irradiation. *See* radiation therapy
scalp ringworm. *See* ringworm; tinea capitis
Schizomycetes, 85–86

Schneller camp (Jerusalem), 257–58, 265–68, 271–72, 282–83
Schöenlein, Johann Lukas, 4, 8*f*
school(s)
  Alliance network, 136, 139–40, 141–42
  Banstead Road School (Sutton, Surrey), 90
  Bridge School (Witham, Essex), 90, 98–100
  Christ's Hospital School (London, England), 80–81, 88
  Ecole des Teigneux (Ecole Lailler), 53–60, 55*f*, 56*f*, 91–92
  hygiene directives, 253
  hygiene rules, 50–51
  isolation from, 332–33, 337, 345, 347
  physicians and teachers in, 50–53
  primary, 50–53
  ringworm, 50–60, 87–93
  ringworm effects, 77, 103–4
Schwartz, Joe, 133–34
screening for ringworm, 50–53, 249*f*
self-confidence, 346
self-image, 345
Serbia (Yugoslavia), 166*f*
  brain tumors, 175–76
  Institute of Public Health, 168–69
  mycological centers, 169
  ringworm elimination campaign (1950s), xi–xii, 16–17, 144, 163–79, 167*f*, 170*f*, 172*f*, 173*f*, 174*f*, 215–16, 270, 341
  ringworm infections, 164, 168–69
  ringworm patient testimonies, 341–42
  thyroid tumors, 175–76
SES (socioeconomic status), 251
Sevo, Goran, 341
Shaar HaAliyah camp (Haifa, Israel)
  closure, 280–81
  immigrants with ringworm, 151
  ringworm treatment protocols, 264, 268, 282–83, 283*t*, 302
Shaar HaAliyah Hospital, 269–77, 278–79, 280–81
  ringworm treatment protocols, 271–73

Tipat Chalav ("a drop of milk") mother and child clinics, 270
UNICEF x-ray machine donations, 270, 275
Shapira, Haim-Moshe, 260–61
Sheba University Medical Center, 266–68
Sheba, Haim, 136–37
shumach, 3
Sick Funds, 260–61
60 Minutes, 224–25, 231*f*, 238n.1
skin cancer, 310–11
skin disease, 81–84
social epithets, 332–33
social isolation, 102–3, 119–20, 205, 248. *See also* ostracism; quarantine conditions
socioeconomic status (SES), 251
Spiro, Shmuel, 152
Staphylococcus aureus, 103–4
Sternberg, Avraham Tuvia, 257
stigma, 205
St. John's Hospital for Disease of the Skin, 83
Stovall, Marilyn, 303
suicide, 341
sulfur salts, 192–93
syphilis, 82–83
Syria
  radiation therapy for ringworm, 215–16
  UNICEF ringworm eradication campaign, 165, 270

Tachkemoni School (Jerusalem), 251
Talmud Torah network, 136
Tangier, 116
teachers, 50–53
teigne. *See* tinea capitis (ringworm of the scalp)
teigne achromateuse (porrigo decalvans de Bateman), 39–40
teigne decalvante, 39–40
teigne mentagre, 39–40
teigne tondante de Mahon (tinea tonsurans), 39–40, 42
Tel Aviv, Israel, 17–18, 258

Tel HaShomer Hospital, 24–25, 266–68, 275, 276, 283, 295, 302
thallium acetate, 60, 94–95, 105–6, 150
Thompson, Elihu, 21–22
thyroid cancer
  early detection of, 236–37
  Michael Reese Hospital campaign about, 219–20
  national campaign about, 225–29, 226f, 229f
  patient testimonies, 342
  radiation-related, xi, 199–203, 204t, 206–7, 216, 217, 219–20, 225–29, 226f, 229f
thyroid tumors, 305–6
Tilbury Fox, William, 83, 84, 86, 87–88
tinea capitis (scalp ringworm), 2, 40–41, 163–64, 250f, See also ringworm; tuberculosis, trachoma, and ringworm (TTT)
  clinical signs of, 332–33
  diagnosis of, 182–86
  disease evolution, 182–86
  early classification of, 7
  empiric treatment of, 35–39
  epidemiology of, 186–90, 187f
  favus, 183–86, 184f, 190–91, 199–208, 204t
  forms of, 39–40
  history of, 1–9, 5f, 32
  human perspective on, 331–51
  Israeli studies (1965–1995), 293–329
  length of hospital stays for, 169
  medical treatment of, 39–46
  microsporic, 183–84, 184f, 185–86, 199–208, 204t
  patient testimonies, 331–51
  prevalence, 189, 190–91, 247–51
  radiation therapy for, xi–xii, 11–30, 61–69, 63f–66f, 94–103, 98f, 99f, 105, 105t, 163–79, 170f, 173f, 190–99, 193f, 194f, 206t
  reinfection, 248–51
  socioeconomic status and, 251
  tonsure, 186, 198–99
  treatment of, xi–xii, 3–4, 5f, 6–7, 11–30, 32, 88–89, 164, 190–99
  trichophytic, 183, 184f, 185–86, 199–208, 204t
  x-ray depilation treatment of, 95–103, 98f, 99f
tinea tonsurans (teigne tondante de Mahon, herpes tonsurant de Cazenave), 39–46, 48–49, 50
tinea vera, 32
Tipat Chalav ("a drop of milk") mother and child clinics, 270
Tomes, Nancy, 105–6
tonsure tinea, 186, 198–99
Towarzystwo Ochrony Zdrowia Ludnos´ci ˙ydowskiej (TOZ), 156n.4, See also Organization for Safeguarding the Health of Jews (OSE)
trachoma, 248. See also tuberculosis, trachoma, and ringworm (TTT)
Trichophyton, 92, 142–43, 183
Trichophyton megninii, 183
Trichophyton megalosporon, 50
Trichophyton mentagrophytes, 92, 183
Trichophyton microsporon, 50
Trichophyton schoenleinii, 183, 196–97, 199
Trichophyton tonsurans, 183, 198–99
Trichophyton violaceum, 164, 183, 198–99
trustee physicians, 136–37
TTT. See tuberculosis, trachoma, and ringworm (*tinea capitis* or teigne)
tuberculosis, 136–37
tuberculosis, trachoma, and ringworm (tinea capitis or teigne) (TTT)
  JDC-Joint and OSE campaign to eradicate, 115–16, 119–20, 135–36
  prevalence of, 134
tumors
  brain, 200–3, 304–5, 306–9, 338–39
  head and neck, 199–200, 304–5, 306–7
  nerve sheath, 306–7
  radiation-induced, 199–203, 304–9, 312
  ringworm patient testimony, 338–39
  risk assessment, 304–12, 322
  salivary gland, 312
  skin, 311
  thyroid, 305–6

Tunisia
  health ministry, 134–35
  Jewish community, 150
  radiation therapy for benign diseases, 215–16
  ringworm treatment, 116, 138, 150–51
Turner, Daniel, 4, 6–7
Turner, Dawson, 100–1
Turner, John P., 92–93
tzaraʽat (leprosy), 2
Tzarfati, Shula, 271

UNICEF
  ringworm elimination campaigns, xi–xii, 135, 144, 163–79, 167*f*, 170*f*, 172*f*, 173*f*, 174*f*, 215–16, 270, 275, 280
  x-ray machine donations, 165, 270, 275
Union OSE, 118–19
United Kingdom. *See also* England; Wales
  ringworm, 77–114
  ringworm schools, 87–93
  ringworm therapy, xi–xii
United States
  campaign about radiation-related thyroid cancer, 225–29, 226*f*
  campaign to warn public, 225–30
  mass schooling, 77
  National Cancer Program (US), 222–24
  ringworm epidemic, 15–16, 92–93, 163–64
  ringworm patient testimonies, 333–38
  ringworm treatment, xi–xii, 15–16, 105–6
  school hygiene directives, 253
  tinea capitis research, 5–6
University College Hospital, 84
University of Chicago, 217
University of Texas M.D. Anderson Cancer Center, 303–4
U.S. Army, 15–16

Vanderbilt University, 11–12
Vaseline, 272

Victorian period, 87–88
visual evoked response (VER), 314–15
Vito, Robert, 222
Volpé, Robert, 236–37

Wales: ringworm cases, 105, 105*t*
Walfish, Paul, 236–37
war, 118
Warshaw-Dadon, Rachel, 219–20
Weinberger, Casper, 230
Weissberger, Yehuda, 273, 277
Werner, Abraham, 294–95
Westminster Hospital (London, England), 92
Wilks, Samuel, 85
Willan, Robert, 4, 7, 78, 79, 80–81
Wilson, Erasmus, 83–84
Windham Community Memorial Hospital (Willimantic, CT), 224
women, 345, 346
World Congress of Dermatology (Paris, 1900), 61
World Health Organization (WHO), 135
World Zionist Movement, 152–53
Wulman, Leon, 117

x-ray epilation. *See* radiation therapy
x-ray machines
  costs, 151, 169
  UNICEF donations, 165, 270, 275
x-rays
  discovery of, 11–12, 61
  indications for, 61
  protection standards, 20–21
  therapeutic, 61–69

Yaski, Haim, 258
Yugoslavia. *See* Serbia

Zaken, Ben, 138
Zambuk, 102
Zamenhof Clinic (Haifa, Israel), 258–59, 300, 303
zinc ointment, 170–71

Made in the USA
Monee, IL
03 May 2026

49437401R00210